T0321157

Clinics in Developmental Medicine No. 188
ALCOHOL, DRUGS AND MEDICATION IN
PREGNANCY: THE LONG-TERM OUTCOME
FOR THE CHILD

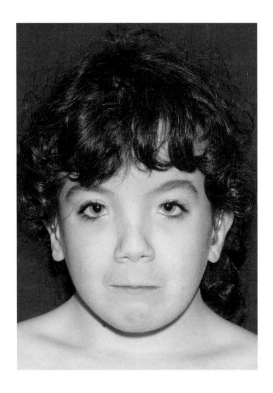

Four-year-old girl with features of fetal alcohol syndrome and mild learning difficulties. She was born at 32 weeks' gestation following a pregnancy in which she was exposed to alcohol and probably also amphetamines. She had multiple small bowel atresias, ventricular septal defect and multiple capillary haemangiomas. She has been treated by bowel excision and entral feeding via a gastrostomy and is now growing between the 9th and 25th centiles. She has suffered from recurrent ear infections and resultant conductive deafness and now uses hearing aids. She is doing well at school with specialist support, and she is currently being evaluated for concentration and attention problems.

Clinics in Developmental Medicine No. 188

Alcohol, Drugs and Medication in Pregnancy: the Long-term Outcome for the Child

Edited by

PHILIP M PREECE
Chesterfield Royal Hospital
Chesterfield, Derbyshire, UK

EDWARD P RILEY
Center for Behavioral Teratology
San Diego State University
San Diego, CA, USA

2011
Mac Keith Press

Distributed by Wiley–Blackwell

© 2011 Mac Keith Press
6 Market Road, London N7 9PW, UK

Editor: Hilary Hart
Managing Director: Caroline Black
Production Manager: Udoka Ohuonu
Project Manager: Pat Chappelle
Indexer: Pat Chappelle

First published in this edition 2011

British Library Cataloguing-in-Publication data
A catalogue record for this book is available from the British Library

ISBN: 978 1 898683 88 9

Printed by Latimer Trend & Company, Plymouth, Devon, UK

Mac Keith Press is supported by Scope

CONTENTS

Colour Plates
1 & 2 between pages 246 & 247, 3 & 4 between pages 262 & 263

AUTHORS' APPOINTMENTS

Gus Baker

Professor of Clinical Neuropsychology, Division of Neurosciences, University of Liverpool; *and* Consultant Clinical Neuropsycholgist, Walton Centre for Neurosciences, Liverpool, UK

Margaret Barrow

Formerly Consultant Clinical Geneticist, Leicester Royal Infirmary, Leicester, UK

David J Bramble

Consultant Child and Adolescent Learning Disability Psychiatrist, Telford and Wrekin Community Services, Monkmoor Multi-Agency Support Services Campus, Shrewsbury, UK

Sara Citron

Graduate Student, Department of Occupational Science and Occupational Therapy, University of Toronto, Toronto, Canada

Jill Clayton-Smith

Professor of Medical Genetics, Manchester Academic Health Sciences Centre; *and* Consultant Clinical Geneticist, St Mary's Hospital, Manchester, UK

Peter A Fried

Professor Emeritus, Distinguished Research Professor, Department of Psychology, Carleton University, Ottawa, Ontario, Canada

Sarah E Fulton

National Children's Study Operational Manager/Communications Coordinator, School of Medicine, Case Western Reserve University, Cleveland, OH, USA

Julie Gelo

Executive Director, NOFAS (Washington State), Bothell, WA; *and* Family Advocate, University of Washington Fetal Alcohol Syndrome Diagnostic and Prevention Network, Seattle, WA, USA

Elizabeth A Godin	Graduate Student, Bowles Center for Alcohol Studies, University of North Carolina, Chapel Hill, NC, USA
Julia E Goodwin	Research Fellow, Institute for Research in Child Development, Department of Psychology, University of East London, London; and Department of Psychiatry, University of Oxford, Oxford, UK
Therese M Grant	Streissguth Endowed Professor in Fetal Alcohol Spectrum Disorders; Associate Professor of Psychiatry and Behavioral Sciences; Director, Fetal Alcohol and Drug Unit; and Director, Washington State Parent–Child Assistance Program, University of Washington School of Medicine, and Adjunct Associate Professor of Epidemiology, University of Washington School of Public Health, Seattle, WA, USA
Ron Gray	Senior Clinical Research Fellow, National Perinatal Epidemiology Unit, University of Oxford, Headington, Oxford, UK
Evelyne Jacqz-Aigrain	Department of Paediatric Pharmacology and Pharmacogenetics, Clinical Investigation Centre – Inserm CIC 9202, Hôpital Robert Debré, Paris, France
Wendy O Kalberg	Educational Diagnosician and Clinical Research Associate, Center on Alcoholism, Substance Abuse and Addictions, University of New Mexico, Albuquerque, NM, USA
Faye Macrory	Consultant Midwife, Manchester Specialist Midwifery Service, Zion Community Centre, Hulme, Greater Manchester, UK
Christie L McGee Petrenko	Postdoctoral Fellow in Psychiatry, The Kempe Center for the Prevention and Treatment of Child Abuse and Neglect, University of Colorado Denver, Denver, CO, USA
Sonia Minnes	Assistant Professor, Mandel School of Applied Social Sciences, Case Western Reserve University, Cleveland, OH, USA

Derek G Moore

Professor and Director, Institute for Research in Child Development, Department of Psychology, University of East London, London, UK

Raja A S Mukherjee

Honorary Senior Lecturer, St George's University, London; *and* Consultant Psychiatrist and Service Manager, Fetal Alcohol Spectrum Disorder Clinic, Surrey and Borders Partnership NHS Foundation Trust, Oxted, Surrey, UK

Michael Murphy

Senior Lecturer, School of Social Work, Psychology and Public Health, University of Salford, Salford, Greater Manchester, UK

Irena Nulman

Associate Professor of Pediatrics, University of Toronto; *and* Staff, Division of Clinical Pharmacology and Toxicology; Program Director, Fellowship Training Program in Clinical Pharmacology; Associate Director, Motherisk Program; and Associate Scientist, Child Health Evaluative Sciences (CHES), The Hospital for Sick Children, Toronto, Canada

Shonagh K O'Leary-Moore

Postdoctoral Fellow, Bowles Center for Alcohol Studies, University of North Carolina, Chapel Hill, NC, USA

Scott E Parnell

Assistant Professor, Department of Cell and Developmental Biology and Bowles Center for Alcohol Studies, University of North Carolina, Chapel Hill, NC, USA

Andrew C Parrott

Professor, Department of Psychology, Swansea University, Swansea, UK

Kate E Pickett

Professor of Epidemiology, Department of Health Sciences, University of York, Heslington, York, UK

Philip M Preece

Consultant Paediatrician, Chesterfield Royal Hospital, Chesterfield, Derbyshire, UK

Edward P Riley

Distinguished Professor of Psychology, and Director, Center for Behavioral Teratology, San Diego State University, San Diego, CA, USA

Lynn T Singer — Professor of Pediatrics, Psychiatry, Psychology and Environmental Health Sciences; and Deputy Provost and Vice President for Academic Affairs, Case Western Reserve University, Cleveland, OH, USA

Ann P Streissguth — Professor Emerita, Department of Psychiatry and Behavioral Sciences, Fetal Alcohol and Drug Unit, University of Washington School of Medicine, Seattle, WA, USA

Kathleen K Sulik — Professor, Department of Cell and Developmental Biology and Bowles Center for Alcohol Studies, University of North Carolina, Chapel Hill, NC, USA

Michelle Todorow — Graduate Student, Department of Psychology, York University, Toronto, Canada

John J D Turner — Principal Lecturer, Recreational Drugs Research Team, Department of Psychology, University of East London, London, UK

Elizabeth Uleryk — Director, Hospital Library, The Hospital for Sick Children, Toronto, Canada

Lauren S Wakschlag — Associate Chair for Scientific Development and Institutional Collaboration, Department of Medical Social Sciences, Feinberg School of Medicine, Northwestern University, Chicago, IL, USA

1
INTRODUCTION

Philip M Preece

It has been almost 70 years since rubella was suspected of being a human teratogen (an agent capable of inducing birth defects), and, in that time, much has been learned about how prenatal influences can affect the normal development of the embryo and fetus (Gregg 1941). In the 1960s and '70s, these concepts were expanded to the field of behavioural teratology, when it was observed that prenatal exposure to certain agents or conditions could influence later behaviour and function in the offspring even in the absence of any obvious physical deficit. More recently, the idea of fetal programming has been proposed, whereby conditions during pregnancy (e.g. undernutrition) can have long-term effects on the health and well-being of the offspring. Such conditions might, for instance, increase the likelihood of diabetes, obesity and cardiovascular disease (Barker 2000, Godfrey and Barker 2001). Clearly, a range of factors can influence embryonic and fetal development, affecting both physical and functional status in the offspring.

Scope of the book

This book firstly documents the consequences of intrauterine exposure to various drugs and substances of abuse. Next, we hope to demonstrate the complexity of the subject, as the raw effects of exposure to such chemicals in utero are modified or influenced by a wide range of pre-, peri- and postnatal factors.

In exploring the range of challenges to understanding this complex subject, we seek to provide the research base available in the literature. This should provide, for the practitioner, the basis for making decisions about the care and management of these children with some security and at as early a time as possible. Professionals need to provide active medical and social interventions, in addition to protective management, to prevent vacillation and delay in the appropriate and effective care of these children (Department for Children, Schools and Families 2008).

Prenatal factors

Children's development and emotional security are intimately connected to parental factors and the circumstances of their birth. A multitude of parameters influence the success of this process in normal circumstances (Fig. 1.1). It is self-evident that many childhood features reflect parental genetic make-up. There are significant risks in a range of conditions in which mothers may need or choose to take medications and drugs in pregnancy. Epilepsy and learning disability (North American terminology: mental retardation) have a variable

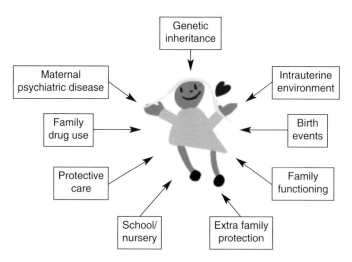

Fig. 1.1. Cumulative effect on infant development.

heritability and may also mean exposure of the infant to maternal medication. Psychiatric disease such as depression and psychosis may require treatment in pregnancy but both of these conditions may also have a significant effect on maternal parenting skills and subsequent infant development, particularly in language development irrespective of any potential intrauterine effect of the drugs used in treatment (Orr and Miller 1995, Murray and Cooper 1997). Maternal ill health and nutritional deficiency during pregnancy can have a significant effect on fetal growth and development, which may be compounded by smoking, drugs of abuse and alcohol use in pregnancy (Maughan et al. 2004).

Parents who take drugs such as opiates or misuse alcohol may have additional difficulties, predisposing them to their choice of lifestyle, including a range of neurodevelopmental and mental health problems (Kennare et al. 2005). Mothers who abuse alcohol and drugs often do not care well for themselves in pregnancy, and their chaotic lifestyles do not allow for optimum health (Guerrini et al. 2009). Such women may also be exposed to blood-borne viral infections such as hepatitis and human immunodeficiency virus, which may be trans-mitted to the fetus (Bell and Harvey-Dodds 2008). Some intrauterine pharmacological agents cause poor fetal growth and premature labour and expose infants to the complications of preterm birth and low birthweight. The effects of smoking, alcohol and drug use may also be cumulative (Riley and McGee 2005).

Postnatal factors
Major concerns arise in infants of drug- and alcohol-abusing mothers. Not only are there the potential risks of intrinsic neurodevelopmental problems, explored in the subsequent chapters of this book, but there are also the real risks of family disharmony, domestic violence, physical and emotional abuse and neglect (Advisory Council on the Misuse of Drugs 2003). Such dysfunctional families provide unique challenges to the statutory agencies

2

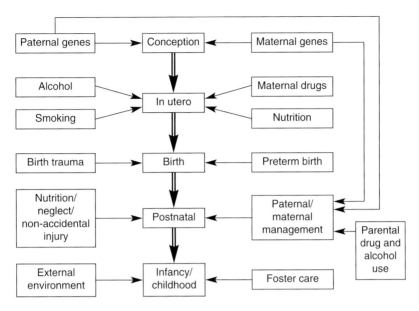

Fig. 1.2. Factors influencing infant development.

designed to protect children. These families move frequently, associate with a wide range of individuals who are often fellow drug abusers, use unsuitable carers, disengage with social and primary health care services, and may obstruct efforts to supervise and protect children (Fig. 1.2).

As will be seen throughout this book, disentangling the primary effects of the intra-uterine exposure from genetic predisposition and the subsequent family environment needs particularly careful research and large numbers of families to study, to control for all the potential confounding factors. For example, very few mothers who abuse drugs do so with single agents, more often mixing these with the effects of alcohol and smoking (see Chapter 8). Recreational drugs are often taken intermittently, making the study of the effects of amphetamines and ecstasy difficult to evaluate, as it is well known that teratogenic effects will vary at different times in gestation. Finally, children cannot be left in the family home if they are at clear risk of further harm. As a result, many studies are compromised by the need to accommodate children at different postnatal stages when home circumstances demand the child be protected.

These vulnerable children are often very difficult to place with suitable foster carers and provide enormous challenges to even the most experienced childcare specialists. The current drive to place children 'looked after' (i.e. fostered) as early as possible in adoptive placements, to minimize the risks of frequent changes of foster carers, may result in placement at an early age when the pattern of neurodevelopmental problems may not be fully expressed. As a result, adoptive placements with well-meaning but frequently inexperienced parents pose further challenges for post-adoption support.

Effect of intrauterine exposure

This book is designed to inform the reader of the potential risks to infants exposed to a range of intrauterine chemicals, which are potentially neuroactive, medicinal drugs such as antiepileptics, antidepressants and antipsychotics, and recreational drugs/drugs of abuse such as alcohol, opiates, cannabis and tobacco. We review the teratogenic action of some of the chemical processes and the relationship to the stage of pregnancy of exposure. Not all of these agents alter anatomical structure, however. Some may alter the chemical balance of neurotransmitters and affect the regulation of brain function in both the short and long term (Stanwood et al. 2001). These changes may have profound effects on children's behaviour and propensity to behavioural disturbances, forcing changes in parental strategies for dealing with potentially challenging behaviours. Birth parents retaining custody of their children, while already struggling to deal with the many challenges in their own lives, often encounter additional difficulties managing an irritable child with potential problems such as the withdrawal symptoms of neonatal abstinence syndrome. Those children who are in the care of statutory agencies will pose different challenges to foster carers who may question their own parenting strategies when confronted with a very difficult child and, if not well informed of the likely effect of the child's previous exposure, may feel inadequate as parents and carers. Some children from very troubled backgrounds will need more than the love and security the average family can provide and need 'super parents' with a wide range of support packages to ensure family stability. We explore strategies to support families with these children and provide statutory agencies with the information to assess when to intervene to protect children from harm.

The following case study illustrates the complexity of the subject. It concerns a child exposed to a potentially toxic agent in utero, describing the impact a wide range of factors had on the individuals in her family and how their lives were affected by the circumstances in which they found themselves, and details the efforts of her parents, advisors and statutory agencies to protect her from a range of potentially damaging factors.

Case history

M was her mother's fifth child. The mother was identified as a heavy drinker and was consuming at least 8 units (64 g) of alcohol per day. At birth (at 38 weeks' gestation) M weighed 1.94 kg and had a ptosis of the right eye and bifid uvula. No other abnormalities were noted at the time. She had mild hypoglycaemia (minimum blood sugar level 2.4 mmol/L) despite tube feeding. Discharge was delayed as the mother appeared drunk on the unit. Enquiry to Social Care revealed two previous children who were in the care of the maternal grandmother, but the parental partnership was strong and there was no reason to further delay discharge from the neonatal unit.

M then had a stormy period of three admissions to hospital within four months with poor weight gain and feeding. On one occasion, the general practitioner queried the quality of home care. The failure to gain weight by 4 months prompted a more detailed look at M, and clinical examination suggested features of fetal alcohol syndrome (FAS) with short palpebral fissures, flat philtrum and thin upper lip associated with faltering growth, ptosis and bifid uvula. Investigations with routine metabolic screen and chromosome analysis were normal, while cerebral ultrasonography revealed an isolated right cerebral cyst. Tube feeding was started and there was an initial weight gain. The mother had been referred to a psychiatrist three months after M's birth for treatment of alcoholism and attended once, but thereafter did not attend.

Following home tube feeding with the supervision of the community paediatric nurse, M's weight and growth improved from the fourth to the sixth month of life. There was one incident when she was seen with an unusual pattern of bruising which was explained by the use of a damaged child's bouncing seat. However, at 6 months growth was again faltering and Social Care had become concerned by the level of care in the home and organized a strategy meeting of all the professionals involved. It was agreed to proceed to a formal child protection conference under the UK Children Act (1989). Before the meeting could take place, an incident occurred at home where the mother was severely injured in a domestic dispute with the father and was admitted to the hospital. The father subsequently disappeared and was found contemplating jumping off a motorway bridge into traffic. M was admitted to hospital care and the opportunity taken to refer her to have a gastrostomy fitted to maintain long-term enteral feeding. The child protection conference agreed that M should be placed in foster care and the two other children at home placed with family members. Developmental assessment at this stage suggested normal psychomotor development. While in foster care, M stayed with the parents six hours per day, four days per week in an attempt to assess maternal function and reintegrate her into the family home. At 13 months she started to have breath-holding attacks and reflex anoxic seizures. She was a very active girl and was on the go continuously once she was independently mobile. She had a very variable sleep pattern and she was transferred to alternative foster carers who could manage better with her continued restlessness. Her mother continued to drink and the home situation continued to cause concern until eventually the siblings, who had returned home, were accommodated with the maternal grandmother.

Detailed developmental assessment at 20 months revealed that while motor development was progressing, other aspects of development, particularly speech, were now seriously delayed, and assessment was severely impaired by poor concentration and hyperactivity. Growth parameters were still below the 0.4th centile for height, weight and head circumference. At this point, Social Care told the parents that reintegration was not a realistic possibility, and the mother decided to make a serious attempt to stop drinking reinforced by regular monitoring of liver function. Social Care now had a dilemma, and the children's guardian ad litem (a court appointment under English law to represent the interests of the child) recommended a last attempt to reintegrate M within the family so long as the mother continued to abstain and could provide a structured home environment. M moved to new foster parents while the reintegration plan was explored, and she was again placed with the birth family at 2 years 6 months and removed from the child protection register. She still presented as a very active child with limited attention span and delayed expressive speech. By the age of 2 years 11 months, a Griffiths developmental assessment demonstrated normal motor development but speech at a 15-month level and hand/eye coordination at an 18-month level.

When M was 3.5 years old her mother relapsed and was warned by Social Care that any deterioration in maternal care would result in the children being removed, once again, from the family home. At 4 years 3 months, one of her siblings was injured and M and her elder brother were removed from the home for their safety to the grandparents' care. Unfortunately, the grandfather died suddenly less than a year later and as her grandmother could not manage M's care on her own she was again placed with foster parents. All the changes in family circumstances had up to now inhibited active management of M's increasingly difficult behaviour. She was placed in a special school for children with moderate learning difficulties. She was described as very active with impulsivity, flitting attention, and autistic features of indiscriminate affection, solitary play and lack of imaginative play thought to be characteristic of the developmental pattern of attachment disorder in the context of FAS.

A formal assessment of attention skills was initiated but a recommendation that medical treatment should be offered was held up, as the parents still retained parental responsibility and Social Care was required to seek their permission.

An application for a freeing order, to allow adoption, was opposed by the family, who made a further application for residence with the grandmother. While this was rejected, it further delayed the opportunity to finalize M's adoptive placement, which was only finally agreed at 6 years 4 months. The foster parents, by now, needed regular respite care, and the prospective adopters withdrew at 6 years 9 months. By this time, M was described as having no awareness of danger, self-harming when frustrated and with an erratic sleep pattern in addition to her other problems. At this stage the foster parents and Social Care agreed to a trial of long-acting methylphenidate with some benefit. Finally, she was confirmed in her long-term placement under special guardianship arrangements and care was transferred to another unit close to the guardian's home and her new school at the age of 7 years 6 months.

Complexities of care

M's story was an enormous education to all the professionals working to protect her future and illustrates vividly the complexities of care for these vulnerable children. She had two parents who were impulsive and volatile even when they were not drinking. They lived a chaotic lifestyle exacerbated by frequent domestic disputes and violence. M also suffered from the teratogenic effects of exposure to alcohol in pregnancy, and then was subjected to physical abuse and neglect. She also was vulnerable in a system which attempted to keep the family together, whereas the parents were too dysfunctional to provide her with the security and structure needed to ameliorate the effects of FAS. Once she became a 'looked after' child, she was moved to a range of carers before eventually finding an adoptive placement at 7 years of age. By this time, many of her behaviour patterns were already ingrained and difficult to change. It is clear that she was a victim not only of FAS but also of a care system which, despite the provision within the Children Act (1989) that "the child's interests are paramount", found it difficult to weigh up the balance between her best interests and the interests of her family and society as a whole. It is clear that she will continue to challenge the support services available even in a highly developed country such as Britain.

How could we have intervened in M's interests at a point when she could be protected from the secondary risks of disadvantaged children? It is possible in some circumstances, when forewarned, to minimize the exposure to alcohol in utero by early work with alcohol-abusing mothers (see Chapter 13). A prebirth child protection case conference would now be the norm in these circumstances, and social care and health workers could devise appropriate strategies to intervene with intensive support and monitoring when M's care fell below acceptable standards (see 'Thresholds for intervention', Chapter 12). Early legal procedures could, using a supervision order, allow her to stay with the family, while maintaining a degree of coercion with clear criteria for intervention. Adoption legislation in England and Wales now allows 'twin tracking' so that time is not lost waiting for circumstances to declare themselves before final decisions about placement are made, and there are now standards regarding timescales to avoid the drift illustrated in this case history. There are still uncertainties in the legal system though, and the presumption of 'kinship placements' within The Children Act (2000) can complicate decisions, as illustrated in M's case. However, a thorough knowledge of the natural history of FAS, as outlined in Chapters 6 and 7, could have predicted her high level of need and the probable failure of her placement with family members who, at best, were not in robust health, and who also had some ambivalence to the parental problems, which clouded their judgement.

Behavioural teratogenesis
Maternal alcohol ingestion represents the archetypal form of behavioural teratogenesis, causing not only physical malformations but also disruption of brain development, significant impairments in behaviour, attention control and language development, and an increased risk of offending behaviour in later life. However, a similar process may occur in a range of circumstances where infants are exposed to a variety of neuroactive substances, therapeutic drugs and drugs of abuse.

Antiepileptic drugs (AEDs) are necessary to control epilepsy in adults, and pregnancy poses additional risks for women with epilepsy (EURAP Study Group 2006). Fetal hydantoin (phenytoin) syndrome has been well described for many years, but the newer range of AEDs is now more commonly used, including carbamazepine and sodium valproate. The long-term outcome for the commonest medications currently in use to treat seizure disorders described in Chapter 4, but we need to continue to monitor the outcome of pregnancies where the newer AEDs such as lamotrigine, topiramate and levetiracetam are being used as 'safer' alternatives in the management of the more complex forms of epilepsy. However, in view of the most recent studies there is a need to consider whether all adolescent girls should consider a switch of treatment from valproate to prevent potential problems, especially since a significant number of pregnancies in young women are unplanned (Tomson 2009).

In the last 20 years, a wide range of medications has been introduced for the management of serious psychiatric diseases such as depression and psychosis, with significant improvement in the quality of life of the sufferers. However, these drugs are complex and may affect fetal development. Their long-term effects are difficult to quantify as they are less understood than other medications. Clearly there is a need to minimize the risk by withdrawal of the medication, if possible, but there are real risks to the mental health of mothers and the safety of the infant postnatally with inadequate treatment. The risk of infanticide, abuse and neglect should not be underestimated (Orr and Miller 1995), and it is probable that the use of medication to minimize symptoms is preferable to the risks of no treatment (see Chapter 5).

FAS has been well described, and the problems of alcohol use were even highlighted in ancient times and graphically illustrated by Hogarth in 18th century London (although there are other interpretations of these works) (Calhoun and Warren 2007). The morphological features and presentation in young children, and the lasting implications and characteristic neurobehavioural patterns in older children and adolescents, are now widely recognized in typical cases. What has only recently started to be understood is the wider spectrum of intrauterine alcohol effects without the characteristic morphological pattern, i.e. fetal alcohol spectrum disorder (Calhoun et al. 2006). The dose and frequency pattern related to severity of effect is still not clearly delineated, and the difficulties of measuring the dose/effect response are elegantly highlighted in Chapter 2. Concerns have been raised about the effect of low levels of alcohol exposure and, more importantly, the effect of binge drinking, resulting in the emerging consensus that there is no 'safe' level of exposure (Department of Health 2007). We are now developing a clearer understanding of the critical effect of alcohol and other teratogens on the developing brain in very early pregnancy before the completion of embryogenesis with resultant structural changes to the brain. We are also developing an understanding of the complex mechanisms for continuing damage in later pregnancy through a host of different mechanisms including dendritic pruning, apoptosis and epigenetic factors (Gemma et al. 2007).

Acute withdrawal effects of opiates are a common reason for admission to neonatal units in developed countries, and the relationship of exposure to cocaine, heroin and methadone use in pregnancy and withdrawal is well understood (Advisory Council on the Misuse of Drugs 2003). Large-cohort studies in some populations are now describing longer-term effects of crack cocaine (Chapter 8), but particular attention needs to be given to potential confounding factors such as exposure to other agents in utero, e.g. cigarettes, alcohol and recreational drugs like cannabis (Chapter 9). Mothers who abuse opiates do not always take care of their own health antenatally (Kennnare et al. 2005), and the infants are often raised in less than ideal family circumstances, with a significant number being accommodated with foster families, further clouding the validity of observational studies (Ornoy et al. 1996, Street et al. 2008). Such factors make it difficult to define the primary effect of the agent under study and the secondary effects of the confounding factors. Most of the work in this area has been done in communities where crack cocaine is the most prevalent agent, but fewer long-term, well-conducted studies in heroin- and methadone-using mothers are available (Ornoy et al. 2001). However, it is now clear that the outcome is significantly affected by socioeconomic factors, and providing a nourishing family atmosphere can be protective against poor outcome (Singer et al. 2008).

Many people regard cannabis as a relatively benign drug of abuse and so less interest has been paid to the long-term effects on individuals regularly exposed in utero. Two large studies have now reported findings over a 20-year period showing clear if subtle long-term effects despite studying two widely differing client populations (Goldschmidt et al. 2000, Fried 2004). These data need to be interpreted in the light of changing patterns of cannabis use, with the development of more potent strains, which is likely to potentiate the effects

(Hardwick and King 2008, Hall and Degenhardt 2009). Other recreational drugs such as amphetamines and ecstasy are even more difficult to study, as use is intermittent and often mixed with other agents, making the effects difficult to quantify (Smith et al. 2006). Only one substantial long-term study of amphetamines is available (Eriksson et al. 2000).

Smoking is a common confounder in many of the studies of potential teratogenic factors in the use of drugs, alcohol and medications used in psychiatric conditions (Chapter 11). Combined with caffeine, it modulates its main effect through reduced birthweight (CARE Study Group 2008).

The different management strategies for these infants exposed to a range of potentially harmful teratogens do have many similarities (Section 3). Limitation of harm by reducing exposure prenatally, early intervention with parenting programmes, and specific management of comorbidities such as attention deficit disorder are important. However, this field is complicated by a range of factors including maternal acceptance of the possibility that the child's problems may be related to their drug taking, whether therapeutic, recreational or addictive, and consequent agreement to participate in programmes to support her in parenting postnatally (Williams-Petersen et al. 1994). The poor social circumstances of some of these families raises the need to protect the child from the risks of physical and emotional abuse and neglect. Social Care services have a duty to protect, but also to attempt to maintain children within their biological families, which is at times an impossible expectation to implement (Chapter 12). Even accommodation with other family members is fraught with difficulties in the midst of the complex relationship between a grandparent and their child whose infant has been exposed to teratogenic influences. It is possible to ameliorate the long-term effects with a combination of highly motivated experienced carers, specific targeted behavioural interventions (Advisory Council on the Misuse of Drugs 2003), and the judicious use of medication, particularly psychostimulants (Chapter 15). These individuals will, however, always remain vulnerable to a range of risks and impairments as they move on into adult life (Williams and Ross 2007).

REFERENCES

Advisory Council on the Misuse of Drugs (2003) *Hidden Harm: Responding to the Needs of Children of Problem Drug Users.* London: Home Office.

Barker DJ (2000) In utero programming of cardiovascular disease. *Theriogenology* **53**: 555–574.

Bell J, Harvey-Dodds L (2008) Pregnancy and injecting drug use. *BMJ* **336**: 1303–1305.

Calhoun F, Warren K (2007) Fetal alcohol syndrome: historical perspectives. *Neurosci Biobehav Rev* **31**: 168–171.

Calhoun F, Attilia ML, Spagnolo PA, et al. (2006) National Institute on Alcohol Abuse and Alcoholism and the study of fetal alcohol spectrum disorders. The International Consortium. *Ann Ist Super Sanita* **42**: 4–7.

CARE Study Group (2008) Maternal caffeine intake during pregnancy and the risk of fetal growth restriction: a large prospective study. *BMJ* **337**: 1334–1338.

Department for Children, Schools and Families (2008) Analysing child deaths and serious injury through abuse and neglect: what can we learn? Research Report DCSF RR023, 70–96.

Department of Health (2007) Updated alcohol advice for pregnant women. London: Department of Health.

Eriksson M, Jonsson B, Zetterström R (2000) Children of mothers abusing amphetamine: head circumference during infancy and psychosocial development until 14 years. *Acta Paediatr* **89**: 1474–1478.

EURAP Study Group (2006) Seizure control and treatment in pregnancy: observations from the EURAP epilepsy pregnancy registry. *Neurology* **66**: 354–360

Fried PA (2004) Pregnancy and effects on offspring from birth through adolescence. In: Grotenhermen F, ed. *Cannabis und Cannabinoide. Pharmakologie, Toxikologie und therapeutisches Potenzial. 2nd edn.* Bern: Verlag Hans Huber, pp. 329–338.

Gemma S, Vichi S, Testai E (2007) Metabolic and genetic factors contributing to alcohol induced effects and fetal alcohol syndrome. *Neurosci Biobehav Rev* **31**: 221–229.

Godfrey KM, Barker DJ (2001) Fetal programming and adult health. *Public Health Nutr* **4**: 611–624.

Goldschmidt L, Day NL, Richardson GA (2000) Effects of prenatal marijuana exposure on child behavior problems at age 10. *Neurotoxicol Teratol* **22**: 325–336.

Gregg NM (1941) Congenital cataract following German measles in the mother. *Trans Ophthalmol Soc Aust* **3**: 35–46.

Guerrini I, Jackson S, Keaney F (2009) Pregnancy and alcohol misuse. *BMJ* **338**: 829–832.

Hall W, Degenhardt L (2009) Adverse health effects of non-medical cannabis use. *Lancet* **374**: 1389–1391.

Hardwick S, King L (2008) *Home Office Cannabis Potency Study.* St Albans, Hertfordshire: Home Office Scientific Development Branch.

Kennare R, Heard A, Chan A (2005) Substance use during pregnancy: risk factors and obstetric and perinatal outcomes in South Australia. *Aust N Z J Obstet Gynaecol* **45**: 220–225.

Maughan B, Taylor A, Caspi A, Moffitt TE (2004) Prenatal smoking and early childhood conduct problems: testing genetic and environmental explanations of the association. *Arch Gen Psychiatry* **61**: 836–843.

Murray L, Cooper P (1997) Effects of postnatal depression on infant development. *Arch Dis Child* **77**: 99–101.

Ornoy A, Segal J, Bar-Hamburger R, Greenbaum C (2001) Developmental outcome of school-age children born to mothers with heroin dependency: importance of environmental factors. *Dev Med Child Neurol* **43**: 668–675.

Ornoy A, Michailevskaya V, Lukashov I, et al. (1996) The developmental outcome of children born to heroin addicted mothers, raised at home or adopted. *Child Abuse Negl* **20**: 385–396.

Orr S, Miller CA (1995) Maternal depressive symptoms and the risk of poor pregnancy outcome. *Epidemiol Rev* **15**: 165–171.

Riley EP, McGee CL (2005) Fetal alcohol spectrum disorders: an overview with emphasis on changes in brain and behaviour. *Exp Biol Med* **230**: 357–365.

Singer LT, Nelson S, Short E, et al. (2008) Prenatal cocaine exposure: drug and environmental effects at 9 years. *J Pediatr* **153**: 105–111.

Smith LM, LaGasse LL, Derauf C, et al. (2006) The infant development, environment, and lifestyle study: effects of prenatal methamphetamine exposure, polydrug exposure, and poverty on intrauterine growth. *Pediatrics* **118**: 1149–1156.

Stanwood GD, Washington RS, Shumsky JS, Levitt P (2001) Prenatal cocaine exposure produces consistent developmental alterations in dopamine-rich regions of the cerebral cortex. *Neuroscience* **106**: 5–14.

Street K, Whitlinggum G, Gibson P, et al. (2008) Is adequate parenting compatible with maternal drug use? A 5 year follow up. *Child Health Care Dev* **34**: 204–206.

Tomson T (2009) Which drug for the pregnant woman with epilepsy? *N Engl J Med* **360**: 1667–1669.

Williams JH, Ross L (2007) Consequences of prenatal toxin exposure for mental health in children and adolescents: a systematic review. *Eur Child Adolesc Psychiatry* **16**: 243–253.

Williams-Petersen MG, Myers BJ, Degen HM, et al. (1994) Drug using and non-using women: potential for child abuse, child rearing attitudes, social support and affection for the expected baby. *Int J Addict* **29**: 1631–1643.

2
EPIDEMIOLOGY OF DRUG AND ALCOHOL USE DURING PREGNANCY

Ron Gray

I begin this chapter by considering the main difficulty in conducting research in this area, the problem of accurate exposure measurement. I then highlight some recent trends in exposure to street drugs and alcohol in women of childbearing age and pregnant women in the USA and Europe. Although there are detailed chapters on the adverse consequences of such exposures later in the book, I briefly highlight some of these in order to illustrate the methodological difficulties involved in making causal inferences from observational studies in humans. Finally I close with some considerations on risk and safety and how these might guide policy-makers in preventative messages.

Clearly both drugs and alcohol may have severe physical and psychosocial consequences for the women using them, irrespective of any damage to the fetus. However, such considerations are beyond the scope of this chapter. Similarly, evidence on the use of prescription medications, on smoking and caffeine consumption, as well as findings from animal models are considered elsewhere in subsequent chapters of this book.

Measurement of exposure of the fetus

The major problem faced by researchers working in the area of alcohol and drug use is how to accurately measure and summarize exposure (Dawson 2003, Greenfield and Kerr 2008). Although there are a number of promising approaches using biomarkers of exposure (Koren et al. 2008), self-report still remains the main method of exposure ascertainment and is likely to remain so. The difficulties involved in measurement may lead to misclassification of consumption level, which may result in bias in observational studies that, for example, associate alcohol with poor health outcome (Dufour 1999).

Self-reported alcohol and drug consumption during pregnancy can be measured retrospectively or prospectively on one or many occasions. The methods for collecting data include diaries, interviews and self-completed questionnaires (Kesmodel and Olsen 2001).

However, self-report relies on several assumptions that have been shown to be problematic. For example, self-report relies on accurately remembering the frequency, quantity, portion size and type of alcohol or drug used over a particular time period. Sometimes the reporters are asked to calculate their average daily or weekly consumption or remember how many times they consumed more than a certain number of drinks. The ability to do this accurately (unless one has made a meticulous contemporaneous record) is doubtful. In addition, there are factors such as shame, fear of disclosure, or the concern about admitting to engaging in socially undesirable behaviour that will affect willingness to report drug or alcohol use accurately. These factors are likely to play an even more important role in pregnancy, where both drinking alcohol and drug use have been associated with harm to the unborn child. On the other hand, it is also possible that some younger women may overestimate their drinking as a sign of bravado. The amount recalled also critically depends on how the question is framed (Stockwell et al. 2004).

Standardization of exposure

Let us assume, though, that we have some rich data, which we feel are an accurate picture of reported consumption over various periods during pregnancy. The next problem is to convert the reported amounts into a standard form for analysis. In the case of alcohol this relies on conversion from reported drink size and type to grams, fluid ounces or a standard measure such as the British Standard Unit. But this is problematic as well. First there are varying strengths of beer, wine and spirits: it may be unclear which strength to apply. Many drinkers are unaware whether they are drinking a standard lager or a strong one. In the case of wine, there have been increases in the sizes of glasses in which wine is served in restaurants and bars and a trend towards increased strength of wines. But perhaps the most difficult thing to quantify accurately is the content of drinks poured at home. It has been shown that the alcohol content of home-poured measures is considerably underestimated (Gill and Donaghy 2004). In an attempt to provide international comparisons, most countries define a 'standard drink' as 10–14 g alcohol. In the USA a 'standard drink' is 14 g. In the UK we use the 'unit' of 8 g, but the 'standard drink' of 125 mL (a small glass) of wine (12% alcohol by volume) or a measure (35 mL) of spirits (40% alcohol by volume) is 1.5 units, i.e. 12 g.

Patterns of exposure

Let us further assume that our rich, accurately reported data have been in turn accurately converted into a standard form. The next issue is how best to summarize this in a simple measure of exposure. Current popular ways to represent this are as average weekly alcohol consumption and as the maximum amount consumed on any one day in the last week. The problem here is that we lose some of the fine detail on the pattern of drinking. For example, we may be interested in the number of days someone consumed more than a certain amount or what period of time they consumed a large quantity over: drinking four pints of beer (eight standard units) uniformly over the course of a day will give rise to very different blood alcohol levels from consuming them within two hours. A further problem here is that asking for weekly total consumption and dividing by seven to get an 'average' daily consumption and then reporting only this measure can mask huge variability (Abel 1998). For example, consuming 20 drinks on a Saturday and abstaining from Sunday to Friday could be construed as having three drinks per day.

In addition to information on quantity and pattern we might also want to know about features of withdrawl, craving, tolerance or dependence.

Although prospectively collecting detailed information using daily diaries would seem a useful method to gauge consumption more accurately, one has to be realistic about what can be collected, analysed, presented and understood for a given purpose. In the case of large population surveys (where quantifying alcohol and drug use is usually only one aim amongst many) there will be limits on the amount of information that can be collected, and its accuracy. The same considerations apply to large cohort studies. However, in studies specifically designed to study the effects of alcohol and/or drugs on the fetus, one could argue that seeking to measure the exposure as accurately as possible (and perhaps using biomarkers to validate this information) is a reasonable requirement. This then enables one to investigate hypotheses on timing of exposure, effects of cumulative exposure and the effects of ceasing exposure at various points in pregnancy. In the case of binge drinking, Henderson et al. (2007b) have argued that collecting information in this way would allow one more adequately to conceptualize what a binge exposure might be and how it relates to other aspects of drinking pattern and quantity.

The complexities around measurement of exposure mean that using terms like 'heavy', 'moderate' and 'light' or 'low to moderate' drinking during pregnancy is also problematic, with no internationally agreed definitions. These terms therefore are rather vaguely quantified. Hereafter, I will refer to *heavy drinking* as that in excess of normally recommended levels for non-pregnant women, *moderate drinking* as consumption of one 'standard drink' (1.5 British Standard Units, i.e. 12 g ethanol) or more per day on average and *low-to-moderate drinking* as anything below this. I recognize the limitations of these arbitrary categories.*

There are some additional difficulties in trying to quantify illicit drug use. For example, the purity of street heroin is highly variable and also varies by the route of administration: heroin that is smoked is very different from injected heroin.

In the following sections the epidemiological trends in drinking and drug use are explored. There are really two populations of interest: women with confirmed pregnancy, and women who may become pregnant or who may already be in the early stages of pregnancy but unaware of this. For all practical purposes this second population includes all women of childbearing age, although this population also includes women who chose not to or cannot become pregnant (e.g. due to contraception or infertility). Another issue to note is that a substantial number of pregnancies (30–40%), particularly in younger women, are unplanned (Dex and Joshi 2005). This means that women may continue to drink unaware of the fact that they are pregnant, resulting in potential harm to the fetus.

It should be noted that there is marked variation between countries (and even between regions of countries) in quantities, patterns and types of alcohol consumed and illicit drugs used. Therefore generalization from one country to another is probably unwise, and researchers, clinicians and policy makers should rely on local estimates rather than extrapolating. Below, I highlight some studies from the UK, USA and Europe, although one cannot hope to be comprehensive. Most regions or countries will have statistical agencies that carry out surveys and publish data. These data are nowadays often published as reports, made publically available on the internet. The information rarely appears in peer-reviewed journals. Therefore, those using these data need to carefully consider how the information was

---

*For the US definition of a 'standard drink', with examples of standard drink equivalents, see: http://www.niaaa.nih.gov/NR/rdonlyres/1D2BE3DF-18D7-47EE-98C5-E907C7611929/0/StandardDrink.pdf.

gathered and collated as well as how comprehensive, valid, timely and comparable it is likely to be.

Alcohol – our favourite drug

Trends in alcohol consumption in the UK from a number of surveys have recently been collated and critically reviewed (Smith and Foxcroft 2009). One interesting trend noted was the increase in drinking amongst women. This was identified consistently across several different surveys and different measures of alcohol consumption. However, part of the trend is accounted for by recent changes in converting reported consumption into units of alcohol in UK surveys. This change in practice mainly affects those consuming wine and therefore has differentially affected women (as women are more likely to consume wine than are men), leading to an apparent increase in women's consumption of around 45% and a reduction in sex differences (Goddard 2007). That there is still a real increase in consumption despite this artefactual consideration is supported by the large increase in alcohol-related harm to women recorded in recent years, including mortality and hospital discharges with an alcohol-related diagnosis (ISD Scotland 2007). Another potential cause of artefact has been an increase in apparent binge drinking related to changes in the definition of a 'binge' for women: the lower threshold has led to more women now being defined as over the binge measure than occurred with the same drink size changes for men (Plant and Plant 2006).

Across Europe, it is clear that although many women stop drinking once pregnant, a significant minority continue to drink with reported levels generally higher than in the USA (Anderson and Baumberg 2006). Based on data from the 2002 Behavioral Risk Factor Surveillance System in the USA it has been reported that 10% of women consumed alcohol during pregnancy and around 2% were drinking in a binge-type pattern. However, of women who might become pregnant, 55% were drinking alcohol with around 12% drinking in a binge pattern (CDC 2004).

Illicit drugs – experimental, recreational and dependent use

While about 5% of the world's population between the ages of 15 and 64 use illicit drugs, only a small proportion of these (0.6%) are considered to be 'problem drug users' (United Nations Office on Drugs and Crime 2008). Illicit drug use has been conceptualized as a spectrum (British Medical Association 1997) with occasional experimental use of 'soft' drugs at one end, which is virtually universal in many developed countries, through to dependent drug use at the other. In the middle is the recreational use of drugs. In most cases this involves weekend use of cannabis, ecstasy and sometimes cocaine by young people. Recreational use tends not to be associated with psychosocial deterioration and tends to tail off in early adulthood. It is frequently accompanied by alcohol use.

RECREATIONAL DRUG USE

During the 1990s a new social movement emerged amongst young people in Europe and the USA, the so-called 'dance club culture'. This seems to have been associated with a parallel increase in recreational drug use (Deehan and Saville 2003). The British Crime Survey uses cross-sectional surveys to estimate prevalence of self-reported drug use over the past year in the UK. Some interesting trends are apparent looking at the results for those in the 16–24 age group between 1995 and 2006/7 (Nicholas et al. 2007). First, the use of drugs in general has declined from 29.7% of those surveyed to 24.1% in this period. The use of ecstasy has remained at between 4% and 7% over this period but the use of cannabis has significantly declined from 26% to 20.9%. There have also been reductions in the use of opiates and hallucinogens, and a large reduction in amphetamines (from 11.8% to 3.5%) during this period. However, the use of cocaine, mainly in the powdered form, has increased fourfold in this time from 1.4% in 1995 to 6.1% in 2006/7.

The European Monitoring Centre for Drugs and Drug Addiction (2005) used data from a number of sources to try and tease apart the patterns of drug use in women across Europe and how they varied by age. The key findings showed that there was marked variation between countries in prevalence and in sex differences. However, the following findings seemed fairly clear. In regard to cannabis use, European Union countries with relatively high prevalence rates showed smaller sex differences than countries with low prevalence rates. These sex differences seem to be larger in older than in younger age-groups. However, sex differences seem to be disappearing over time with a trend towards equality. The findings on prevalence for ecstasy use were of smaller magnitude than those for cannabis and showed more variability, but similar trends were apparent.

There have been very few studies investigating prevalence of illicit drug use in pregnant women. The US National Pregnancy and Health Survey (National Institute on Drug Abuse 1996) gathered self-report data from a national sample of 2613 women who delivered babies in 52 urban and rural hospitals during 1992 in the USA. The study's findings were that 5.5% of pregnant women used illicit drugs while pregnant: 11.3% of African-American women, 4.4% of white women, and 4.5% of Hispanic women. A similar overall figure of 4.7% using any illicit drugs in the first trimester was found using the national Household Survey on Drug Abuse data for 1996–1998 in the USA (Ebrahim and Gfroerer 2003). More recent estimates (Substance Abuse and Mental Health Services Administration 2007) based on the SAMHSA Office of Applied Studies National Survey on Drug Use and Health, 2003, 2004, 2005 and 2006, indicate that although around 10% of the non-pregnant female reproductive-age population in a US sample were using illicit drugs, in the pregnant group this prevalence fell to 4.6% in 2003–2004 and to 4% in 2005–2006. Use of cannabis accounted for about three-quarters of this (3.6% and 3.0% of drug use in these respective periods). There was marked variation by age: the 2005–2006 prevalence estimate was 15.5% in those aged 15–17, falling to 6.5% in those aged 18–25 and to 1.8% in those aged 26–44. There was also variation by trimester with prevalence rates of 5.4%, 3.6% and 2.7% during the first, second and third trimesters respectively.

Studies using meconium and/or other analyses of biological samples suggest that the figures above may be underestimates at least in some geographical areas. For example, a study in Glasgow (Williamson et al. 2006) analysing meconium from 400 infants found cannabinoids in 13.25%, cocaine in 2.75%, and amphetamine in 1.75%. Similarly, a study of 974 mother–infant dyads from Barcelona (Lozano et al. 2007) detected cannabis in 5.3% of meconium samples and noted that only 1.7% of the participating mothers disclosed

15

gestational drug use. Another recent study (Azadi and Dildy 2008) determined the prevalence of substance abuse in 416 women from New Orleans in 2005 at delivery admission by universal urine toxicology screening. Some 19% screened positive for one or more substances, including cocaine (3.1%), amphetamines (2.4%), barbiturates (2.1%), opiates (2.6%), cannabis (17.2%) and benzodiazepine (5.7%). A similar study focusing on early pregnancy found that of 807 consecutive positive pregnancy test urine samples taken in south London (Sherwood et al. 1999), cannabis was detected in 14.5%.

DEPENDENT DRUG USE

In contrast to the recreational use of drugs, the dependent drug user is likely to be socially excluded, subject to domestic abuse, in poor general health, and often involved in criminal activity or prostitution to subsidize the drug use. Thus, although a numerically much smaller group, in general their pregnancy outcomes are much worse than those only involved in recreational drug use. While some of this increased risk of poor outcome can be attributed to the drugs used, much of it is related to coexisting factors such as poverty, poor nutrition, poor mental and physical health, and smoking during pregnancy. For this reason many areas have set up specialized maternity services to manage this group of women and in particular to try to stabilize drug use during pregnancy by using methadone (Winklbaur et al. 2008). Estimates of prevalence from the Northern and Yorkshire Region of the UK (Grandey et al. 2002) suggest a rate of 7.9 [95% confidence interval (CI) 7.2–8.8] per 1000 deliveries, i.e. 0.79%.

In addition to regional variation in drug (and alcohol) use, there is also considerable variation within a population. For example, drug use is much more common in certain population groups, predominating in those with low socio-economic status. Similarly, both heavy drinking and abstinence are also more associated with low socio-economic status, whereas light-to-moderate patterns of consumption are more likely in those with higher socio-economic status. For example, a study comparing pregnant teenagers with pregnant adults indicated that while use of cannabis and cocaine decreased during pregnancy for both teenagers and adults, offspring of teenagers were at higher risk for intermittent high peak alcohol exposure later in pregnancy than offspring of older women (Cornelius et al. 1994).

In summary, prevalence estimates of drug use vary widely geographically, and estimation of local rates as well as types of drug used are essential. Self-reported rates drop during pregnancy but are likely to be an underestimate by a factor of 2 or 3.

Outcomes

ALCOHOL

For heavy drinking during pregnancy, a number of studies have demonstrated associations with spontaneous abortion, stillbirth, preterm birth, infants who are small for gestational age, and birth defects (including fetal alcohol syndrome), while other studies have failed to find any associations or found negative associations. These studies (up to the mid-1990s) have been collated and reviewed by Abel (1998), who sees the association with heavy or binge drinking as being a "universal organizing principle". For moderate drinking the evidence is much more contested. In the USA, the National Institute on Alcohol Abuse and

Alcoholism (NIAAA 2004) concluded that low-to-moderate drinking "does not seem to be associated with an increased risk of fetal physical malformations but may have behavioral or neurocognitive consequences." A more recent systematic review on the effects of low-to-moderate alcohol consumption during pregnancy reached similar conclusions (Henderson et al. 2007a). Evidence from two meta-analyses on moderate drinking (defined as between two drinks per day and two drinks per week) also suggest that moderate drinking is not associated with deficits in growth or birth defects although it may be associated with spontaneous abortion. Polygenis et al. (1998) conducted a meta-analysis of moderate alcohol consumption during pregnancy and the incidence of fetal malformations. Moderate consumption was defined as the range >2 drinks per week and <2 drinks per day (24–168 g per week). The meta-analysis included 130 810 pregnancy outcomes and reported a relative risk for fetal malformation of 1.01 (95% CI, 0.94–1.08). Makarechian et al. (1998), using the same definition of moderate, found the odds ratio for spontaneous abortion was 1.35 (95% CI, 1.09–1.67), for stillbirth was 0.65 (95% CI, 0.46–0.91), and for preterm birth was 0.95 (95% CI, 0.79–1.15). The result for stillbirth was considered unstable and inconclusive because of the small number of studies, and significant heterogeneity existed among the individual odds ratios for spontaneous abortion. However, a more recent study has found a three-fold increase in risk of stillbirth in women drinking five or more drinks weekly (Kesmodel et al. 2002). These issues are explored in more detail in Chapters 6 and 7.

The long-term neurobehavioural consequences of drinking during pregnancy that have been demonstrated include neurodevelopmental delay, global and specific cognitive impairments and behaviour disorders as well as increased risk of psychiatric disorder (Riley and McGee 2005). Again the evidence for the effects seems much more secure at higher levels of consumption. Nevertheless, there is a growing belief that there may be effects at low-to-moderate levels of consumption, which has led to a more cautious approach advising pregnant women to avoid alcohol during pregnancy. This is an area where more research is urgently required.

DRUGS

In contrast to the effects of heavy drinking on birth outcomes the effects of illicit drugs are much less clear (Schempf 2007) despite popular characterizations such as 'crack babies' (Haasen and Krausz 2001). Although a number of reviews have concluded that the main groups of drugs – cannabis, cocaine, amphetamine and opiates – can all have adverse effects in the perinatal period and on the fetus (Kuczkowski 2007), the effects seem much clearer for cocaine than for opiates (Shankaran et al. 2007), with prenatal cannabis exposure appearing to have little effect if any (Fried 2002).

In terms of neurodevelopmental effects, the evidence of effect is stronger but rather difficult to interpret. Undoubtedly there are associations between illicit drug use and later cognitive and behavioural problems, but these may, to a greater extent, be due to the adverse effects of the associated postnatal environment rather than to a teratogenic effect of the drug. The work of Singer and colleagues, for example (see Chapter 8), suggests that although prenatal cocaine exposure has teratogenic effects on neurodevelopment, likely mediated through impairment of fetal brain growth, the effects are greatly attenuated in those who are subsequently adopted (Singer et al. 2004, 2008). As mentioned below, further work incorporating such natural experiments as adoption or comparing serial pregnancies in women, which are concordant or discordant for exposure, are required.

Methodological issues in moving from association to causation

As outlined above, findings from human observational studies provide good evidence of associations between drug and alcohol use during pregnancy and subsequent adverse pregnancy outcome and impaired neurodevelopment. However, before making strong claims about causation it is important to point out the limitations of these studies (Huizink and Mulder 2006). These limitations include small sample sizes, problems in measuring and classifying exposure in an accurate way, and the presence of factors that confound the associations between exposure and outcome and may be measured imperfectly (Olsen and Basso 1999) or in some cases not measured at all (Fewell et al. 2007). This creates problems for causal inference given that many of the associations are weak (Florey 1988) in any case or found inconsistently.

These problems are not peculiar to observational studies in the area of prenatal exposures to toxins, but certain problems have been pointed out repeatedly (Verkerk 1992, Jacobson and Jacobson 2005, Smith 2008). Of course the wealth of consistently replicated findings from animal studies (Driscoll et al. 1990, Zajac and Abel 1992, Cudd 2005) also provides good evidence, but this is largely because such studies follow the experimental design (i.e. random manipulation of exposure leads to a change in outcome), which observational studies clearly do not. Randomized controlled trials in humans are not affected by confounding (if large enough sample sizes are used), and findings from other areas of medicine have shown how one can be persuaded of a causal effect from observational studies only to be repudiated by results from well-designed randomized controlled trials (Smith and Ebrahim 2002). However, it would be unethical to carry out controlled experiments in humans to investigate the behavioural and cognitive effects.

Whilst there is no ideal solution to this problem, there are some potential ways forward. The first is to take a Bayesian type of approach to the synthesis of the available evidence (Cooper et al. 2002). This might start with elucidating the key policy and public health decisions to be made, followed by eliciting a range of prior opinions on likely sizes of effects (and of biases) and then synthesizing evidence from a range of studies while explicitly taking the prior beliefs into account in the analysis. A second approach is the use of natural experiments (Rutter 2007, Gray et al. 2009) such as adoption or mendelian randomization (Smith and Ebrahim 2005).

Risk, safety and the precautionary principle

The use of any illicit drugs is by definition not recommended at any time and I therefore confine discussion to alcohol. Clearly those women who use alcohol regularly and in large amounts during pregnancy are placing not only themselves but also their fetus at risk of harm (Abel 1998). Those drinking at moderate levels potentially place their offspring at risk of adverse neurodevelopmental outcome (Jacobson and Jacobson 2002). For those drinking less than this, the evidence of harm is much less consistent and compelling, with many studies showing no effect and those that have generally showing a rather weak association (Gray and Henderson 2006). However, there is a need for further studies to clarify this, and pending these studies it would be unwise to interpret the absence of strong evidence as evidence of no effect and hence 'safety'. Therefore, advice that women are best to avoid alcohol during pregnancy, if they can, may be warranted until such time as we know more – the precautionary principle (Grandjean 2008). Equally, though, if a concerned woman retrospectively reports occasional low-to-moderate drinking during her pregnancy, it seems reasonable to reassure her that the risk, if any, is likely to be low.

Preventative messages and their limitations

Even assuming that we consider the harms from alcohol and drugs during pregnancy to be worthy of issuing public health advice to pregnant women (or women who may become pregnant), there remain three important issues. The first is how best to get the message across, the second is the limited impact of public health messages, and the third is to consider the evidence on reducing alcohol consumption in the general population (of which pregnant women and women of childbearing age are part).

There is a whole body of literature on how best to communicate risk to the public (Calman and Royston 1997, Lipkus 2007). Key findings are that the public has particular difficulties in comprehending small risks (i.e. less than 1%) and that better ways for presenting risk magnitudes in an easily understandable form are required. One of the critical issues is to frame risk in absolute as well as in relative terms, while contextualizing the risk by comparison with other risks. The way the message is disseminated, and by whom, is also important. Perhaps as wide dissemination as possible using a variety of media and methods would help, e.g. labelling of bottles, use of the internet and physicians/midwives, general practitioners, etc. Other more innovative approaches to dissemination (Choi 2005) could be investigated, but all need to be thoroughly evaluated.

Naive assumptions that giving a message results in it being received, understood and believed in such as way as to alter not only attitudes but crucially behaviour as well need to be challenged. This so-called cognitive–rational paradigm needs to be updated or else replaced with better models that capture both the complexity and non-linear aspects of behaviour change in individuals and in populations (Resnicow and Vaughan 2006). Related to this last point, it is clear that educational strategies alone, including advertising campaigns, labelling alcoholic beverages with warning statements and education in schools, are likely to be popular but ineffective. Such strategies in the past have improved knowledge and influenced attitudes but have failed to change behaviour (Room et al. 2005). That is not to say that educational strategies should not be tried – more that we should be aware of the limitations of this approach and use it only as part of a more comprehensive public health strategy.

ACKNOWLEDGEMENTS

I would like to thank Lesley Smith and Jo Neale at Oxford Brookes University and Moira Plant at the University of the West of England for helpful comments on an earlier draft of this chapter.

REFERENCES

Abel E (1998) *Fetal Alcohol Abuse Syndrome.* New York: Plenum Press.

Anderson P, Baumberg B (2006) *Alcohol in Europe: A Public Health Perspective.* London: Institute of Alcohol Studies.

Azadi A, Dildy GA (2008) Universal screening for substance abuse at the time of parturition. *Am J Obstet Gynecol* **198**: e30–e32.

British Medical Association (1997) *The Misuse of Drugs.* London: Routledge.

Calman KC, Royston GH (1997) Risk language and dialects. *BMJ* **315**: 939–942.

CDC (2004) Alcohol consumption among women who are pregnant or who might become pregnant—United States, 2002. *MMWR Morb Mortal Wkly Rep* **53**: 1178–1181.

Choi BCK (2005) Innovative ideas needed for timely and effective public health information dissemination. *J Epidemiol Community Health* **59**: 259.

Cooper NJ, Sutton AJ, Abrams KR (2002) Decision analytical economic modelling within a Bayesian framework: application to prophylactic antibiotics use for caesarean section. *Stat Methods Med Res* **11**: 491–512.

Cornelius MD, Richardson GA, Day NL, et al. (1994) A comparison of prenatal drinking in two recent samples of adolescents and adults. *J Stud Alcohol* **55**: 412–419.

Cudd TA (2005) Animal model systems for the study of alcohol teratology. *Exp Biol Med* **230**: 389–393.

Dawson DA (2003) Methodological issues in measuring alcohol use. *Alcohol Res Health* **27**: 18–29.

Deehan A, Saville E (2003) Calculating the risk: recreational drug use amongst clubbers in the South East of England. Home Office Online Report 43/03.

Dex S, Joshi H (eds) (2005) *Children of the 21st Century: From Birth to Nine Months.* Bristol: Policy Press.

Driscoll CD, Streissguth AP, Riley EP (1990) Prenatal alcohol exposure: comparability of effects in humans and animal models. *Neurotoxicol Teratol* **12**: 231–237.

Dufour MC (1999) What is moderate drinking? Defining "drinks" and drinking levels. *Alcohol Res Health* **23**: 5–14.

Ebrahim SH, Gfroerer J (2003) Pregnancy-related substance use in the United States during 1996–1998. *Obstet Gynecol* **101**: 374–379.

European Monitoring Centre for Drugs and Drug Addiction (2005) *Differences in Patterns of Drug Use Between Women and Men.* Lisbon: European Monitoring Centre for Drugs and Drug Addiction.

Fewell Z, Davey Smith G, Sterne JA (2007) The impact of residual and unmeasured confounding in epidemiologic studies: a simulation study. *Am J Epidemiol* **166**: 646–655.

Florey CD (1988) Weak associations in epidemiological research: some examples and their interpretation. *Int J Epidemiol* **17**: 950–954.

Fried PA (2002) Conceptual issues in behavioral teratology and their application in determining long-term sequelae of prenatal marihuana exposure. *J Child Psychol Psychiatry* **43**: 81–102.

Gill JS, Donaghy M (2004) Variation in the alcohol content of a 'drink' of wine and spirit poured by a sample of the Scottish population. *Health Educ Res* **19**: 485–491.

Goddard E (2007) *Estimating Alcohol Consumption from Survey Data: Updated Method of Converting Volumes to Units. National Statistics Methodology Series NSM 37.* London: Office of National Statistics.

Grandey M, Cresswell T, Duerden J, Mannion K (2002) *Drug Misuse in Pregnancy in the Northern and Yorkshire Region. Occasional Paper No. 06.* Durham: Northern & Yorkshire Public Health Observatory.

Grandjean P (2008) Late insights into early origins of disease. *Basic Clin Pharmacol Toxicol* **102**: 94–99.

Gray R, Henderson J (2006) *Review of the Fetal Effects of Prenatal Alcohol Exposure. Report to the Department of Health.* Oxford: National Perinatal Epidemiology Unit.

Gray R, Mukherjee RA, Rutter M (2009) Alcohol consumption during pregnancy and its effects on neurodevelopment: what is know and what remains uncertain. *Addiction* **104**: 1270–1273.

Greenfield TK, Kerr WC (2008) Alcohol measurement methodology in epidemiology: recent advances and opportunities. *Addiction* **103**: 1082–1099.

Haasen C, Krausz M (2001) Myths versus evidence with respect to cocaine and crack: learning from the US experience. *Eur Addict Res* **7**: 159–60.

Henderson J, Gray R, Brocklehurst P (2007a) Systematic review of effects of low-moderate prenatal alcohol exposure on pregnancy outcome. *Br J Obstet Gynaecol* **114**: 243–252.

Henderson J, Kesmodel U, Gray R (2007b) Systematic review of the fetal effects of prenatal binge-drinking. *J Epidemiol Community Health* **61**: 1069–1073.

Huizink AC, Mulder EJ (2006) Maternal smoking, drinking or cannabis use during pregnancy and neurobehavioral and cognitive functioning in human offspring. *Neurosci Biobehav Rev* **30**: 24–41.

ISD Scotland (2007) *Alcohol Statistics 2007*. Edinburgh: ISD Publications.

Jacobson JL, Jacobson SW (2002) Effects of prenatal alcohol exposure on child development. *Alcohol Res Health* **26**: 282–286.

Jacobson JL, Jacobson SW (2005) Methodological issues in research on developmental exposure to neurotoxic agents. *Neurotoxicol Teratol* **27**: 395–406.

Kesmodel U, Olsen SF (2001) Self reported alcohol intake in pregnancy: comparison between four methods. *J Epidemiol Community Health* **55**: 738–745.

Kesmodel U, Wisborg K, Olsen SF, et al. (2002) Moderate alcohol intake during pregnancy and the risk of stillbirth and death in the first year of life. *Am J Epidemiol* **155**: 305–312.

Koren G, Hutson J, Gareri J (2008) Novel methods for the detection of drug and alcohol exposure during pregnancy: implications for maternal and child health. *Clin Pharmacol Ther* **83**: 631–634.

Kuczkowski KM (2007) The effects of drug abuse on pregnancy. *Curr Opin Obstet Gynecol* **19**: 578–585.

Lipkus IM (2007) Numeric, verbal, and visual formats of conveying health risks: suggested best practices and future recommendations. *Med Decis Making* **27**: 696–713.

Lozano J, García-Algar O, Marchei E, et al. (2007) Prevalence of gestational exposure to cannabis in a Mediterranean city by meconium analysis. *Acta Paediatr* **96**: 1734–1737.

Makarechian N, Agro K, Devlin J, et al. (1998) Association between moderate alcohol consumption during pregnancy and spontaneous abortion, stillbirth and premature birth: a meta-analysis. *Can J Clin Pharmacol* **5**: 169–176.

National Institute on Drug Abuse (1996) *1992–93 National Pregnancy and Health Survey: Drug Use Among Women Delivering Livebirths*. Rockville, MD: US Department of Health and Human Services.

NIAAA (2004) *State of the Science Report on the Effects of Moderate Drinking*. Bethesda, MD: National Institute on Alcohol Abuse and Alcoholism.

Nicholas S, Kershaw C, Walker A (eds) (2007) *Crime in England and Wales 2006/07*. London: Home Office.

Olsen J, Basso O (1999) Re: Residual confounding. *Am J Epidemiol* **149**: 290.

Plant M, Plant M (2006) *Binge Britain: Alcohol and the National Response*. Oxford: Oxford University Press.

Polygenis D, Wharton S, Malmberg C, et al. (1998) Moderate alcohol consumption during pregnancy and the incidence of fetal malformations: a meta-analysis. *Neurotoxicol Teratol* **21**: 61–67.

Resnicow K, Vaughan R (2006) A chaotic view of behavior change: a quantum leap for health promotion. *Int J Behav Nutr Phys Act* **12**: 25.

Riley EP, McGee CL (2005) Fetal alcohol spectrum disorders: an overview with emphasis on changes in brain and behavior. *Exp Biol Med* **230**: 357–365.

Room R, Babor T, Rehm J (2005) Alcohol and public health. *Lancet* **365**: 519–530.

Rutter M (2007) Proceeding from observed correlation to causal inference: the use of natural experiments. *Perspect Psychol Sci* **2**: 377–395.

Schempf AH (2007) Illicit drug use and neonatal outcomes: a critical review. *Obstet Gynecol Surv* **62**: 749–757.

Shankaran S, Lester BM, Das A, et al. (2007) Impact of maternal substance use during pregnancy on childhood outcome. *Semin Fetal Neonatal Med* **12**: 143–150.

Sherwood RA, Keating J, Kavvadia V, et al. (1999) Substance misuse in early pregnancy and relationship to fetal outcome. *Eur J Pediatr* **158**: 488–492.

Singer LT, Minnes S, Short E, et al. (2004) Cognitive outcomes of preschool children with prenatal cocaine exposure. *JAMA* **291**: 2448–2456.

Singer LT, Nelson S, Short E, et al. (2008) Prenatal cocaine exposure: drug and environmental effects at 9 years. *J Pediatr* **153**: 105–111.

Smith GD (2008) Assessing intrauterine influences on offspring health outcomes: can epidemiological studies yield robust findings? *Basic Clin Pharmacol Toxicol* **102**: 245–256.

Smith GD, Ebrahim S (2002) Data dredging, bias, or confounding. *BMJ* **325**: 1437–1438.

Smith GD, Ebrahim S (2005) What can mendelian randomisation tell us about modifiable behavioural and environmental exposures? *BMJ* **330**: 1076–1079.

Smith L, Foxcroft D (2009) *Drinking in the UK: An Exploration of Trends*. York: Joseph Rowntree Foundation.

Stockwell T, Donath S, Cooper-Stanbury M, et al. (2004) Under-reporting of alcohol consumption in household surveys: a comparison of quantity-frequency, graduated-frequency and recent recall. *Addiction* **99**: 1024–1033.

Substance Abuse and Mental Health Services Administration (2007) *2006 National Survey on Drug Use and Health: Detailed Tables*. Rockville, MD: Office of Applied Studies.

United Nations Office on Drugs and Crime (2008) *2007 World Drug Report.* Vienna: United Nations Office on Drugs and Crime.

Verkerk PH (1992) The impact of alcohol misclassification on the relationship between alcohol and pregnancy outcome. *Int J Epidemiol* **21** Suppl 1: S33–S37.

Williamson S, Jackson L, Skeoch C, et al. (2006) Determination of the prevalence of drug misuse by meconium analysis. *Arch Dis Child Fetal Neonatal Ed* **91**: F291–F292.

Winklbaur B, Kopf N, Ebner N, et al. (2008) Treating pregnant women dependent on opioids is not the same as treating pregnancy and opioid dependence: a knowledge synthesis for better treatment for women and neonates. *Addiction* **103**: 1429–1440.

Zajac CS, Abel EL (1992) Animal models of prenatal alcohol exposure. *Int J Epidemiol* **21** Suppl 1: S24–S32.

3
NORMAL AND ABNORMAL EMBRYOGENESIS OF THE MAMMALIAN BRAIN

Kathleen K Sulik, Shonagh K O'Leary-Moore, Elizabeth A Godin and Scott E Parnell

This chapter provides a description of normal and abnormal embryonic development of the mammalian brain. For abnormal brain development, focus is on the consequences to the embryo of maternal alcohol use and maternal treatment with the anticonvulsant valproic acid.

Since much of the existing knowledge regarding both normal and abnormal human brain development has been extrapolated from studies of other species, data from animal experiments, in addition to those from humans, are presented. In the scientific literature, normal and abnormal development of the mouse brain is particularly well documented. This is largely because of the ability of mice to be manipulated both genetically and with environmental agents. Indeed, most of the experimental studies described in this chapter have employed this species.

The developmental stage-dependency of various neuroteratogenic outcomes is emphasized. Therefore, it is important to appreciate how human pregnancies are typically dated and staged and also how the stages of human development correlate to those in animal models. Figure 3.1 provides developmental timelines for both the mouse and humans. For humans, it is common for clinicians to use the last normal menstrual period as the reference point for the beginning of pregnancy. This adds approximately two weeks to the post-fertilization age of the conceptus. In this chapter, all human prenatal ages are referenced to the time of fertilization, not the last normal menstrual period, with the normal gestation period being 38 weeks.

It is generally accepted that major structural birth defects (malformations), including those of the brain, are the result of environmental insult or genetic damage occurring during the period of embryogenesis. The embryonic period comprises weeks 3 through 8 of human development. The fetal period follows, ending at birth. With human pregnancy commonly being divided into trimesters, each of approximately 12 weeks, the first trimester includes both the embryonic period and the early fetal period. As shown in Figure 3.1, in the mouse the embryonic period extends through approximately the 13th day of a 20-day gestation period. At birth, mice are relatively immature, being roughly equivalent in their development to mid-second trimester humans. The stages of development that correspond to the last half

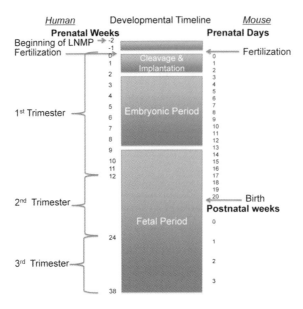

Fig. 3.1. Comparison of human prenatal and mouse developmental timelines illustrates that mice, which have a 20-day gestation period, are born at stages that occur during the human second trimester. Also shown is that the human embryonic period encompasses the majority, but not all, of the first trimester. The human fetal period extends from the ninth week until term (38 weeks).

of the second trimester and the third trimester in humans occur after birth in mice. Therefore, many studies of environmental teratogens that employ rodents (especially those studies investigating functional deficits that occur in the absence of overt malformations) are conducted postnatally. In this chapter, neuroteratogenic insult occurring during the period of embryogenesis is emphasized. For consideration of a broader period of insult, the reader is directed to recent publications by others (e.g. Miller 2006, Young and Olney 2006, Thompson et al. 2009). For additional description and illustration of early mammalian embryogenesis and mouse/human comparisons, the following websites are useful: http://embryology.med.unsw.edu.au, http://www.med.unc.edu/embryo_images and http://www.translatingtime.net.

Morphogenesis of the normal mammalian brain
During the first two weeks following fertilization in humans, the cells of the embryo divide and differentiate into those that will form the embryo proper and those that will contribute to its supporting tissues (non-maternal portions of the placenta). By the end of the second week, the cells of the embryo proper have become arranged as a bilayered disc. The dorsal or upper layer of the disc includes those cells that will eventually form the central nervous system (CNS; brain and spinal cord).

As the embryo enters its third week, it becomes possible to identify its rostral (head) and caudal (tail) ends, as well as its right and left sides. This is due to the formation of a

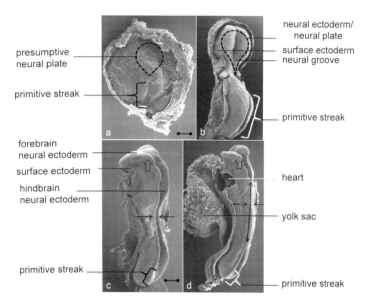

Fig. 3.2. Scanning electron micrographs of human embryos at 17 (a), 19 (b), 21 (c) and 22 (d) days post-fertilization illustrate changes in form that allow initial identification of the developing central nervous system. The neural plate [dashed area in (a) and (b)] becomes the brain and spinal cord. Folding of the neural plate brings the neural folds together dorsally, to form the neural tube. The first site of neural fold union [arrows in (c)] occurs near the brain/spinal cord junction. Fusion proceeds in both a rostral and caudal direction [double-headed arrow in (d)]. The open arrows in (c) and (d) indicate the position of the midbrain (mesencephalic) neural folds. Bar in (a) = 0.05 mm; bar in (c) = 0.1 mm.

midline groove called the primitive streak, which occupies the caudal half of the embryo's dorsal midline (Fig. 3.2a). During the third week, the embryonic disc acquires a middle layer, and the three definitive germ layers – ectoderm, mesoderm and endoderm – can be identified. It is the ectoderm (the dorsal germ layer) from which the CNS develops. In Figure 3.2a, which is a scanning electron micrograph of the dorsal (ectodermal) side of a mid-third week human embryo, the developing brain and spinal cord cannot yet be distinguished. However, fate mapping (i.e. tracing the developmental history of cells) and gene expression studies in experimental animals show that it is the ectoderm located rostral to the primitive streak that will form the CNS. This is the neuroectoderm, as opposed to other (surface) ectodermal cells that are located more peripherally as well as caudally. At this early primitive streak stage of development, the human embryo is approximately 0.5mm in diameter. By the end of the third week, the embryo has elongated considerably in the rostro-caudal direction. At this time, the developing brain is evidenced as bilateral elevations on each side of a median neural groove (Fig. 3.2b). These neuroectodermal elevations are termed the neural plate.

As human embryogenesis continues into the fourth week, the neural groove deepens as the right and left halves of the neural plate (neural folds) bend toward each other (Fig. 3.2c). Approximation and union of the neural folds (i.e. neural tube closure) first occur very

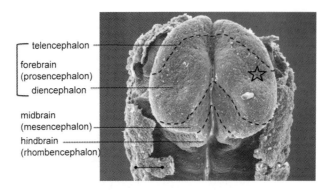

telencephalon
forebrain
(prosencephalon)
diencephalon
midbrain
(mesencephalon)
hindbrain
(rhombencephalon)

Fig. 3.3. Illustrated in a scanning electron micrograph of the rostral neural folds of the 21-day human embryo shown in Figure 3.2c are the regions that comprise the developing forebrain (prosencephalon; telencephalon plus diencephalon), midbrain (mesencephalon), and hindbrain (rhombencephalon). The optic sulcus (developing eye) on the embryo's right side is indicated by a star. Bar = 0.1 mm.

close to the junction of the developing brain and spinal cord, and then extend both rostrally and caudally (Fig. 3.2d). By the time that neural tube closure begins, regional variations in the shape and size of the portion of the neural folds that will form the brain are evident. Thus, the future forebrain (prosencephalon), midbrain (mesencephalon) and hindbrain (rhombencephalon) can be distinguished morphologically. In addition to identification of these three main subdivisions of the brain, at the time that the neural tube begins to close, it is possible to define the tissues that will become the telencephalic and the diencephalic portions of the forebrain (Fig. 3.3). The telencephalon (which will become the cerebrum) is most rostrally positioned and, at this stage of development, comprises relatively little tissue compared with the rest of the developing brain. The adjacent diencephalon (portions of which will form the thalamus and hypothalamus) is characterized by the presence of the optic primordia.

Closure of the rostral (cranial) portion of the neural tube is complete by the 25th to 26th day of human development, i.e. before the end of the fourth week. As illustrated in Figure 3.4, the rostral progression of closure through the hindbrain and midbrain region is accompanied by a change in orientation (from eversion to inversion) of the forebrain neural folds, allowing their median apposition. Closure of the diencephalic portion of the forebrain continues to progress rostrally as the growth of the telencephalic folds advances from the opposite direction. The site of final closure of the cranial neural folds (anterior neuropore) appears to approximate the junction of the telencephalon and diencephalon (Fig. 3.5), and, with reference to the developing face, is in the midline just below the level of the developing eyes.

Dorsal (Fig. 3.4a,c) and side views (Figs. 3.4b,d and 3.5b) of the cranial end of 24- and 25-day embryos illustrate the relationship between the major brain segments and the developing face and neck. The tissue surrounding the forebrain is termed the frontonasal prominence. Its major derivatives are the tissues of the upper midface, i.e. the nose, median aspect of the upper lip (philtrum), the (alveolar) ridge in which the upper incisors form,

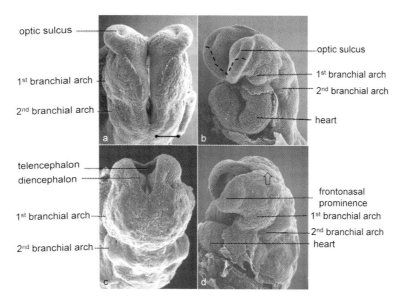

Fig. 3.4. Progression of rostral (cranial) neural tube closure is illustrated in scanning electron micrographs of human embryos at 24 (a,b) and 25 days (c,d) of development. As shown in the dorsal view of the 24 day embryo, the neural tube remains open rostral to the level of the middle of the hindbrain (corresponding to the level of the second branchial arch). As closure progresses toward the forebrain, the rostral-most neural folds change from an everted [shown in (b)] to an inverted [shown in (d)] conformation. The open arrow in (d) indicates the position of the midbrain. Bar in (a) = 0.1 mm.

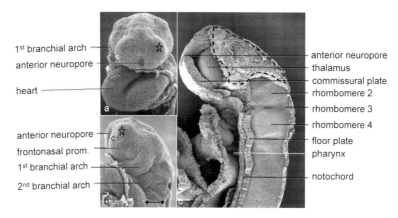

Fig. 3.5. Frontal (a) and lateral (b) views of an embryo just prior to complete closure of the anterior neuropore (at 25 days), along with a midsagittal view of an embryo at this same developmental stage (c). In (c), the ventricular surface of the forebrain and hindbrain is clearly seen, while that for the midbrain is obscured by tissue that was not removed (dashed line). The first branchial arch, from which the lower jaw will form, is shown in (a) and (b) and is at the level of rhombomere 2, while the second branchial arch [shown in (b)] is at the level of rhombomere 4. The position of the developing eye is indicated with a star. Bar in (b) = 0.1 mm.

27

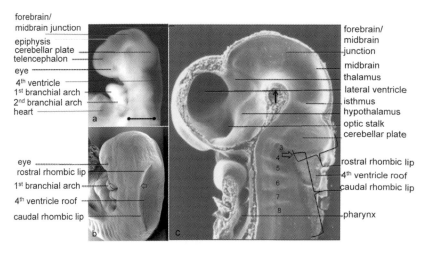

forebrain/
midbrain junction

epiphysis
cerebellar plate
telencephalon
eye
4th ventricle
1st branchial arch
2nd branchial arch
heart

a

eye
rostral rhombic lip
1st branchial arch
4th ventricle roof
caudal rhombic lip

b

c

forebrain/
midbrain
junction

midbrain
thalamus
lateral ventricle
isthmus
hypothalamus
optic stalk
cerebellar plate

rostral rhombic lip
4th ventricle roof
caudal rhombic lip

pharynx

Fig. 3.6. Light microscopic (a) and scanning electron microscopic (b) images of a human day 32 embryo illustrate the features of the developing face and brain. Particularly notable is the thin roof of the fourth ventricle, which appears somewhat collapsed in (b). In (c), a midsagittal cut through the head of a comparably staged mouse embryo shows the ventricular surface of each of the brain segments. The open arrow indicates the junction of the rostral and caudal rhombic lip. The solid arrow indicates the site of the mesencephalic (midbrain) flexure. Bar in (a) = 1 mm.

and the antero-median aspect of the hard palate (the primary palate). The first and second branchial arches, which will contribute to the lower jaw, ear and upper neck region, are evident bilaterally and are at the level of the hindbrain. As further described below, recognition of the relationship between the early development of the brain and the face aids in understanding the basis for their frequent, concurrent insult.

A midsagittal cut (Fig. 3.5c) through the head and neck of an embryo that is at the final stages of anterior neuropore closure (25th day) shows the central cavity or ventricular space and interior walls of the neural tube. At this time, the telencephalic portion of the forebrain remains relatively small. Its midline cell population is termed the commissural plate and is that region which is later traversed by fibres of the corpus callosum as they pass between the two cerebral hemispheres. Also evident are the prominent thalamic portion of the diencephalon and the segments of the hindbrain, i.e. the rhombomeres. The first two rhombomeres comprise the metencephalic portion of the hindbrain (that which will form the pons and cerebellum). This portion of the hindbrain is in register with the first branchial arch. The more caudal rhombomeres comprise the myelencephalon (the progenitor of the medulla oblongata). Rhombomere 4, which is in register with the second branchial arch, is particularly prominent at this time. By the end of the fourth week, the caudal-most rhombomeres (5–8) become evident.

As illustrated in Figure 3.6 (a,b), by the fifth week of human development the ventricles have expanded considerably. Expansion of the lateral ventricles is accompanied by dorsolateral expansion of the cerebral hemispheres, while expansion of the fourth ventricle is

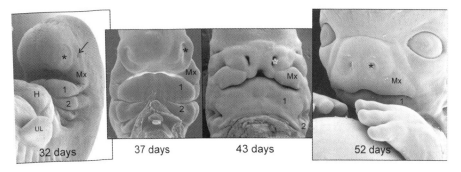

Fig. 3.7. Scanning electron micrographs illustrate facial morphogenesis from 32 to 52 days of human development. Notable is a relative change in position of the developing nostrils (asterisk) and eyes (arrow) from the lateral to the anterior (ventral) aspect of the head. As development proceeds, the nostrils deepen, with tissues medial to them contributing to the nasal tip and the upper lip. Also contributing to the upper lip are the bilateral maxillary prominences (Mx). The lower jaw and part of the ear are derived from the first branchial arch (1), while the second arch (2) contributes to part of the ear and the upper (hyoid) portion of the neck. H = heart; UL = upper limb.

accompanied by thinning of the rhombencephalic roof plate. The lateral-most extension of this rhomboid-shaped roof plate is at the level of the junction between the first and second branchial arches. At this stage, the morphology of the human brain is remarkably similar to that of a day 10 mouse embryo (Fig. 3.6c). Particularly notable are the following: the thalamic and hypothalamic regions of the diencephalon; clear demarcation of the forebrain/midbrain (diencephalic/mesencephalic) junction at the apex of the mesencephalic flexure; demarcation of the junction of the midbrain and rhombencepahlon by the isthmus; formation of the cerebellar plate which is bounded at its junction with the roof of the fourth ventricle by the rostral rhombic lip; and association of the caudal rhombic lip with the segments of the hindbrain that comprise the myelencephalon. Cellular derivatives of the rhombic lip are highly migratory, typically streaming tangentially, contributing to the cerebellum and forming the dentate, pontine and inferior olivary nuclei.

As development progresses from early in the fifth week toward the end of the embryonic period, the face acquires a recognizably human character (Fig. 3.7). This occurs as the developing nostrils, which are initially evident on the lateral aspects of the frontonasal prominence, assume a relatively more medial position. Olfactory nerves, which form from the ectoderm lining the nostrils, extend toward the brain, a process required for formation of the olfactory bulbs. Tissue located medial to the nostrils contributes to the nasal tip and the centre (philtrum) of the upper lip. Forming the more lateral aspects of the upper lip are bilateral maxillary prominences. The latter also form the majority of the upper jaw and the secondary palate. As previously noted, the lower jaw is derived from the first branchial arch. This arch, along with the second, forms the external ear and the bones of the middle ear. The second arch also forms the upper (hyoid) portion of the neck. With eyelid formation just beginning, the eyes remain open for a few more weeks. Later, the eyelids will fuse and remain so throughout the second trimester.

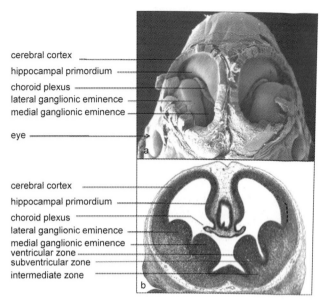

cerebral cortex
hippocampal primordium
choroid plexus
lateral ganglionic eminence
medial ganglionic eminence

eye

cerebral cortex
hippocampal primordium
choroid plexus
lateral ganglionic eminence
medial ganglionic eminence
ventricular zone
subventricular zone
intermediate zone

Fig. 3.8. Removal of the lateral walls of the cerebral cortex of a gestational day 13 mouse embryo allows visualization of the ventricular surface of the medial wall and basal aspect of each hemisphere (a). Prominent features of the medial walls are the hippocampal primordium and choroid plexus, and in the basal forebrain are the ganglionic eminences. These structures are also notable in a histological section made in the frontal plane through the forebrain (b). The dashed line in (b) indicates the margin between the ventricular zone and the preplate of the cerebral cortex.

In a mouse embryo, at a stage comparable to that of a 7-week human fetus, removal of the tissue above the eyes, including the lateral walls of the cerebral hemispheres, allows examination of the interior of the telencephalon (Fig. 3.8a). As also seen in a histological section (Fig. 3.8b), apparent at this time are the hippocampal primordia, which comprise the medial walls of the cerebral hemispheres. Additionally, at the ventral aspect of the cerebrum are bilateral elevations termed ganglionic eminences that will form the corpus striatum (globus pallidus, putamen, caudate nucleus) and amygdaloid nuclei. The ventricular zone (germinal epithelium) of the ganglionic eminences gives rise to cells that become interneurons and undergo tangential migration into the olfactory bulb, cerebral cortex and hippocampus (Wonders and Anderson 2006). The developing cerebral cortex also has a ventricular zone. At this stage in development, the layer adjacent to the ventricular zone is termed the primordial plexiform layer (preplate). Bystron et al. (2006) report that the first cells residing in the primordial plexiform layer of the human cortex are present as early as week 5, having emigrated from the medial and lateral ganglionic eminences. Neurons that arise in the cortical ventricular zone migrate radially, forming the cortical plate. The cortical plate is first evident late in the seventh to early in the eighth week (Bystron et al. 2008, O'Rahilly and Muller 2008) and is the progenitor of layers 2–6 of the cerebral cortex.

Neuronal populations of the cerebellum are also derived from a combination of

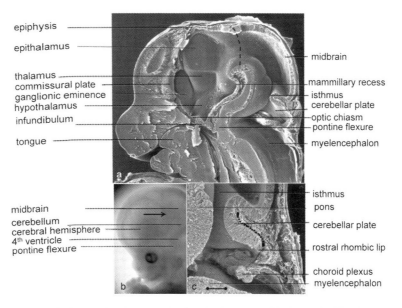

epiphysis

epithalamus

midbrain

thalamus

commissural plate

ganglionic eminence

hypothalamus

infundibulum

mammillary recess

isthmus

cerebellar plate

optic chiasm

pontine flexure

tongue

myelencephalon

a

midbrain

cerebellum

cerebral hemisphere

4th ventricle

pontine flexure

isthmus

pons

cerebellar plate

rostral rhombic lip

choroid plexus

myelencephalon

b

c

Fig. 3.9. At early fetal stages in the mouse (a,c), as in the human (b), the cerebral hemispheres extend caudally only as far as the midbrain (the arrow in b indicates the border between these two brain regions; the dashed line in a indicates the forebrain/midbrain junction). A midsagittal view (a) illustrates subsegments of the diencephalon, the large ventricular space in the midbrain, and the cerebellar plate and choroid plexus (also shown at higher magnification in c) extending into the space of the fourth ventricle. The dotted line along the dorsal aspect of the cerebellar plate indicates the path of migration from the rhombic lip of cells that will form the external germinal layer of the cerebellum. Bar in (c) = 0.1 mm.

tangentially and radially migrating cells. The former arise from the rostral rhombic lip, migrate subpially, and by the beginning of the fetal period form the external germinal layer of the cerebellar plate (Fig. 3.9c). The granule cells of the cerebellum arise from this layer. As in the cerebral cortex, cells in the ventricular layer of the cerebellar plate undergo radial migration. They give rise to the deep cerebellar nuclei as well as Purkinje cells. It is estimated that the peak of neurogenesis for these radially migrating populations occurs during the seventh prenatal week in humans.

As illustrated in Figure 3.9, by the end of the embryonic period (end of the human eighth week; 14th gestational day in mice) a prominent pontine flexure distinguishes two major subdivisions of the hindbrain, the more rostrally positioned metencephalon and the more caudally positioned myelencephalon. Extending from the rhombencephalic roof plate, the choroid plexus has become a significant feature within the fourth ventricle. At this time, the ventricular space within the midbrain remains relatively large. While the cerebral hemispheres are expanding posteriorly, they have not yet extended beyond the forebrain/midbrain junction.

Early in the human fetal period (by week 13) the cerebral hemispheres expand to cover the midbrain, with resulting close approximation of the occipital portion of the cerebrum

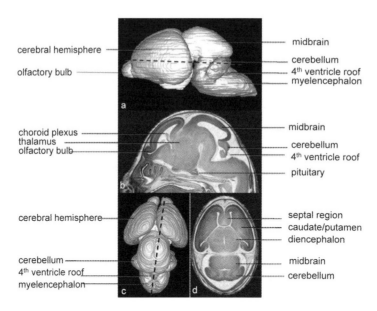

cerebral hemisphere —

olfactory bulb —

— midbrain

— cerebellum

— 4th ventricle roof

— myelencephalon

a

choroid plexus —

thalamus —

olfactory bulb —

— midbrain

— cerebellum

— 4th ventricle roof

— pituitary

b

cerebral hemisphere —

cerebellum —

4th ventricle roof —

myelencephalon —

— septal region

— caudate/putamen

— diencephalon

— midbrain

— cerebellum

c

d

Fig. 3.10. Individual high-resolution magnetic resonance images (b,d), as well as 3D reconstructions made from a series of these scans (a,c) illustrate the morphology of the fetal mouse brain. As compared with the human brain, the olfactory bulbs are relatively large and extend rostral to the cerebral cortex (a). Scans made in sagittal [(b); location indicated by dotted line in (c)] and horizontal planes [(d); location indicated by dotted line in (a)] illustrate the internal features of the brain.

with the cerebellum. At this period of development in the mouse, as shown in a reconstructed 17th gestational day (early fetal) mouse brain (Fig. 3.10), the midbrain remains visible between the cerebral hemispheres and cerebellum. In the mouse, this remains the case throughout adulthood. Other differences between mouse and human brain morphology that become apparent at early fetal stages are the relatively large size of the olfactory bulbs in the former, and the presence of a lateral sulcus bounded by the temporal and frontal lobes of the cortex in the latter. Continued cerebral cortical growth results in the formation of gyri by approximately the middle of human gestation, i.e. by approximately one-third of the way through the fetal period. In the mouse, the cerebral cortex remains smooth, even in adulthood.

Teratogen-induced brain dysmorphogenesis

As early as the third week of human gestation, when the embryo is at the primitive streak stage (i.e. prior to the appearance of morphologically identifiable brain structures, corresponding to gestational day 7 in the mouse), the CNS is vulnerable to teratogenic insult. Among the agents that are known to cause brain defects following maternal intake at this time in development in animal models are retinoic acid, cholesterol biosynthesis inhibitors and alcohol (Shenefelt 1972, Sulik and Johnston 1982, Webster et al. 1983, Sulik 1984, Schambra et al. 1990, Sulik et al. 1995, Dehart et al. 1997, Lanoue et al. 1997). Of these,

32

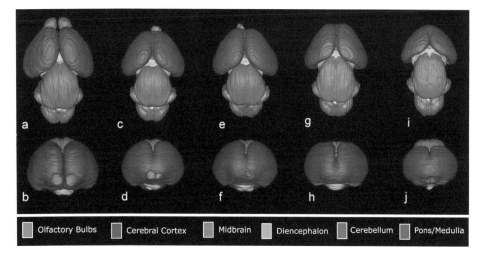

| Olfactory Bulbs | Cerebral Cortex | Midbrain | Diencephalon | Cerebellum | Pons/Medulla |

Fig. 3.11. Colour-coded magnetic resonance imaging reconstructions of control (a,b) and alcohol-exposed brains (c–j) illustrate increasing degrees of severity of holoprosencephaly in the latter. As viewed from the dorsal side (a,c,e,g,i), it is apparent that the major effect of alcohol-exposure is on the forebrain. Frontal views of the same brains (b,d,f,h,j) illustrate varying degrees of rostral union of the cerebral hemispheres and olfactory bulb deficiency or absence in the affected fetal brains. (Modified by permission from Godin et al. 2010.) For colour version of this figure, see plate section at end of book.

alcohol is undoubtedly the most common teratogen to which human pregnancies are exposed. Shown in Figure 3.11 are three-dimensional brain reconstructions from normal and abnormal fetal mice, the latter of which were exposed to high doses of alcohol for a short period of time when they were at the early primitive streak stage of development. The variability in degree of effect can be accounted for, in part, by slightly varying stages of development during which the alcohol exposure occurred. The defects shown fall within the severe end of a spectrum termed holoprosencephaly. Milder manifestations of this same spectrum are also commonly induced by teratogen exposure at this early stage of development.

In addition to environmental agents, mutation in a number of different genes that are required for normal neural plate morphogenesis can yield holoprosencephaly in humans and other species (Muenke and Beachy 2000, Cohen 2006, Schachter and Krauss 2008). Notably, holoprosencephaly represents the most common congenital birth defect of the human forebrain, occurring in 1 in 250 conceptuses. However, very few affected individuals survive to term, resulting in a holoprosencephaly incidence of approximately 1 in 12 000 live births (Croen et al. 1996, Rasmussen et al. 1996). The holoprosencephaly spectrum ranges from severe alobar forms (Fig. 3.11i,j) in which the cerebral hemispheres lack separation by an interhemispheric fissure, the thalami and corpora striata are united in the midline, and the olfactory tracts and bulbs and corpus callosum are missing; to intermediate semilobar forms (Fig. 3.11c,d) in which the cerebral hemispheres are separate caudally and are united rostrally, accompanied by median rostral forebrain deficiencies; to milder lobar forms in which there are is a complete interhemispheric fissure, and in which the olfactory

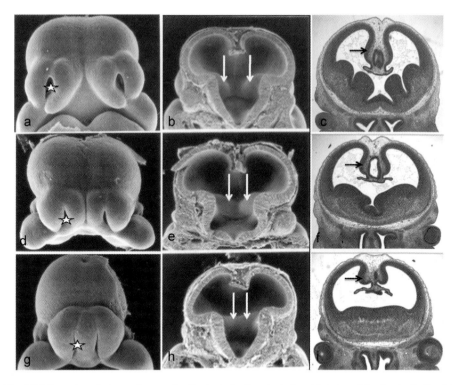

Fig. 3.12. Scanning electron micrographs illustrate the face (a,d,g) and interior of the forebrain (b,e,h) of control (a,b) and alcohol-exposed (d–h) GD11 mouse embryos. Varying degrees of median facial deficiency [evidenced by closely-spaced nostrils (star)] is accompanied by similar reduction in the forebrain [evidenced by variable degrees of union of the ganglionic eminences (white arrows), associated with loss of the septal region]. This is also notable in histological sections of control (c) and alcohol-exposed (f,i) GD13 mouse embryos. Additionally, in the alcohol-exposed embryos, reduction in the size of the hippocampus is apparent (black arrows).

tracts and bulbs as well as the corpus callosum may be absent or hypoplastic (Demyer and Zeman 1963, Cohen 2006). At the less severe end of the holoprosencephaly spectrum, affected individuals may have mild or moderate learning disability and may have sufficient cognitive ability to live freely in society.

The graded series of brain defects in the holoprosencephaly spectrum are accompanied by median upper facial deficiencies. Demyer et al. (1964) noted that in holoprosencephaly, frequently (though not always) the face 'predicts' the brain – i.e. that the severity of craniofacial and brain dysmorphology are often directly correlated. Study of the genesis of alcohol-induced holoprosencephaly in mice has confirmed this premise (Sulik and Johnston 1982). Maternal ethanol exposure limited to the seventh day of pregnancy in mice can result in variable degrees of tissue deficiency concurrently involving the frontonasal prominence/upper midface and brain. As in the developing human face (Fig. 3.7), in normal mouse embryos the nostrils are initially widely spaced (Fig. 3.12a). By day 11–12 of gestation in the mouse,

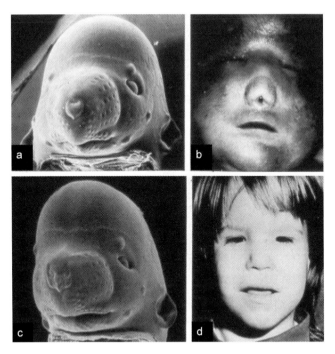

Fig. 3.13. Scanning electron micrographs of fetal mice (a,c) illustrate varying degrees of severity of alcohol-induced facial abnormality, defects that can be correlated to humans with a severe form of holo-prosencephaly (b), and fetal alcohol syndrome (d). (Modified by permission from Sulik et al. 1982.)

following alcohol insult at early primitive streak stages (gestational day 7) it is apparent that the nostrils of some affected embryos are too closely approximated (Fig. 3.12d,e). In these individuals, the concurrent loss of median forebrain tissue is evidenced by midline approximation or union of the ganglionic eminences (indicated by white arrows in Fig. 3.12e,h). In mice, as in humans with holoprosencephaly, the median tissue deficiency can be severe enough that the eyes are closely positioned (hypoteloric) to the point of being united (syn-ophthalmic). Similarly, the midline tissue deficiency may yield a nose that forms with no tissue between the nostrils, resulting in a single central opening (Fig. 3.13a,b). The upper lip, lacking its medial (philtral) component, is smooth and has a narrow vermilion border. In less severely affected individuals, while the nostrils remain separate, the nose is small and the upper lip, though more subtly dysmorphic, still shows evidence of philtral deficiency (Fig. 3.13c,d). This is expanded on in later chapters. In addition to being commonly noted in individuals with holoprosencephaly, the latter facial phenotype has also been reported to result from ethanol exposure on days 19 and 20 of gestation in non-human primates (corres-ponding to the primitive streak stage) (Astley et al. 1999), and is considered characteristic of fetal alcohol syndrome (FAS).

In addition to facial phenotypes that are common to both FAS and holoprosencephaly, brain abnormalities in the holoprosencephaly spectrum have been documented in humans

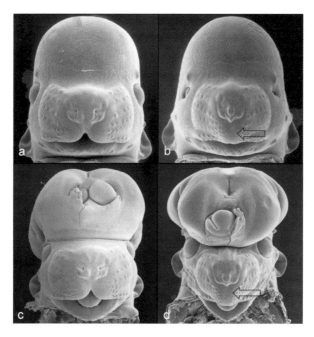

Fig. 3.14. Illustrated are control (a) and alcohol-exposed (b–d) mouse fetuses having normal (a,c) and alcohol-induced abnormal facies (b,d). The latter are characterized by a small nose and long upper lip (open arrowhead). Animals with either normal or abnormal facies may present with exencephaly (c,d).

with FAS. In the first FAS autopsy case report, Jones and Smith (1975) described corpus callosum agenesis. Other autopsies revealed olfactory bulb and tract deficiencies and pituitary abnormalities (Peiffer et al. 1979, Majewski 1981). The advent of clinical magnetic resonance imaging has made in vivo structural analyses of the brains of those with defects resulting from prenatal alcohol exposure possible. With identification of the corpus callosum as being deficient in living individuals with FAS (Mattson et al. 1992, Johnson et al. 1996, Swayze et al. 1997), this region of the brain has recently been the focus of detailed analyses (Bookstein et al. 2001; Sowell et al. 2001, 2008; Ma et al. 2005; Wozniak et al. 2006; Lebel et al. 2008; Fryer et al. 2009). While it is recognized that median forebrain deficiencies, especially those involving the corpus callosum, can result from ethanol insult at developmental stages other than early primitive streak stages, a combination of this type of brain defect and the typical FAS face is expected to result only from insult that occurs very early in embryonic development.

Besides the defects described above, early alcohol exposure in mice (gestational day 7 or 8; equivalent to human week 3–4) can cause a variety of other structural abnormalities of the face and brain. The facial defects include clefts (median or lateral cleft lip as well as median cleft face and cleft palate) and a small lower jaw (micrognathia) (Sulik et al. 1988, Kotch and Sulik 1992a, Godin et al. 2010). Defects of the brain include cortical and ventricular heterotopias (Jones and Smith 1975, Clarren et al. 1978, Majewski 1981, Sulik

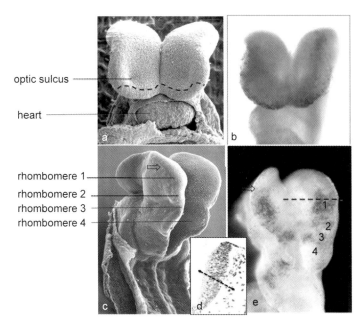

optic sulcus

heart

rhombomere 1
rhombomere 2
rhombomere 3
rhombomere 4

Fig. 3.15. Prenatal alcohol exposure results in excessive cell death (apoptosis) in selected cell populations as shown in gestational day 8 mouse embryos. This is evidenced by stain uptake in (b) and (e) (darkly stained cells are undergoing cell death). The telencephalon [that area rostral to the dashed line in (a)] is particularly sensitive (b), as is the alar portion of rhombomeres 1–3 (c–e). The open arrows in (c) and (e) indicate the midbrain/hindbrain junction. The dashed line in (e) indicates the plane of section for (d). In (d), the dashed line indicates the division between the apoptosis-prone alar plate and the death-free basal plate.

1984, Komatsu et al. 2001, Sakata-Haga et al. 2004, O'Leary Moore et al. 2009, Godin et al. 2010), hippocampal and cerebellar deficiencies (Schambra et al. 1990, Parnell et al. 2009), ventricular enlargement (Parnell et al. 2009), and neural tube closure defects (Fig. 3.14) (Sulik et al. 1988, Kotch and Sulik 1992a). In contrast to fetuses with normal neural tube closure, maternal alcohol administration on gestational day 7 or 8 in mice can cause the anterior neuropore to fail to close, resulting in a condition termed exencephaly. Subsequent deterioration of the abnormally exposed brain tissue leads to the neural tube defect termed anencephaly. Some affected individuals present with concurrent facial abnormalities involving the upper midface and lower jaw. The pathogenesis involved in the alcohol-induced neural tube closure failure and the accompanying upper midfacial abnormalities includes excessive cell death in cell populations at the periphery of the neural plate (Fig. 3.15b) (Sulik et al. 1988, Kotch and Sulik 1992a, Sulik and Sadler 1993).

Another human teratogen that causes neural tube defects, the pathogenesis of which has been shown in animal models to include excessive cell death, is valproic acid (Nau et al. 1991, Sulik and Sadler 1993, Nau 1994). This anticonvulsant is associated with both anencephaly and spina bifida, as well as with other structural anomalies, and is now considered to have the highest teratogenic potential of all antiepileptic agents (reviewed by Ornoy

2006). Of interest, children with 'valproate syndrome' present with facial dysmorphism manifested by midfacial hypoplasia, a short nose, a thin upper lip and micrognathia, as in FAS. Work regarding valproate teratogenesis in rodent models has shown that in addition to neural tube defects, insult during embryogenesis yields hindbrain defects. More specifically, research conducted by Rodier and her coworkers (Rodier et al. 1997, Ingram et al. 2000) has shown that valproic acid administered to pregnant rats near the time of neural tube closure in the pups yields shortening of the brainstem accompanied by loss of motor neurons, along with cerebellar deficiencies. These authors have pointed out commonalities in the hindbrain defects in this model and those seen in autistic individuals (Rodier et al. 1996).

Similar to prenatal valproic acid exposure, maternal alcohol administration on the eighth day of pregnancy in mice adversely affects the hindbrain (Kotch and Sulik 1992b, Dunty et al. 2002, Parnell et al. 2009). This is evidenced by excessive cell death in selected hindbrain cell populations (Fig. 3.15e), disrupted rhombomere development, aberrant hindbrain-associated cranial nerves, and a small cerebellum. Importantly, excessive cell death is also a significant pathogenic feature of later alcohol exposures. This has been well demonstrated by Olney and coworkers in perinatal rodents (reviewed by Olney et al. 2000). These investigators have shown that in infant animals (corresponding to late fetal stages in humans), a rise in blood ethanol to a level in the region of 50 mg/dL for a duration of 30–45 minutes is sufficient to trigger excessive neuronal cell death (Young and Olney 2006). This group has also recently shown that the ethanol-induced cell death can be prevented with lithium co-administration (Young et al. 2008).

In addition to lithium, other compounds have also been shown, in experiments employing animal models, to be capable of reducing ethanol's teratogenesis. Included are antioxidants (Cohen-Kerem and Koren 2003, Chen et al. 2004, Dong et al. 2008), choline (Thomas et al. 2000, 2004, 2007; Ryan et al. 2008), and cholesterol (Li et al. 2007). With regard to the last of these, it is noteworthy that, as with ethanol exposure, cholesterol deficiency in mouse embryos leads to excessive cell death in cells of the hindbrain alar plate (Homanics et al. 1995, Dehart et al. 1997). Outcomes that appear to be directly related to this excessive cell death are narrowing of the isthmus of the cerebral aqueduct and subsequent hydrocephalus (Fig. 3.16b).

Along with studies of pathogenesis and structural defects that result from teratogen exposure in animal models, there are numerous reports of long-term behavioural consequences (Driscoll et al. 1990, Riley 1990, Riley and McGee 2005, Guerri et al. 2009). However, relatively few behavioural studies have specifically focused on the impact of exposures restricted to early gestation. Noteworthy findings from these few existing studies include the observation that alcohol exposure limited to gestational day 8 in the rat (during early primitive streak stages) causes delays in surface righting and suckling when tested during the neonatal period. This study also showed persistence into periadolescence of functional damage following early prenatal insult (Vigliecca et al. 1986). Also, with alcohol exposure limited to early primitive streak stages, studies of rats (Minetti et al. 1996) as well as of mice (Dumas and Rabe 1994) have illustrated long-term deficits in the retention of previously learned tasks. Though the duration of early prenatal alcohol exposure is longer than in the previously mentioned rodent studies, studies employing non-human primates (rhesus

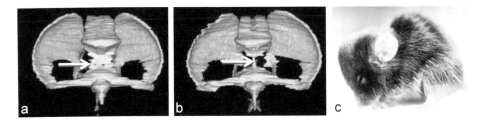

Fig. 3.16. Reconstructed magnetic resonance images of control (a) and alcohol-affected (b) ventricles, as seen in a posterior view, illustrate narrowing of the aqueductal isthmus (arrow) in the latter. Aqueductal stenosis is a causal basis for hydrocephaly, the condition evidenced by the enlarged head in the mouse in (c). Yellow = lateral ventricles; blue = mesencephalic (cerebral aqueduct) and fourth ventricle; orange = third ventricle. For colour version of this figure, see plate section at end of book.

monkeys) have shown that exposure to moderate alcohol levels at times spanning the first trimester of pregnancy (days 0 through 50 of a 164-day gestation period) are related to lower scores on neurobehavioural tests (specifically, orientation and motor maturity scores) in infants. The behavioural defects apparent among offspring that were exposed to alcohol at early gestational stages did not differ from those of others that had late or continuous pre-natal exposure (Schneider et al. 2001). In another study employing non-human primates (pigtail macaques), Clarren et al. (1992) demonstrated that a once-a-week binge ethanol exposure from weeks 1 to 6 in pregnancy was as detrimental as drinking for the entire 24-week gestational period. Findings included marked hyperactivity during free play in animals exposed from weeks 1 to 6 of gestation. Additional studies directed toward further defining developmental stage-dependent behavioural endpoints and the associated changes in the structure of the brain that result from alcohol insult as well as from other teratogenic agents are needed. It is expected that, just as various environmental exposures or genetic abnormalities acting at specific stages in development can yield similar structural birth defects, behavioural abnormalities will also be overlapping for a number of neuroteratogens.

While diagnostic challenges can result from the fact that a variety of different teratogens and also genetic abnormalities can yield similar developmental endpoints, these similarities can be helpful in determining teratogenic mechanisms, defining critical developmental periods, and developing treatment and prevention strategies. For example, as previously noted, in addition to the teratogens mentioned above, the holoprosencephaly spectrum is recognized to result from mutations in several different genes (reviewed by Cohen 2006). Among these is sonic hedgehog (*Shh*), as well as some of the downstream genes in the Shh signalling pathway. Even at very early developmental stages (as early as the third week in the human), proper Shh signalling is required for normal brain development. Importantly, recent studies have shown that the signalling cascade is dependent upon modification by cholesterol of the *Shh*-encoded protein; ethanol affects Shh signalling (Ahlgren et al. 2002, Aoto et al. 2008, Loucks and Ahlgren 2009), and, in animal models, this effect can be diminished with cholesterol supplementation (Li et al. 2007). This exemplifies establishment of the biological basis for a potential nutritional intervention that may reduce alcohol teratogenesis in humans. While molecular mechanism(s) through which ethanol affects Shh signalling remain to be identified, it is noteworthy that besides its morphogenic activity, Shh protein is recognized as a survival factor (e.g. Cai et al. 2008, Mille et al. 2009). Of interest will be studies directed at determining whether ethanol-mediated reduction in this survival factor may underlie excessive apoptotic cell death and subsequent birth defects.

Conclusion

It is clear that, from its earliest stages (stages occurring prior to the time that human pregnancies are typically recognized), the developing brain is sensitive to teratogenic insult. In addition to identification of critical developmental periods, research employing animal models has advanced our knowledge of the cellular mechanisms and subsequent pathology associated with human neuroteratogens. Appreciation of these findings, not only by the research community but also by physicians and other health advisors, parents and future parents, is key to the prevention of birth defects.

REFERENCES

Ahlgren SC, Thakur V, Bronner-Fraser M (2002) Sonic hedgehog rescues cranial neural crest from cell death induced by ethanol exposure. *Proc Natl Acad Sci U S A* **99**: 10476–10481.

Aoto K, Shikata Y, Higashiyama D, et al. (2008) Fetal ethanol exposure activates protein kinase A and impairs SHH expression in prechordal mesendoderm cells in the pathogenesis of holoprosencephaly. *Birth Defects Res A Clin Mol Teratol* **82**: 224–231.

Astley SJ, Magnuson SI, Omnell LM, Clarren SK (1999) Fetal alcohol syndrome: changes in craniofacial form with age, cognition, and timing of ethanol exposure in the macaque. *Teratology* **59**: 163–172.

Bookstein FL, Sampson PD, Streissguth AP, Connor PD (2001) Geometric morphometrics of corpus callosum and subcortical structures in the fetal-alcohol-affected brain. *Teratology* **64**: 4–32.

Bystron I, Rakic P, Molnar Z, Blakemore C (2006) The first neurons of the human cerebral cortex. *Nat Neurosci* **9**: 880–886.

Bystron I, Blakemore C, Rakic, P (2008) Development of the human cerebral cortex: Boulder Committee revisited. *Nat Rev Neurosci* **9**: 110–122.

Cai C, Thorne J, Grabel L (2008) Hedgehog serves as a mitogen and survival factor during embryonic stem cell neurogenesis. *Stem Cells* **26**: 1097–1098.

Chen SY, Dehart DB, Sulik KK (2004) Protection from ethanol-induced limb malformations by the superoxide dismutase/catalase mimetic, EUK-134. *FASEB J* **18**: 1234–1236.

Clarren SK, Alvord EC, Sumi SM, et al. (1978) Brain malformations related to prenatal exposure to ethanol. *J Pediatr* **92**: 64–67.

Clarren SK, Astley SJ, Gunderson VM, Spellman D (1992) Cognitive and behavioral deficits in nonhuman primates associated with very early embryonic binge exposures to ethanol. *J Pediatr* **121**: 789–796.

Cohen MM (2006) Holoprosencephaly: clinical, anatomic, and molecular dimensions. *Birth Defects Res A Clin Mol Teratol* **76**: 658–673.

Cohen-Kerem R, Koren G (2003) Antioxidants and fetal protection against ethanol teratogenicity. I. Review of the experimental data and implications to humans. *Neurotoxicol Teratol* **25**: 1–9.

Croen LA, Shaw GM, Lammer EJ (1996) Holoprosencephaly: epidemiologic and clinical characteristics of a California population. *Am J Med Genet* **64**: 465–472.

Dehart DB, Lanoue L, Tint GS, Sulik KK (1997) Pathogenesis of malformations in a rodent model for Smith–Lemli–Opitz syndrome. *Am J Med Genet* **68**: 328–337.

Demyer W, Zeman W (1963) Alobar holoprosencephaly (arhinencephaly) with median cleft lip and palate: clinical, electroencephalographic and nosologic considerations. *Confin Neurol* **23**: 1–36.

Demyer W, Zeman W, Palmer CG (1964) The face predicts the brain: diagnostic significance of median facial anomalies for holoprosencephaly (arhinencephaly). *Pediatrics* **34**: 256–263.

Dong J, Sulik KK, Chen SY (2008) Nrf2-mediated transcriptional induction of antioxidant response in mouse embryos exposed to ethanol in vivo: implications for the prevention of fetal alcohol spectrum disorders. *Antioxid Redox Signal* **10**: 2023–2033.

Driscoll CD, Streissguth AP, Riley EP (1990) Prenatal alcohol exposure: comparability of effects in humans and animal models. *Neurotoxicol Teratol* **12**: 231–237.

Dumas RM, Rabe A (1994) Augmented memory loss in aging mice after one embryonic exposure to alcohol. *Neurotoxicol Teratol* **16**: 605–612.

Dunty WC, Zucker RM, Sulik KK (2002) Hindbrain and cranial nerve dysmorphogenesis result from acute maternal ethanol administration. *Dev Neurosci* **24**: 328–342.

Fryer SL, Schweinsburg BC, Bjorkquist OA, et al. (2009) Characterization of white matter microstructure in fetal alcohol spectrum disorders. *Alcohol Clin Exp Res* **33**: 514–521.

Godin EA, O'Leary-Moore SK, Khan AA, et al. (2010) Magnetic resonance microscopy defines ethanol-induced brain abnormalities in prenatal mice: Effects of acute insult on gestational day 7. *Alcohol Clin Exp Res* **34**: 98–111.

Guerri C, Bazinet A, Riley EP (2009) Foetal alcohol spectrum disorders and alterations in brain and behaviour. *Alcohol Alcohol* **44**: 108–114.

Homanics GE, Maeda N, Traber MG, et al. (1995) Exencephaly and hydrocephaly in mice with targeted modification of the apolipoprotein B (Apob) gene. *Teratology* **51**: 1–10.

Ingram JL, Peckham SM, Tisdale B, Rodier PM (2000) Prenatal exposure of rats to valproic acid reproduces the cerebellar anomalies associated with autism. *Neurotoxicol Teratol* **22**: 319–324.

Johnson VP, Swayze VW, Sato Y, Andreasen NC (1996) Fetal alcohol syndrome: craniofacial and central nervous system manifestations. *Am J Med Genet* **61**: 329–339.

Jones KL (1975) The fetal alcohol syndrome. *Addict Dis* **2**: 79–88.

Jones KL, Smith DW (1975) The fetal alcohol syndrome. *Teratology* **12**: 1–10.

Komatsu S, Sakata-Haga H, Sawada K, et al. (2001) Prenatal exposure to ethanol induces leptomeningeal heterotopia in the cerebral cortex of the rat fetus. *Acta Neuropathol* **101**: 22–26.

Kotch LE, Sulik KK (1992a) Experimental fetal alcohol syndrome: proposed pathogenic basis for a variety of associated facial and brain anomalies. *Am J Med Genet* **44**: 168–176.

Kotch LE, Sulik KK (1992b) Patterns of ethanol-induced cell death in the developing nervous system of mice; neural fold states through the time of anterior neural tube closure. *Int J Dev Neurosci* **10**: 273–279.

Lanoue L, Dehart DB, Hinsdale ME, et al. (1997) Limb, genital, CNS, and facial malformations result from gene/environment-induced cholesterol deficiency: further evidence for a link to sonic hedgehog. *Am J Med Genet* **73**: 24–31.

Lebel C, Rasmussen C, Wyper K, et al. (2008) Brain diffusion abnormalities in children with fetal alcohol spectrum disorder. *Alcohol Clin Exp Res* **32**: 1732–1740.

Li YX, Yang HT, Zdanowicz M, et al. (2007) Fetal alcohol exposure impairs Hedgehog cholesterol modification and signaling. *Lab Invest* **87**: 231–240.

Loucks EJ, Ahlgren SC (2009) Deciphering the role of Shh signaling in axial defects produced by ethanol exposure. *Birth Defects Res A Clin Mol Teratol* **85**: 556–567.

Ma X, Coles CD, Lynch ME, et al. (2005) Evaluation of corpus callosum anisotropy in young adults with fetal alcohol syndrome according to diffusion tensor imaging. *Alcohol Clin Exp Res* **29**: 1214–1222.

Majewski F (1981) Alcohol embryopathy: some facts and speculations about pathogenesis. *Neurobehav Toxicol Teratol* **3**: 129–144.

Mattson SN, Riley EP, Jernigan TL, et al. (1992) Fetal alcohol syndrome: a case report of neuropsychological, MRI and EEG assessment of two children. *Alcohol Clin Exp Res* **16**: 1001–1003.

Mille F, Thibert C, Fombonne J, et al. (2009) The Patched dependence receptor triggers apoptosis through a DRAL-caspase-9 complex. *Nat Cell Biol* **11**: 739–46.

Miller MW (2006) *Brain Development: Normal Processes and the Effects of Alcohol and Nicotine.* Oxford: Oxford University Press.

Minetti A, Arolfo MP, Virgolini MB, et al. (1996) Spatial learning in rats exposed to acute ethanol intoxication on gestational day 8. *Pharmacol Biochem Behav* **53**: 361–367.

Muenke M, Beachy PA (2000) Genetics of ventral forebrain development and holoprosencephaly. *Curr Opin Genet Dev* **10**: 262–269.

Nau H (1994) Valproic acid-induced neural tube defects. *Ciba Found Symp* **181**: 144–152; discussion 152–160.

Nau H, Hauck RS, Ehlers K (1991) Valproic acid-induced neural tube defects in mouse and human: aspects of chirality, alternative drug development, pharmacokinetics and possible mechanisms. *Pharmacol Toxicol* **69**: 310–321.

41

Olney JW, Ishimaru MJ, Bittigau P, Ikonomidou C (2000) Ethanol-induced apoptotic neurodegeneration in the developing brain. *Apoptosis* **5**: 515–521.

O'Rahilly R, Muller F (2008) Significant features in the early prenatal development of the human brain. *Ann Anat* **190**: 105–118.

Ornoy A (2006) Neuroteratogens in man: an overview with special emphasis on the teratogenicity of antiepileptic drugs in pregnancy. *Reprod Toxicol* **22**: 214–226.

Parnell SE, O'Leary-Moore SK, Godin EA, et al. (2009) Magnetic resonance microscopy defines ethanol-induced brain abnormalities in prenatal mice: effects of acute insult on gestational day 8. *Alcohol Clin Exp Res* **33**: 1001–1011.

Peiffer J, Majewski F, Fischbach H, et al. (1979) Alcohol embryo- and fetopathy. Neuropathology of 3 children and 3 fetuses. *J Neurol Sci* **41**: 125–137.

Rasmussen SA, Moore CA, Khoury MJ, Cordero JF (1996) Descriptive epidemiology of holoprosencephaly and arhinencephaly in metropolitan Atlanta, 1968–1992. *Am J Med Genet* **66**: 320–333.

Riley EP (1990) The long-term behavioral effects of prenatal alcohol exposure in rats. *Alcohol Clin Exp Res* **14**: 670–673.

Riley EP, McGee CL (2005) Fetal alcohol spectrum disorders: an overview with emphasis on changes in brain and behavior. *Exp Biol Med* **230**: 357–365.

Rodier PM, Ingram JL, Tisdale B, et al. (1996) Embryological origin for autism: developmental anomalies of the cranial nerve motor nuclei. *J Comp Neurol* **370**: 247–261.

Rodier PM, Ingram JL, Tisdale B, Croog VJ (1997) Linking etiologies in humans and animal models: studies of autism. *Reprod Toxicol* **11**: 417–422.

Ryan SH, Williams JK, Thomas JD (2008) Choline supplementation attenuates learning deficits associated with neonatal alcohol exposure in the rat: effects of varying the timing of choline administration. *Brain Res* **1237**: 91–100.

Sakata-Haga H, Sawada K, Ohnishi T, Fukui Y (2004) Hydrocephalus following prenatal exposure to ethanol. *Acta Neuropathol* **108**: 393–398.

Schachter KA, Krauss RS (2008) Murine models of holoprosencephaly. *Curr Top Dev Biol* **84**: 139–170.

Schambra UB, Lauder JM, Petrusz P, Sulik KK (1990) Development of neurotransmitter systems in the mouse embryo following acute ethanol exposure: a histological and immunocytochemical study. *Int J Dev Neurosci* **8**: 507–522.

Schneider ML, Moore CF, Becker EF (2001) Timing of moderate alcohol exposure during pregnancy and neonatal outcome in rhesus monkeys (Macaca mulatta). *Alcohol Clin Exp Res* **25**: 1238–1245.

Shenefelt RE (1972) Morphogenesis of malformations in hamsters caused by retinoic acid: relation to dose and stage at treatment. *Teratology* **5**: 103–118.

Sowell ER, Mattson SN, Thompson PM, et al. (2001) Mapping callosal morphology and cognitive correlates: effects of heavy prenatal alcohol exposure. *Neurology* **57**: 235–244.

Sowell ER, Johnson A, Kan E, et al. (2008) Mapping white matter integrity and neurobehavioral correlates in children with fetal alcohol spectrum disorders. *J Neurosci* **28**: 1313–1319.

Sulik KK (1984) Critical periods for alcohol teratogenesis in mice, with special reference to the gastrulation stage of embryogenesis. *Ciba Found Symp* **105**: 124–141.

Sulik KK, Johnston MC (1982) Embryonic origin of holoprosencephaly: interrelationship of the developing brain and face. *Scan Electron Microsc* **1**: 309–322.

Sulik KK, Sadler TW (1993) Postulated mechanisms underlying the development of neural tube defects. Insights from in vitro and in vivo studies. *Ann N Y Acad Sci* **678**: 8–21.

Sulik KK, Cook CS, Webster WS (1988) Teratogens and craniofacial malformations: relationships to cell death. *Development* **103** Suppl: 213–231.

Sulik KK, Dehart DB, Rogers JM, Chernoff N (1995) Teratogenicity of low doses of all-trans retinoic acid in presomite mouse embryos. *Teratology* **51**: 398–403.

Swayze VW, Johnson VP, Hanson JW, et al. (1997) Magnetic resonance imaging of brain anomalies in fetal alcohol syndrome. *Pediatrics* **99**: 232–240.

Thomas JD, La Fiette MH, Quinn VR, Riley EP (2000) Neonatal choline supplementation ameliorates the effects of prenatal alcohol exposure on a discrimination learning task in rats. *Neurotoxicol Teratol* **22**: 703–711.

Thomas JD, Garrison M, O'Neill TM (2004) Perinatal choline supplementation attenuates behavioral alterations associated with neonatal alcohol exposure in rats. *Neurotoxicol Teratol* **26**: 35–45.

Thomas JD, Biane JS, O'Bryan KA, et al. (2007) Choline supplementation following third-trimester-equivalent alcohol exposure attenuates behavioral alterations in rats. *Behav Neurosci* **121**: 120–130.

Thompson BL, Levitt P, Stanwood GD (2009) Prenatal exposure to drugs: effects on brain development and implications for policy and education. *Nat Rev Neurosci* **10**: 303–312.

Vigliecca NS, Ferreyra Moyano H, Molina JC (1986) Acute prenatal alcohol exposure in rats: a behavioral study. *Acta Physiol Pharmacol Latinoam* **36**: 463–472.

Webster WS, Walsh DA, McEwen SE, Lipson AH (1983) Some teratogenic properties of ethanol and acetaldehyde in C57BL/6J mice: implications for the study of the fetal alcohol syndrome. *Teratology* **27**: 231–243.

Wonders CP, Anderson SA (2006) The origin and specification of cortical interneurons. *Nat Rev Neurosci* **7**: 687–696.

Wozniak JR, Mueller BA, Chang PN, et al. (2006) Diffusion tensor imaging in children with fetal alcohol spectrum disorders. *Alcohol Clin Exp Res* **30**: 1799–1806.

Young C, Olney JW (2006) Neuroapoptosis in the infant mouse brain triggered by a transient small increase in blood alcohol concentration. *Neurobiol Dis* **22**: 548–554.

Young C, Straiko MM, Johnson SA, et al. (2008) Ethanol causes and lithium prevents neuroapoptosis and suppression of pERK in the infant mouse brain. *Neurobiol Dis* **31**: 355–360.

4
EPILEPSY IN PREGNANCY AND THE EFFECT OF PRENATAL ANTIEPILEPTIC MEDICATION

Jill Clayton-Smith and Gus Baker

Epilepsy is a common condition affecting around 1 in 200 people in the general population. The majority of these individuals will require long-term medication with antiepileptic drugs (AEDs). A significant proportion will be women in their childbearing years. It is well established that the incidence of major and minor malformations is increased in the offspring of women who take medication for epilepsy during pregnancy, particularly the older generation of AEDs (Samren et al. 1997, Kaneko et al. 1999, Artama et al. 2006, Morrow et al. 2006). Concerns that some of the AEDs in use may be teratogenic were first raised as early as 1968 (Meadow 1968). Studies of these risks have differed substantially in methodology, however, and figures given for malformation rates have varied. Perucca (2005) critically reviewed the literature in this area and compared findings from both retrospective and prospective studies. Overall, exposure to AEDs in pregnancy gives rise to an approximately three-fold increased risk of malformations, relative to the general population risk of 2–3%. There is also evidence of adverse effects on neurological and cognitive development of children exposed to AEDs in pregnancy (Adab et al. 2004, Vinten et al. 2005). In addition to teratogenicity of AEDs, the occurrence of frequent or severe seizures during pregnancy, socio-economic factors and genetic predisposition may also impact on the child, and it is difficult to assess the influence of these confounding factors. This chapter summarizes the main physical and neurodevelopmental problems that have been observed in children born to mothers with epilepsy and draws upon our own experience from a current prospective study where we have documented both the physical and neurodevelopmental findings in a cohort of over 300 children born to mothers with epilepsy and a similar number of control children.

Epilepsy and pregnancy

The management of epilepsy in pregnancy has been well reviewed by Adab and Chadwick (2006). Whilst in most cases women with epilepsy will have complication-free pregnancies and normal offspring, there are definite increased risks for both the mother and the child, and optimal management of the mother's seizure disorder during pregnancy has to be balanced against the risk of teratogenicity of the AEDs used. Approximately one-third of women will experience an increase in their seizure frequency during pregnancy, and a confidential enquiry into maternal deaths during pregnancy has shown that maternal epilepsy is one of the most common causes of mortality (CEMACH 2004). The physiological changes associated with pregnancy affect the metabolism and serum levels of AEDs and make monitoring of serum levels unhelpful, with management being guided by the seizure frequency. Nonconvulsive seizures are not thought to pose a risk to the fetus, but it has been suggested that prolonged tonic–clonic seizures may lead to fetal hypoxia and should be minimized (Yerby 2000). The choice of drug for treatment of epilepsy during pregnancy usually depends mainly on the type of seizures present, but there is now firm evidence to suggest that some AEDs are more teratogenic than others and this should also be taken into account when prescribing (Holmes et al. 2001). Sodium valproate, in particular, has been associated with higher congenital malformation rates and greater adverse effects on cognitive outcome (Morrow et al. 2006). Risks are higher for pregnancies exposed to polytherapy (Pennell 2008). Thus, women with epilepsy should be offered preconceptual advice so that the pregnancy can be planned and any modifications of treatment made before pregnancy if possible. Although the benefits of high-dose folic acid remain unclear, folic acid is usually prescribed at a higher dose of 5 mg daily from before the time of conception in women with epilepsy. Polytherapy is best avoided, and any changes in medication should be made in consultation with a specialist. Although counselling of the mother should include information on the teratogenic risks of AEDs, it is extremely important to emphasize that medication should not be stopped suddenly before or during pregnancy because of the significant risk uncontrolled seizures would pose to both mother and baby.

Teratogenic effects of antiepileptic drugs

The teratogenic effects of AEDs can be divided into the three broad categories of major congenital malformations, minor congenital malformations including dysmorphic features, and neurodevelopmental effects. Major malformations are primary errors in morphogenesis that have serious medical or cosmetic consequences and require treatment (e.g. cleft palate). Minor malformations are structural anomalies that do not require treatment (e.g. facial features). They may be part of normal variation, e.g. a single palmar crease or epicanthic folds, and some of them will resolve spontaneously with age. Although minor malformations are not significant in themselves, the presence of two or more is unusual and may be a pointer to other problems such as cognitive deficits. The neurodevelopmental effects seen with exposure to AEDs have not been studied in as much depth as malformations but include delayed milestones, learning disability and behaviour problems. Both major and minor malformations may occur in association with neurodevelopmental impairment as part of a recognizable fetal anticonvulsant syndrome (Moore et al. 2000) (also discussed in Chapter 3).

MAJOR MALFORMATIONS

Anecdotal reports of major malformations occurring in infants exposed to AEDs have been made from the mid-1970s since the first description of fetal hydantoin syndrome (Hanson and Smith 1975). Overall the types of malformation seen are similar to those that occur

45

TABLE 4.1

Malformations seen in association with prenatal antiepileptic drug exposure

Drug	Malformation rate	Major malformations	Minor malformations	Effect on development	Main references
All monotherapy	3.7%				Morrow et al. (2006)
All polytherapy	6.0%			Yes, especially if valproate included	Morrow et al. (2006)
Phenytoin	3.7%	Cardiac defects, cleft lip/palate, microcephaly	Nail hypoplasia, facial dysmorphism	Yes. Lowering of IQ	Scolnik et al. (1994), Morrow et al. (2006)
Phenobarbitone	6.5%	Congenital heart defects most common		Yes	Koch et al. (1999), Dessenset al. (2000), Holmes et al. (2004)
Valproate	6.2–20%	Neural tube defects, heart defects, radial ray defects, optic nerve hypoplasia, abdominal wall defects, genito-urinary abnormalities	Facial dysmorphism, trigonocephaly, joint laxity, overlapping toes, myopia, laryngomalacia	Yes. Lowering of verbal IQ, impaired memory, autistic features	Adab et al. (2001, 2004), Holmes et al. (2004), Vajda and Eadie (2005), Vinten et al. (2005), Meador et al. (2006, 2009), Bromley et al.(2008)
Carbamazepine	2.2–5%	Cleft lip/palate, neural tube defects, heart defects	Nail hypoplasia, mild facial dysmorphism	No significant effect on IQ	Kini et al. (2006), Morrow et al. (2006)
Lamotrigine	1–3.2%	Possible increase in cleft palate, bowel atresias	No obvious facial dysmorphism reported	No significant effect on IQ at 3 years	Cunnington et al. (2005), Meador et al. (2006, 2009)
Topiramate	4.8–7.1%	Cleft lip/palate, hypospadias	Not studied	Not yet studied	Morrow et al. (2006), Hunt et al. (2008)
Levetiracetam	Low, ? population risk	Not yet studied	Not studied	Not yet studied	Morrow et al. (2006)

46

most commonly in the general population and include neural tube defects, congenital heart defects, hypospadias and cleft palate. Some malformations occur at a particularly high incidence after AED exposure, most notably spina bifida, observed in up to 1–2% of infants exposed to sodium valproate and in a lower percentage of infants exposed to carbamazepine (Lindhout and Omtzigt 1994). The defects often specifically involve the lower part of the neural tube in the lumbosacral area, and it is thus important that this region of the spine is checked specifically on antenatal scans. Cardiac malformations, both complex and simple septal defects, have also been reported after exposure to several AEDs, including sodium valproate, phenytoin and carbamazepine (Clayton-Smith and Donnai 1995). Sodium valproate, phenytoin, carbamazepine and lamotrigine have all been associated with orofacial clefting, though with both valproate and lamotrigine clefting is specifically confined to the palate and very rarely involves the lip. Table 4.1 outlines the frequencies and types of major malformation seen with specific drug exposures.

A prospective study from the UK Epilepsy and Pregnancy Register (Morrow et al. 2006) showed that the overall rate of major congenital malformations (MCMs) in pregnancies exposed to AEDs was 4.2%, compared with a risk of 3.5% in women with epilepsy who had not taken AEDs. The risk of MCMs in children exposed to sodium valproate was 6.2% vs 2.2% in carbamazepine-exposed infants. These findings were comparable to those of other similar studies. Risks of MCM with exposure to phenytoin, one of the older AEDs, have usually been quoted as lower than those for sodium valproate, and Holmes et al. (2001) found an overall MCM risk of 3.4% in a cohort of 87 infants. There have been fewer studies of children exposed to the newer AEDs but an MCM rate of 3.2% was reported in a cohort of 647 children exposed to lamotrigine (Morrow et al. 2006) and one of 4.8% in a cohort exposed to topiramate (Hunt et al. 2008). Risks with polytherapy have been high in several studies, especially if the polytherapy includes sodium valproate.

MINOR MALFORMATIONS

Minor malformations are common within the general population but occur at a higher frequency and are more likely to be multiple in infants exposed to AEDs. Common minor anomalies seen in association with AEDs include minor limb anomalies, nail hypoplasia, joint laxity and dysmorphic facial features. Whilst some facial features are shared across children with different drug exposures, others are more specific to a particular drug, such as the ridged metopic suture giving rise to trigonocephaly with valproate exposure (Clayton-Smith and Donnai 1995). It has been postulated that some of the facial features, such as a broad, flat nasal bridge and short nose, could be attributed to vitamin K deficiency, which occurs at an increased frequency in mothers on some AEDs, as other conditions associated with maternal vitamin K deficient states are associated with similar facial chracteristics (Howe et al. 1995). Kini et al. (2006) reviewed the facial features of a retrospective cohort of children exposed to AEDs in pregnancy and concluded that children exposed to sodium valproate had the most recognizable facial gestalt but that carbamazepine exposure, too, was associated with subtle but recognizable differences in facial features. Many of the minor dysmorphic features seen in AED-exposed infants were also observed in normal unexposed infants and in infants with other prenatal exposures such as fetal alcohol syndrome.

Some single-gene disorders, e.g. Cornelia de Lange syndrome, also share overlapping facial dysmorphism. Kini et al. cautioned against making a diagnosis of a fetal anticonvulsant syndrome on facial features alone. In their valproate-exposed cohort the facial gestalt was more easily recognizable in children exposed to higher doses and there was a correlation between the presence of facial dysmorphism and learning disability. For all drugs, the facial features are usually recognized more easily in younger children and tend to normalize with age. Thus it is useful to see earlier photographs when considering a diagnosis of fetal anticonvulsant syndrome.

NEUROPSYCHOLOGICAL AND BEHAVIOURAL CONSEQUENCES
There has been little research on the long-term effects of exposure to AED treatment in respect of the more subtle neurological and cognitive development, although many of the early anecdotal reports of fetal anticonvulsant syndromes listed developmental delay as a feature. Studies of this area are difficult because of the many factors contributing to normal intellectual development, particularly in children of mothers with epilepsy (Titze et al. 2008). Koch et al. (1999) carried out a retrospective study in schoolchildren and demonstrated a lowering of IQ in children exposed to primidone in utero. Animal studies have demonstrated neurocognitive impairment with exposure to several different AEDs (Holmes et al. 2007). For the last 10 years, the Liverpool and Manchester Neurodevelopment Group have been investigating the potential effects of exposure to AED treatment in utero on neuro-development. The first study conducted involved a retrospective survey of women between the ages of 16 and 40 years registered at the Mersey Region Epilepsy Clinic. Each mother was asked to complete a postal questionnaire concerning the experience of pregnancy and the subsequent schooling of the liveborn child. The results of this study highlighted that monotherapy or polytherapy with valproate during pregnancy carries particular risks for the development of children exposed in utero. Children exposed to sodium valproate were more likely to attend special school and to be referred for "statementing of special education needs" (Adab et al. 2001). The retrospective nature of this study meant that the results had to be treated with caution; in order to understand the potential neuropsychological effects in more detail the group recruited, between January 2000 and May 2001, women with epilepsy who had children aged 6 months to 16 years and who were attending epilepsy and antenatal clinics in the Liverpool and Manchester region. Each mother underwent a clinical assessment, and both the mother and child underwent neuropsychological testing. The findings of this study demonstrated that children exposed to sodium valproate may show a more specific pattern of impairment for verbal abilities and that the mothers of children exposed to sodium valproate were more likely to report delayed development in speech and language in their children (Adab et al. 2004, Vinten et al. 2005). We identified using multiple statistical analyses that the risk of developmental delay was associated with exposure to sodium valproate, maternal IQ and more than five generalized seizures during pregnancy. Again, the retrospective nature of the study left it open to methodological criticism, particularly in respect of selection bias, and in order to obtain information on the absolute risk a prospective study that minimized confounding factors was necessary.

In 2000 the Liverpool and Manchester Neurodevelopment Group initiated a prospective study; to date we have recruited 632 children from antenatal clinics in both Liverpool and Manchester. Of those recruited, 336 children were born to mothers without epilepsy and form an important control group. The primary outcome measures include the outcome of pregnancy, the physical, cognitive and behavioural development of the child, and the results of genetic investigations. In addition we have initiated further research based on clinical experience, to examine language functioning of the child at age 6. In 2002 we joined with an American prospective study, the NEAD study group (Meador et al. 2006), and as a consequence are now currently following up 333 children from sites in the USA and UK, exposed to AEDs in utero. The UK study is likely to be concluded in 2010. A report on the cognitive outcome of children in this study at the age of 3 years has shown that exposure to sodium valproate, especially at high doses, has a significant impact on the subsequent IQ of the child, with verbal IQ being specifically affected (Meador et al. 2009). On average, children exposed to valproate had an IQ 9 points lower than those exposed to lamotrigine and 6 points lower than those exposed to carbamazepine.

In the conduct of our research it became obvious that some of the children assessed were exhibiting symptoms associated with autism. Analysis of findings from our cohort demonstrated a significant association between exposure to sodium valproate and an increase in the incidence of autism spectrum disorders (Bromley et al. 2008). Poorer adaptive behaviour and impaired socialization have also been reported in association with valproate exposure in pregnancy (Vinten et al. 2009). It is clear that many of the effects seen are subtle and may not become apparent until school age or even later.

There is a continuing need for large high-quality prospective studies that investigate in detail the neurodevelopmental effects (educational, occupational, social and relationship attainments) of exposure to AEDs in utero. Without such data information about the absolute risk of developmental delay cannot be communicated to the women with epilepsy considering childbirth.

FETAL ANTICONVULSANT SYNDROMES

Specific patterns of malformations, growth and development have been defined in association with some of the more commonly used AEDs; these are referred to as fetal anticonvulsant syndromes. Though some features are common to exposure to several AEDs, some are associated with only one particular drug, e.g. a short, anteverted nose has been associated with exposure to phenytoin, carbamazepine and sodium valproate, while radial ray defects are specifically associated with valproate exposure (Sharony et al. 1993).

Fetal hydantoin syndrome was first described in 1975 in phenytoin-exposed children who presented with hypertelorism, broad nasal bridge, short nose and facial hirsutism (Hanson and Smith 1975). Major malformations, which occurred with an increased incidence, included congenital heart disease, cleft lip and palate, and optic nerve hypoplasia. Nail hypoplasia and hypoplastic distal phalanges are prominent with phenytoin exposure, and stippled epiphyses may be seen on radiography. These latter features have been attributed to maternal vitamin K deficiency (Howe et al. 1995) as mentioned above. Phenytoin (hydantoin) was the first AED to be associated with a specific pattern of problems in offspring, and clinicians have subsequently been very wary of the teratogenic effects. As

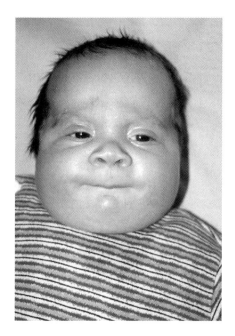 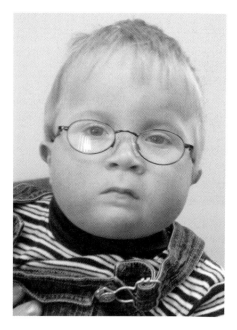

Fig. 4.1. Fetal valproate syndrome: infant facies. Note anteverted nares, small, downturned mouth with flat philtrum, thin upper lip and infra-orbital grooves.

Fig. 4.2. Fetal valproate syndrome: childhood facies. Note short nose, broad nasal bridge and neat, arched eyebrows. Mouth is downturned with thin upper lip and everted lower lip.

regards malformation rates, phenytoin appears to be safer to use in pregnancy than some other drugs but some studies have suggested an adverse effect on neurodevelopment (Scolnik et al. 1994). This needs further exploration in larger studies as phenytoin remains in current use as an AED.

Valproic acid is arguably the best drug for treatment of primary generalized epilepsy and has therefore been a popular AED, particularly in the UK, for the last 30 years. *Fetal valproate syndrome* (FVS) was delineated by Di Liberti et al. (1984). They pointed out that infants exposed to valproate in utero had a specific pattern of facial features which included a broad nasal bridge, short anteverted nose, infraorbital grooves, and small, downturned mouth with thin upper lip and flattening of the philtrum (Figs. 4.1, 4.2). These facial features usually occurred in association with other major and minor malformations. Debate has continued as to whether the facial features of FVS are specific to valproate alone or similar to those seen with other AED exposure, but it is generally agreed that the facial features seen after valproate exposure are often more striking than with other drugs. Trigonocephaly due to ridging of the metopic suture is a particularly prominent feature of FVS and may require surgery for correction. Several major malformations occur with increased frequency in FVS. There is a particularly high risk of neural tube defect, usually spina bifida (Fig. 4.3), and various types of congenital heart defect have been described ranging from complex

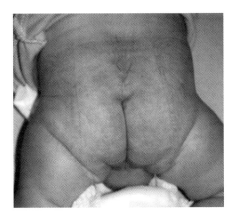

Fig. 4.3. The neural tube defects associated with fetal valproate syndrome usually affect the lumbosacral region.

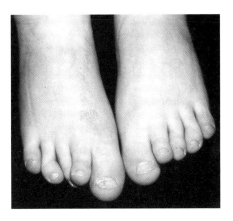

Fig. 4.4. Fetal valproate syndrome: typical appearance of feet with hypoplastic, overlapping toes.

defects, which may be fatal, to minor septal defects. Genito-urinary malformations, abdominal wall defects and hypospadias occur, and isolated cleft palate, but not cleft lip, is increased in frequency. Optic atrophy and septo-optic dysplasia have been noted. A number of limb defects occur after valproate exposure. The commonest are generalized joint laxity, talipes deformity and hypoplastic, overlapping toes. Nail hypoplasia is not as common as with other AEDs. Several exposed infants have had radial ray defects ranging from minor hypoplasia of the thumbs and flattening of the thenar eminence to complete absence of the radius (Sharony et al. 1993). Radial ray defects are important to note because even the mild ones can cause significant functional problems, e.g. with writing. Animal studies have shown that the radial ray defects can be reproduced after valproate exposure, and downregulation of genes involved in limb patterning has been demonstrated (Faiella et al. 2000). Lower-limb defects are not as common but have been reported (Cole et al. 2009) (Fig. 4.4). Although growth retardation was noted in some cases of FVS early on, most recent reports have not confirmed this and some have suggested that macrosomia may be more common (Kozma 2001). In contrast to phenytoin-exposed children, head circumference is usually normal. There may be neonatal withdrawal symptoms after birth but thereafter most infants will feed and grow well. Medical problems seen with an increased frequency include otitis media, an increased incidence of myopia, and laryngeal stridor in infancy (Moore et al. 2000). Motor milestones may be delayed due to joint laxity, and both nocturnal and diurnal enuresis occur at a higher frequency than in the general population, possibly related to low muscle tone.

Recent concerns regarding exposure to sodium valproate during pregnancy have focused on the effects on neurodevelopment, and adverse effects on IQ have been seen in several studies (Adab et al. 2001, 2004; Vinten et al. 2005). These studies also point out more subtle effects on memory, behaviour and concentration. The increased incidence of autism spectrum disorder, as part of the FVS, was reported anecdotally by Rasalam et al. (2005), and the observations cited above by Bromley et al. (2008) confirm this finding. Our own observations suggest that children with FVS are also socially immature for their age, and this can affect their peer group relationships and self-esteem. Thus, FVS presents a complex pattern of problems, but if recognized and managed appropriately children with this condition can do well.

Carbamazepine is usually used to treat focal epilepsies (Marson et al. 2007) and may also be used for the treatment of other neurological and non-neurological disorders. The effects of carbamazepine exposure in utero are subtle but a specific fetal carbamazepine syndrome has been suggested (Jones et al. 1989, Moore et al. 2000, Kini et al. 2006). Descriptions of the face in carbamazepine-exposed children have differed, but the most convincing is perhaps that of Kini et al. (2006) who described and illustrated a "doll-like" face with small mouth and chin, short anteverted nose and a long philtrum. Neural tube defects, cleft palate, congenital heart defects and hypoplastic nails complete the picture, but malformation rates, although increased above those in the general population, are lower than for some other drugs. Earlier reports suggested that developmental delay may be associated with carbamazepine exposure but this has not been convincingly borne out by later, and better designed studies.

Lamotrigine has been used increasingly over the past few years as an alternative to sodium valproate for the treatment of primary generalized epilepsy, though seizure control may not be quite so good. As it is a relatively new AED compared with other drugs, data on long-term follow-up of infants exposed to lamotrigine are limited. Limited information regarding the occurrence of major malformations after lamotrigine exposure has been obtained from pregnancy registries, and quoted malformation rates for lamotrigine have been consistently lower than for valproate and carbamazepine at around 2–2.5% (Morrow et al. 2006, Pennell 2008). No consistent malformations have been observed, though Holmes et al. (2008) reported an increase in orofacial clefting. This has not been borne out in subsequent studies (Dolk et al. 2008). No specific facial dysmorphology has been reported so far in infants exposed to lamotrigine in utero, and there are no published data on long-term cognitive outcomes following lamotrigine exposure.

Phenobarbitone is still used for treatment of maternal epilepsy in some countries, and major malformation rates after exposure have differed. In the largest registry-based study Holmes et al. (2004) found an MCM rate of 6.5%. There does not appear to be a specific fetal barbiturate syndrome but congenital heart defects have been reported relatively frequently. Dessens et al. (2000) reported impaired cognitive outcome after phenobarbitone exposure in a retrospective study.

Hunt et al. (2008) reported the outcome of 70 pregnancies exposed to *topiramate* monotherapy. There were three MCMs in this group, giving a malformation rate of 4.8%. When topiramate was used as part of polytherapy the malformation rate was 11.2%, with orofacial clefts and hypospadias being observed most frequently. These results were at odds with those reported by Ornoy et al. (2008), where growth retardation was more frequent but MCMs were not increased. Though further studies are needed, these observations give some cause for concern. Cognitive outcomes after topiramate are as yet unknown.

Many other new AEDS have come on to the market in recent years and their safety record is as yet unknown. Monitoring of pregnancy outcomes through pregnancy registers and well-designed prospective follow-up studies will continue to be needed, though adverse effects on cognition, behaviour and the implications for adulthood and employment will not be known for some years to come.

Folic acid: impact on teratogenicity

The use of folic acid supplementation in the general population has significantly reduced the incidence of neural tube defects and may have impacted also on other types of malformation. Folic acid deficiency is thought to be involved in causation of MCMs because of the role of folic acid in DNA synthesis and methylation and the association of folic acid deficiency with raised levels of homocysteine, which is toxic to the fetus. Women taking some AEDs, including carbamazepine and phenytoin, are at increased risk of folic acid deficiency because of lower absorption rates. In view of the known association of folic acid deficiency with neural tube defects and the increased incidence of neural tube defects with AED exposure, these women are advised to take folic acid at the higher dose of 5 mg daily during pregnancy. In truth, it is unknown whether the neural tube defects occurring with AED exposure are caused by the same mechanism as those in the general population. A recent study by Morrow et al. (2009) showed no protective effect of folic acid amongst women on the UK pregnancy register, yet other studies, for example that reported by Dean et al. (2007), have suggested that there may be a link between impaired folic acid metabolism and the occurrence of MCMs in the offspring of women with epilepsy by demonstrating that affected children were more likely to be homozygous for the low-activity allele of the *MTHFR* gene, which encodes an enzyme integral to normal folate metabolism. Again, most studies in this area have been underpowered, and the results of larger studies or meta-analyses are awaited. Until then, it seems sensible to continue to advise mothers with epilepsy to take folic acid at either the normal or higher dose (Adab and Chadwick 2006). Morrow's study showed that uptake of folic acid supplementation at any dose pre-conception was still less than 50%; further effort is needed to improve this figure.

Conclusion

There is no doubt that our knowledge of the risks of adverse outcomes on offspring of women with epilepsy has increased considerably over the last 10 years, and this has led to major changes in prescribing habits during pregnancy and a much greater emphasis on pre-conception counselling. Perhaps the most important finding has been the confirmation from several studies that sodium valproate used either as monotherapy or in combination with other drugs is associated both with higher MCM rates than for other drugs and with neurodevelopmental problems. It is also apparent that neurodevelopmental problems can be subtle and may not become apparent until school age or later. Management of women with epilepsy has now changed to reflect the importance of counselling for a range of malformations, not just neural tube defects, and for the risk of learning disability (Adab and Chadwick 2006). Solutions to the problems of teratogenicity are not always easy; for many women sodium valproate may be the only AED that controls their seizures, and changing to another drug or reducing or withdrawing valproate involves major lifestyle changes, e.g. not driving, or can lead to an increase in seizure frequency with all the risks that this entails, especially for mothers looking after small children. One strategy that might be adopted is that of considering a change of medication from sodium valproate to another drug in late adolescence as teenagers leave paediatric care, because many pregnancies in the 16–25 age group are not planned. The recent study by Meador et al. (2009) suggests that lamotrigine is a safer alternative as regards prognosis for development, although further follow-up on this newer AED is still needed. One important development has been the recognition that studies of AED teratogenicity need to be well designed to avoid potential confounding factors, such as selection bias, effect of other medications, parental IQ and social class. The move to obtaining information from prospective studies with matched controls and the setting up of population-based pregnancy registers has facilitated collection of more meaningful data. These will continue to be important for evaluation of newer AEDs and for long-term follow-up studies in years to come.

REFERENCES

Adab N, Chadwick DW (2006) Management of women with epilepsy during pregnancy. *Obstetrician Gynaecologist* **8**: 20–25.

Adab N, Jacoby A, Chadwick D, Smith D (2001) Additional educational needs in children born to mothers with epilepsy. *J Neurol Neurosurg Psychiatry* **70**: 15–21.

Adab N, Kini U, Vinten J, et al. (2004) The longer term outcome of children born to mothers with epilepsy. *J Neurol Neurosurg Psychiatry* **75**: 1575–1583.

Artama M, Ritvanen A, Gissler M, et al. (2006) Congenital structural anomalies in offspring of women with epilepsy – a population-based cohort study in Finland. *Int J Epidemiol* **35**: 280–287.

Bromley RL, Mawer G, Clayton-Smith J, et al. (2008) Autism spectrum disorders following in utero exposure to antiepileptic drugs. *Neurology* **71**: 1923–1924.

CEMACH (2004) *Why Mothers Die 2000–2002. The Sixth Report of Confidential Enquiries into Maternal Deaths in the United Kingdom.* London: RCOG Press.

Clayton-Smith J, Donnai D (1995) The fetal valproate syndrome. *J Med Genet* **32**: 724–727.

Cole RL, Van Ross ER, Clayton-Smith J (2009) Fibular aplasia in a child exposed to sodium valproate in pregnancy. *Clin Dysmorphol* **18**: 37–39.

Cunnington M, Tennis P, International Lamotrigine Pregnancy Registry Scientific Advisory Committee (2005) Lamotrigine and the risk of malformations in pregnancy. *Neurology* **64**: 955–960.

Dean J, Robertson Z, Reid V, et al. (2007) Fetal anticonvulsant syndromes and polymorphisms in MTHFR, MTR and MTRR. *Am J Med Genet A* **143A**: 2303–2311.

Dessens AB, Cohen-Kettenis PT, Mellenburgh GJ, et al. (2000) Association of prenatal phenobarbital and phenytoin exposure with small head size at birth and with learning problems. *Acta Paediatr* **89**: 533–541.

DiLiberti JH, Farndon PA, Dennis NR, Curry CJ (1984) The fetal valproate syndrome. *Am J Med Genet* **19**: 473–481.

Dolk H, Jentink J, Loane M, et al. (2008) Does lamotrigine use in pregnancy increase oro-facial cleft risk relative to other malformations. *Neurology* **71**: 714–22.

Faiella A, Wernig B, Consalez GG, et al. (2000) A mouse model for valproate teratogenicity: parental effects, homeotic transformations, and altered HOX gene expression. *Hum Mol Genet* **9**: 227–236.

Hanson JW, Smith DW (1975) The fetal hydantoin syndrome. *J Pediatr* **87**: 285–290.

Holmes GL, Harden C, Liporace J, Gordon J (2007) Postnatal concerns in children born to women with epilepsy. *Epilepsy Behav* **11**: 270–276.

Holmes LB, Harvey EA, Coull BA, et al. (2001) The teratogenicity of anticonvulsant drugs. *N Engl J Med* **344**: 1132–1138.

Holmes LB, Wyszynski DF, Lieberman E (2004) The AED (antiepileptic drug) pregnancy registry. A six year experience. *Arch Neurol* **61**: 673–678.

Holmes LB, Baldwin EJ, Smith CR, et al. (2008) Increased frequency of isolated cleft palate in infants exposed to lamotrigine during pregnancy. *Neurology* **70**: 2152–2158.

54

Howe AM, Lipson AH, Sheffield LJ, et al. (1995) Prenatal exposure to phenytoin, facial development, and a possible role for vitamin K. *Am J Med Genet* **58**: 238–44.

Hunt S, Russell A, Smithson WH, et al. (2008) Topiramate in pregnancy: preliminary experience from the UK Epilepsy and Pregnancy Register. *Neurology* **71**: 272–276.

Jones KL, Lacro RV, Johnson KA, Adams J (1989) Pattern of malformations in the children of women treated with carbamazepine during pregnancy. *N Engl J Med* **320**: 1661–1666.

Kaneko S, Battino D, Andermann E, et al. (1999) Congenital malformations due to antiepileptic drugs. *Epilepsy Res* **33**: 145–158.

Kini U, Adab N, Vinten J, et al. (2006) Dysmorphic features: an important clue to the diagnosis and severity of the fetal anticonvulsant syndromes. *Arch Dis Child Fetal Neonatal Ed* **91**: F90–F95.

Koch S, Titze K, Zimmermann RB, et al. (1999) Long term neuropsychological consequences of maternal epilepsy and anticonvulsant treatment during pregnancy for school-age children and adolescents. *Epilepsia* **40**: 1237–1243.

Kozma C (2001) Valproic acid embryopathy: report of two siblings with further expansion of the phenotypic abnormalities and a review of the literature. *Am J Med Genet* **98**: 168–175.

Lindhout D, Omtzigt JG (1994) Teratogenic effects of antiepileptic drugs: implications for the management of epilepsy in women of childbearing age. *Epilepsia* **35** Suppl 4: S19–S28.

Marson AG, Appleton R, Baker GA, et al. (2007) A randomised controlled trial examining the longer-term outcomes of standard versus new antiepileptic drugs. The SANAD trial. *Health Technol Assess* **11**: iii–iv; ix–x; 1–134.

Meador K, Baker GA, Finnell RH, et al. (2006) In utero antiepileptic drug exposure: fetal death and malformations. *Neurology* **67**: 407–412.

Meador KJ, Baker GA, Browning N, et al. (2009) Cognitive function at 3 years of age after fetal exposure to antiepileptic drugs. *N Engl J Med* **360**: 1597–605.

Meadow SR (1968) Anticonvulsant drugs and congenital anomalies. *Lancet* **2**: 1296.

Moore SJ, Turnpenny P, Quinn A, et al. (2000) A clinical study of 57 children with fetal anticonvulsant syndromes. *J Med Genet* **37**: 489–97.

Morrow J, Russell A, Guthrie E, et al. (2006) Malformation risks of anti-epileptic drugs in pregnancy. A prospective study from the UK Epilepsy and Pregnancy Register. *J Neurol Neurosurg Psychiatry* **77**: 193–198.

Morrow JI, Hunt SJ, Russell AJ, et al. (2009) Folic acid use and major congenital malformations in offspring of women with epilepsy. A prospective study from the UK Epilepsy and Pregnancy Register. *J Neurol Neurosurg Psychiatry* **80**: 506–511.

Ornoy A, Zvi N, Arnon J, et al. (2008) The outcome of pregnancy following topiramate treatment: a study on 52 pregnancies. *Reprod Toxicol* **25**: 388–389.

Pennell PB (2008) Antiepileptic drugs during pregnancy. What is known and which AEDs appear to be safest? *Epilepsia* **49** Suppl 9: 43–55.

Perucca E (2005) Birth defects after pre-natal exposure to anti-epileptic drugs. *Lancet Neurol* **4**: 781–786.

Rasalam AD, Hailey H, Williams JH, et al. (2005) Characteristics of fetal anticonvulsant syndrome associated autistic disorder. *Dev Med Child Neurol* **47**: 551–555.

Samrén EB, van Duijn CM, Koch S, et al. (1997) Maternal use of antiepileptic drugs and the risk of major congenital malformations; a joint European prospective study of human teratogenesis associated with maternal epilepsy. *Epilepsia* **38**: 981–990.

Scolnik D, Nulman I, Rovet J, et al. (1994) Neurodevelopment of children exposed in utero to phenytoin and carbamazepine monotherapy. *JAMA* **271**: 767–770.

Sharony R, Garber A, Viskochil D, et al. (1993) Preaxial ray reduction defects as part of valproic acid embryofetopathy. *Prenat Diagn* **10**: 909–918.

Titze K, Koch S, Helge H, et al. (2008) Prenatal and family risks of children born to mothers with epilepsy: effects on cognitive development. *Dev Med Child Neurol* **50**: 117–122.

Vajda FJ, Eadie MJ (2005) Maternal valproate dosage and fetal malformations. *Acta Neurol Scand* **112**: 137–142.

Vinten, J, Adab N, Kini U, et al. (2005) Neuropsychological effects of exposure to anticonvulsant medication in utero. *Neurology* **64**: 949–954.

Vinten J, Bromley RL, Taylor J, et al. (2009) The behavioral consequences of exposure to antiepileptic drugs in utero. *Epilepsy Behav* **14**: 197–201.

Yerby MS (2000) Quality of life, epilepsy advances, and the evolving role of anticonvulsants in women with epilepsy. *Neurology* **55** Suppl 1: 21–31.

5
NEURODEVELOPMENT OF CHILDREN EXPOSED TO ANTIDEPRESSANT AND ANTIPSYCHOTIC MEDICATIONS DURING PREGNANCY

Irena Nulman, Sara Citron, Michelle Todorow and Elizabeth Uleryk

Psychiatric disorders are common in pregnancy. When untreated, they are associated with increased maternal morbidity, adverse perinatal outcomes, risk for future child psychopathology and impaired neurodevelopment. Pharmacotherapy during gestation involves weighing possible risk of fetal exposure to psychotropic medication against the potential adverse effects of untreated maternal mental disorder to both mother and child. While the majority of studies focus on the immediate pregnancy outcome following exposure to psychotropic drugs, the long-term outcomes, although of equally paramount importance, have received limited attention. The reproductive safety of psychotropic medications cannot be assured without considering potential behavioural teratogenicity. We have reviewed the available publications on neurodevelopmental outcomes of children exposed in utero to antidepressant and antipsychotic medication, and translated this knowledge into an evidence-based summary.

Depression in women
Depression presents a significant health care concern, affecting up to 25% of women, peaking during childbearing age (Evans et al. 2001), and rising as high as 51% in specific populations (Halbreich 2004). A cluster of depressive symptoms, called a depressive episode, may last for weeks, months or even years if not effectively treated. Depression has a morbidity rate comparable to hypertension and angina, and 15% of patients may die if untreated (Bostwick and Pankratz 2000). Around 10–16% of pregnant women fulfill the DSM-IV diagnostic criteria for major depression and require pharmacotherapy (Burke et al. 1991). Depression during gestation is more common than in the postnatal period (Lappin 2001) and can significantly increase the risk for postpartum depression (Troutman and Cutrona 1990, Stowe and Nemeroff 1995). Postpartum depression affects 10–22% of women and up to 26% of pregnant adolescents (Troutman and Cutrona 1990, Stowe and Nemeroff 1995). The decision to initiate or continue pharmacotherapy during pregnancy is complicated by the need to balance maternal well-being with fetal safety.

Uncontrolled depression poses risks not only to the mother but also to her fetus and the child's future development. A lack of social support, teenage pregnancy, single motherhood, unplanned pregnancies and low socio-economic status are all risk factors for the occurrence of depression during gestation (O'Hara 1986, 1994; Gotlib et al. 1989; Rosenfeld and Everett 1996). Depression in pregnancy has been associated with poor self- and prenatal care, inadequate nutrition and weight gain, sleep disturbances, emotional deterioration and suicide attempts, an increase in obstetric complications and risk for postpartum depression (Kumar and Robson 1984, Zuckerman et al. 1989, Bolton et al. 1998, Morse et al. 2000, O'Keane and Marsh 2007). Moreover, depression is associated with increased anxiety and stress, and frequently precedes substance-abusive behaviour (Zilberman et al. 2003).

The effect of depression on the fetus is often neglected in research. Stress associated with maternal depression can lead to the dysregulation of the autonomic nervous system and hypothalamic, pituitary, adrenal and placental axes, and may have an adverse effect on fetal development, whether attributed to direct action of endogenous biological factors or to indirect exposure to poor maternal health habits (Zuckerman et al. 1989, Field 1995, Bernstein 2000, Newport et al. 2001, Field et al. 2004, Lazinsky et al. 2008). Fetal exposure to stress-induced maternal behaviour was found to be associated with impaired fetoplacental function, increased rates of malformations, intrauterine growth retardation, stillbirth and perinatal complications (Orr and Miller 1995, Hansen et al. 2000, Wisborg et al. 2008). Preterm delivery and low birthweight are among the leading causes of infant mortality in the USA, and maternal stress is considered to be the leading proposed causal mechanism (Meaney et al. 1994, McLean et al. 1995, Hobel et al. 1999, Bernstein 2000, Taylor et al. 2000). Indeed, an impressive body of literature repeatedly demonstrates a strong association between preterm birth and the child's long-term neurocognitive development. Maternal stress and anxiety during pregnancy was linked with lower cognitive and motor development scores in a study of 8-month-old infants (Huizink et al. 2003), and postpartum stressors have been associated with impaired child behaviour and temperament (Susman et al. 2001). These effects should be seriously considered in the management of maternal depression.

Elevated corticotropin-releasing hormone and cortisol levels associated with preterm delivery may identify women at high risk of preterm labour at 18–20 weeks of gestation (Yim et al. 2009). Neonates of depressed mothers display irritability, excessive crying, hypotonia and lethargy (Field 1995), dysregulated attention, arousal and insecure attachment with later disruptions of performance on non-social learning tasks and of ability to process information, and an increased risk of adverse long-term neurobehavioural outcomes in children (Murray 1992, Murray et al. 1996).

A substantial body of literature has evaluated the impact of maternal postnatal depression on children. Studies of 12- to 21-month-old children of mothers who experienced postnatal depression show poorer outcomes on cognitive and behavioural measures and object concept tasks, and an increased incidence of temper tantrums, separation problems and insecure attachment (Lyons-Ruth et al. 1986, Teti and Gelfand 1991, Murray 1992, Deave et al. 2008) when compared with children from a non-depressed comparison group. Upon evaluation of children's cognitive outcome, Hay and Kumar (1995) found postnatal depression to be associated with impaired cognitive outcomes, difficulties in mathematical reasoning and a higher prevalence of special education needs in 4-year-old children with impaired adaptive functioning and anxiety, attention deficit and conduct disorders. Preschool children with depressed mothers display negative internalizing and externalizing (aggressive, disruptive) behaviour, poor self-control, passivity and non-compliance (Kuczynksi and Kochanska 1990, Murray et al. 1996). They also present with difficulties in cognitive functioning (Murray 1992, Sharp et al. 1995) and in social interaction with parents and peers (Kuczynksi and Kochanska 1990, Murray et al. 1996). Disruption in mother–child interaction and attachment may have a profound impact on children, who are more likely to have behavioural problems and impaired cognitive and emotional development (Jameson et al. 1997, Murray and Cooper 1997, Lyons-Ruth et al. 2000). Maternal depression can also impinge on family interpersonal relationships.

The effects of maternal depression on an adolescent's developmental outcome are exhibited through learning disabilities, psychosocial maladjustment, higher risk for psychopathology, elevated cortisol levels (Halligan et al. 2004) and substance abuse (Beardslee et al. 1983, 1998; Weissman and Olfson 1995; Weissman et al. 1997).

DEPRESSION AND PHARMACOTHERAPY

While depression can have detrimental consequences for both mother and fetus, it is also one of the most treatable mental health disorders. There are more than 20 effective anti-depressant drugs available, belonging to one of eight pharmacologically distinct classes (Preskorn 1999). Despite general agreement that maternal depression should be controlled during pregnancy, depression in many women goes unrecognized, and those who are diagnosed are frequently under-treated (Hirschfeld et al. 1997) or discontinue their medication because of fear of teratogenicity (Einarson et al. 2001), leading to an increased risk of postpartum depression and relapses, and of becoming refractory to pharmacotherapy (Cohen et al. 2006). Treatment of a psychiatric illness during pregnancy involves weighing potential risk of fetal exposure to psychotropic medication against adverse effects of an untreated disorder on mother and fetus.

Tricyclic antidepressants

Tricyclic antidepressants (TCAs) are very effective, and although indicated for depression, are also used for chronic pain, migraine, incontinence and insomnia. However, TCAs have a narrow therapeutic index, are cardiotoxic, and life-threatening in overdose. Their severe anticholinergic effect leads to poor compliance, under-treatment and premature discontinuation of therapy. Nevertheless, TCAs have been in use for about 50 years, with no confirmation of any specific pattern of congenital malformation related to the drug. Both prospective and retrospective studies of thousands of women have failed to associate the drugs with impaired organogenesis or long-term neurodevelopment (Misri and Sivertz 1991; Pastuszak et al. 1993; Altshuler et al. 1996; McElhatton et al. 1996; Nulman et al. 1997, 2002; Simon et al. 2002). Transient neonatal toxicity (urinary retention and functional bowel obstruction) and withdrawal symptoms (irritability, jitteriness, seizures) were observed in newborn infants when TCAs were used in late pregnancy and near term (Shearer et al. 1972, Webster

1973, Falterman and Richardson 1980, Cowe et al. 1982, Schimmell et al. 1991, Bromiker and Kaplan 1994, McElhatton et al. 1996).

Newer antidepressant medications
The newer generation of selective reuptake inhibitors is currently the most widely prescribed category of antidepressants (Pincus et al. 1998). When compared with older TCAs, newer antidepressant medications have a more tolerable side-effect profile, a lower risk of overdose and more selectivity over central nervous system transmitters (Ferguson 2001). Newer antidepressants, referenced in this review under the umbrella term of selective serotonin reuptake inhibitors (SSRIs), comprise citalopram, fluoxetine, fluvoxamine, paroxetine and sertraline; the serotonin and norepinephrine reuptake inhibitor, venlafaxine; the serotonin (5-HT2A and 2C) and alpha-2 norepinephrine receptor blocker, mirtazapine; and the dopamine and norepinephrine reuptake inhibitor, bupropion. All have emerged as standard medications for the treatment of depression, and are widely prescribed in the USA (Ferguson 2001). Although the selectivity of SSRIs to serotonin reuptake channels reduces their potential to produce adverse effects on the central nervous system, studies have shown that SSRIs can also influence other neurotransmitter transporters, including norepineprhine and dopamine (Rice and Barone 2000) and differ in their receptor affinity. Paroxetine is a potent inhibitor of norepinephrine transport; sertraline is a potent inhibitor of dopamine transport (Tatsumi et al. 1997). Fluoxetine, fluvoxamine and sertraline display a moderate effect at these receptors as well (Owens et al. 1997).

The use of antidepressant medications during pregnancy exposes the fetal brain to psychoactive substances at a time of maximal central nervous system (CNS) development, and can potentially influence neurotransmitter binding in an immature brain. Children's long-term developmental assessment should therefore test outcomes that can be influenced not only by serotonergic but also by dopaminergic and noradrenergic neurotransmitter systems, such as attention, impulse control, aggression, affect regulation, cognition and motor performance (Schore 1994, Netter et al. 1996, Plitzka et al. 1996, Coull 1998, Stokes et al. 1999, Vallone et al. 2000). The safety of antidepressant medications use in pregnancy cannot be assured until possible neurodevelopmental consequences are studied.

Studies examining the neurocognitive development of children exposed prenatally to antidepressants are still sparse in number because of numerous methodological issues associated with conducting the studies. Because randomized trials have limited applicability in studies of pregnant women, the data rely on retrospective reports and few prospective studies. These studies have serious methodological limitations: they are underpowered, not designed to study neurodevelopmental outcomes, and lack comparison groups and control for confounders, all of which limits interpretation of the results. Factors modifying the child's long-term neurodevelopment are pharmacokinetic properties of the drug, time of exposure, dose and rate of administration, comorbidity, severity of maternal depression, stress-associated teratogenicity, maternal and fetal genetic characteristics, interaction with environmental factors, exposure to polytherapy and drugs of abuse, delivery/labour and fetal/neonatal complications, maternal and child infections, socio-economic status and child placements. All these factors should be considered when such studies are designed.

Neonatal effects

An increasing body of research has reported that the use of SSRIs during the third trimester or prior to delivery is associated with clinical neonatal signs involving the respiratory, digestive and central nervous systems. Chambers et al. (1996) reported that 23 out of 73 neonates who had been exposed to fluoxetine during the third trimester exhibited respiratory difficulties, cyanosis on feeding and jitteriness, and termed this group of nonspecific signs 'poor neonatal adaptation syndrome' (PNAS). Self-limited PNAS includes symptoms of irritability, constant crying, shivering, increased muscle tone, eating and sleeping difficulties, and convulsions. An increased requirement for neonatal intensive care occurs in approximately 30% of the neonatal population exposed to SSRIs in late gestation (Nordeng and Spigset 2005, Sivojelezova et al. 2005, Maschi et al. 2008). Little consideration has been given to the long-term neurocognitive outcomes of children presenting with PNAS, as the research is scarce, and studies designed to directly assess these effects are lacking.

Long-term neurodevelopment of infants and children exposed to selective serotonin reuptake inhibitors and tricyclic antidepressants (Tables 5.1, 5.2)

Oberlander et al. (2002) found reduced behavioural pain response and increased para-sympathetic cardiac modulation on the second day of life in infants exposed to prolonged prenatal SSRI medication. This cohort was reassessed at the age of 2 months, showing the same autonomic abnormalities in exposed children. Neurodevelopmental assessment with the Bayley Scales of Infant Development (Bayley 1993) at age 2 and 8 months did not show differences among the groups on Mental Development and Psychomotor Developmental Indices when compared with healthy controls (Oberlander et al. 2004, 2005).

Misri and Sivertz (1991) reported 18 children, prospectively collected and exposed to TCAs during either the first trimester (n=9, age range 6–36 months) or the second and third trimesters (n=9, age range 3–18 months). A total of 15 children were exposed to imipramine, and three were exposed to clomipramine. The imipramine dose ranged from 100 to 250 mg/day, while clomipramine was administered at 200 mg/day. Children were assessed for physical health and neurodevelopment every six months. Although not showing the neurodevelopmental test results, the authors reported developmental progress as normal for chronological age. The Child Behavior Checklist (Achenbach 1991), revised McCarthy Scales of Child Ability (McCarthy 1972), and the Stanford–Binet (revised) test (Roid 2003) were used. Strengths of the report include its prospective, longitudinal design with the exclusion of polytherapy and comorbidity (which may adversely affect the child's outcome), and controls with untreated depression. The study was limited by sample size.

Nulman et al. (1997), using a prospectively collected Motherisk database, designed a study to identify the neurocognitive development of children exposed to fluoxetine in the first trimester (n=37) and throughout pregnancy (n=18), and compared the outcomes with two comparison groups: children exposed to TCAs (n=80), and children not exposed to teratogens born to healthy mothers with no history of psychiatric illness (n=84). Of the 80 children exposed to TCAs, 29 were exposed to amitriptyline, 20 to imipramine, 10 to clomipramine, 9 to desipramine, 8 to nortriptyline, and 1 each to maprotiline, doxepin, amoxapine and trimipramine. Excluded were children exposed to polytherapy and drugs of abuse. Children's ages ranged from 15 to 71 months, and they were tested by a psychometrist (masked to the child's grouping) using standardized, age-appropriate psychological tests, which included neurocognitive development, temperament and behavioural tests (Bayley Scales of Infant Development, McCarthy Scales of Children's Abilities, Carey Temperament Scale, Child Behavior Checklist and the Reynell Developmental Language Scale). Multiple regression analysis of the effect of the duration of antidepressant drug therapy (first trimester vs the entire pregnancy) revealed no significant differences on any of the neurobehavioural tests. No statistically significant differences were found between children exposed and unexposed to antidepressants in utero on the primary outcomes. There were also no significant differences in temperament in either drug group when compared to the controls; likewise, no significant differences in mood scores, arousability, activity level, distractability or behavioural problems were noted. The study results did not show an association between antidepressants and neurotoxicity.

Nulman et al. (2002) utilized a similar design to assess 40 children between the ages of 15 and 71 months, exposed to fluoxetine throughout gestation, and 46 children exposed to TCAs (18 to amitriptyline, 12 to imipramine, 7 to clomipramine, 3 to desipramine, 8 to nortriptyline, 2 to doxepin, and 1 to maprotiline) throughout gestation. Using standardized psychological tests, it was reported that exposure to antidepressants had no adverse affect on a child's global IQ, language or behaviour development when compared with 36 unexposed children of healthy non-depressed mothers. Moreover, no differences among the SSRI, TCA and control groups were detected across the nine temperament scales or three behavioural scales of the Child Behavior Checklist. However, the duration of maternal depression and number of depressive episodes after delivery were negative significant predictors for child's cognitive index and language scores, respectively. In contrast, treatment for maternal depression was a significant positive predictor for language development.

Heikkinen et al. (2002) assessed the effect on children exposed to citalopram in utero and during lactation using a prospectively designed study. Eleven children exposed to citalopram throughout gestation were matched to 10 children from a comparison group with no medication exposure. Ten of the mothers were taking citalopram prior to conception, while one started medication at 20 weeks of pregnancy. Developmental assessments were performed by physiotherapists and paediatricians at 2 weeks, 2, 6 and 12 months, and neurological development for all infants was normal at 1 year of age. Heikkinen et al. (2003) assessed children exposed to 20–40 mg/day of fluoxetine during pregnancy and lactation. Ten women "not taking psychotropic medications" were prospectively matched for confounding obstetric characteristics (age, gravidity, parity, gestational weeks and mode of delivery) and served as a control group. Tested with a modified Gesell developmental schedule (Gesell and Amatruda 1941), including gross/fine motor functioning, tonus, speech development, sensory screening and social behaviour, children were examined at 2, 6 and 12 months of age, and results revealed that there were no neurological differences between the control group children and exposed children. While the studies were limited by small sample size, the finding that therapeutic doses of citalopram and fluoxetine deliver safe outcomes during the first year of life is reassuring.

In a study by Reebye et al. (2002), 24 mother–infant pairs exposed to SSRI monotherapy for depression (paroxetine n=13, fluoxetine n=7, setraline n=4) were assessed. Fourteen additional mother–child pairs were exposed to an SSRI and clonazepam (paroxetine + clonazepam, n=12; fluoxetine + clonazepam, n=2) for depression and anxiety. A group of 23 healthy mother–infant pairs, unexposed to any pharmacotherapy, were assessed as controls. At age 2 months all children were assessed using the Bayley Scales of Infant Development, and no differences were seen on the Mental Development and Psychomotor Development indices. Mothers with depression and anxiety from the SSRIs + clonazepam group reported more infants in the 'difficult' temperament category and fewer in the 'easy' category of the Early Infancy Temperament Questionnaire (Carey and McDevitt 1978) when compared with SSRI and control groups. Lastly, more "sober" behaviour was observed in infants from the control group during feeding when compared with the infants in both drug-exposed groups.

The impact of prenatal SSRI and TCA exposure on infant development was assessed by Simon et al. (2002), drawing samples from Group Health Cooperative, a prepaid health plan database. All children were between 4 and 6 months of age. One hundred and eighty-five children were exposed to SSRIs (129 to fluoxetine, 32 to sertraline, and 28 to paroxetine) with some exposed to polytherapy; 209 children were exposed to TCAs, including 66 exposed to amitriptyline, 49 to imipramine, 36 to doxepin, 33 to nortriptyline, and 22 to desipramine. Both groups with antidepressant exposure were matched to comparison groups unexposed to SSRIs and TCAs (185 and 209, respectively). Mothers in all four groups were matched for age at delivery, and neonates were matched for gestational age. The cohorts exposed to antidepressants were matched for "lifetime use of antidepressants" and "lifetime history of psychiatric treatment". Antidepressant-exposed participants were frequency matched to unexposed comparison groups by maternal age. While SSRI exposure in late pregnancy was associated with shorter duration of gestation and lower Apgar scores, there was no association between SSRI or TCA exposure and developmental delay when compared with unexposed controls. When comprehending the study results, consideration should be given to the use of a database for drug dispensing records, which may present compliance issues; paediatrician reports relying on routinely collected data used in place of standardized psychological tests; and a failure to account for confounders.

Yaris et al. (2004) followed 17 infants with exposure in the first trimester to antidepressants, antipsychotics and antiepileptic polytherapy for up to one year (see Table 5.1 for drug description). Using the Revised Denver Developmental Screening Test (DDST-R) (Frankenburg et al. 1970) for mental and motor development, the authors found no developmental or congenital abnormalities in any of the children. Results should be accepted cautiously because of small sample size, use of different antipsychotic drugs, polytherapy, and the lack of a comparison group. Using a prospective cohort, Yaris et al. (2005) followed 80 women exposed to psychotropic drug polytherapy: 53 were exposed to antipsychotics, 58 to anxiolytics, 59 to TCAs, 74 to SSRIs, and 7 to monoamine oxidase inhibitors (see Table 5.1). Although the authors reported that no mental or motor developmental abnormality was found using the DDST-R in children followed up to 1 year of age, results cannot be applied to individual drug groups.

Oberlander et al. (2004) evaluated the outcome of 46 newborn infants with prenatal exposure to an SSRI alone (paroxetine n=17, fluoxetine n=7, sertraline n=4) or in combination

TABLE 5.1

Summary of studies describing no negative effects of antidepressant exposure in utero

Study	Participants/exposure	Age of children tested (months)	Drug and dose (mg/day)	Results
Misri and Sivertz (1991)	Women who conceived on TCAs, n=9 (group 1) Women treated with TCAs during pregnancy, n=9 (group 2) Women prescribed TCAs during lactation, n=20 Women who refused treatment during lactation but were clinically depressed, n=5	6–36	TCAs (n=18), 125–250	Developmental processes were normal for chronological age; CBCL, McCarthy Scales of Child Ability (revised) and Stanford–Binet (revised) were administered. Group 1 – imipramine (n=8) – clomipramine (n=1) Group 2 – imipramine (n=7) – clomipramine (n=2)
Nulman et al. (1997)	Mother–child pairs exposed to fluoxetine throughout gestation, n=55 Mother–child pairs exposed to TCAs throughout gestation, n=80 Mother–child pairs not exposed to teratogens, n=84	16–86	TCAs (n=80) – amitriptyline (n=29) – imipramine (n=20) – clomipramine (n=10) – desipramine (n=9) – nortriptyline (n=8) – maprotiline (n=1) – doxepin (n=1) – amoxapine (n=1) – trimipramine (n=1) Fluoxetine (n=55) Dosages not specified	Children were given age-appropriate versions of the BSID, McCarthy Scales of Children's Abilities, Carey Temperament Scales, Achenbach Behavior Checklist, and Reynell Developmental Language Scales. There were no significant differences in temperament, mood, activity level, behaviour, language development or global IQ between the three groups of children
Heikkinen et al. (2002)	Mothers taking citalopram, n=11 Control group, no medication, n=10	12	Citalopram (n=11), 20–40	Physiotherapist and paediatrician clinical examination showed normal development in exposed children followed up to 1 year of age
Nulman et al. (2002)	Mother–child pairs exposed to fluoxetine throughout gestation, n=40 Mother–child pairs exposed to TCAs throughout gestation, n=46 Mother–child pairs not exposed to teratogens, n=36	15–71	TCAs (n=46) – amitriptyline (n=18) – imipramine (n=12) – clomipramine (n=7) – desipramine (n=3) – nortriptyline (n=8) – doxepin (n=2) – maprotiline (n=1) Fluoxetine (n=40), 20–80	Neither TCAs nor fluoxetine were significantly associated with child's behaviour, language development or global IQ. BSID-II, McCarthy Scales of Children's Abilities, Toddler Temperament Scale, Reynell Language Development Scale, and CBCL were used to test outcomes in children

[continues over]

TABLE 5.1
(continued)

Study	Participants/exposure	Age of children tested (months)	Drug and dose (mg/day)	Results
Reebye et al. (2002)	SSRIs alone, n=24 SSRIs+, n=14 Healthy women and their healthy infants, n=23 Various exposures in pregnancy and within 3 months postpartum	2	SSRIs alone (n=24) – paroxetine (n=13) – fluoxetine (n=7) – sertraline (n=4) Mean dose: 20 SSRIs+ (n=14) – paroxetine+rivotril (n=18) – fluoxetine+rivotril (n=2) – sertraline+rivotril (n=1) Mean dose: 19	No differences found between the three groups on BSID at age 2 months
Simon et al. (2002)	Exposed to SSRIs, n=185 Exposed to TCAs, n=209 Filled or refilled prescriptions during the 360 days before delivery. Two matched unexposed groups: Not exposed group 1, n=185 Not exposed group 2, n=209	36	TCAs: – amitriptyline (n=66) – imipramine (n=49) – doxepin (n=36) – nortriptyline (n=33) – desipramine (n=22) SSRIs: – fluoxetine (n=129) – sertraline (n=32) – paroxetine (n=28) Dosage not specified	Neither TCA nor SSRI exposure was significantly associated with developmental delays. Motor and speech delay examined through standardized physical examination records from paediatric health monitoring visits
Heikkinen et al. (2003)	Mothers taking fluoxetine during pregnancy, n=11 Mothers unexposed to psychotropic medication during pregnancy, n=10	2–12	Fluoxetine (n=11), 20–40	Modified Gesell developmental schedules showed normal development in exposed children
Oberlander et al. (2004)	Pregnant women exposed to SSRIs alone or SSRIs + benzodiazepines: Exposed, n=46 Not exposed, n=23	2–8	SSRI only (n=28): – paroxetine (n=17) – fluoxetine (n=7) – sertraline (n=4)	No significant differences noted between exposed and not exposed groups on BSID performed at 2 and 8 months of age

[continues over]

Study		Population	Drugs/doses	Findings
		Majority exposed in first trimester and continued throughout pregnancy	SSRI+benzodiazepine (n=18): – paroxetine (n=16) – fluoxetine (n=2) Clonazepam dose range: 0.25–1.75 Paroxetine mean dose: 21.2 Fluoxetine mean dose: 16.5 Sertraline mean dose: 68.8	
Yaris et al. (2004)	12	Women on newer antidepressants for major depressive disorder (n=21) in first trimester	Venlafaxine (n=10) dose range: 75–225 Mirtazapine/+ (n=8) dose range: 30–60 Nefazodone (n=2) dose: 200, 400 Venlafaxine + mirtazapine (n=1)	No association found between exposure to newer antidepressants and developmental outcomes using the DDST-R
Yaris et al. (2005)	12	Women exposed to psychotropic drugs during pregnancy for depression, anxiety and psychotic disorders Exposed, n=80 Unexposed, n=248	TCAs (n=59): – clomipramine (n=13) – amytriptyline (n=27) – maprotiline (n=3) – opipramol (n=8) – mianserin (n=5) – tianeptine Na (n=2) – trazodone (n=1) MAO inhibitors (n=7) – moclobamide (n=7) SSRIs (n=74) – fluoxetine (n=17) – sertraline (n=16) – venlafaxine (n=11) – fluvoxamine (n=9) – citalopram (n=7) – mirtazapine (n=7) – paroxetine (n=4) – nefazodone (n=2) – escitalopram (n=1)	No cognitive or motor developmental abnormality was found using DDST-R

TABLE 5.1
(continued)

Study	Participants/exposure	Age of children tested (months)	Drug and dose (mg/day)	Results
Misri et al. (2006)	During pregnancy, n=22 Not exposed, n=14	48–60	Paroxetine (n=14) mean dose: 23.57 Fluoxetine (n=5) mean dose: 18.00 Sertraline (n=3) mean dose: 91.67	CBCL (internalizing behavior subscales) and Child–Teacher Report Form revealed exposure to psychotropic medication during pregnancy was not associated with increased reports of internalizing behaviours at 4 years of age
Oberlander et al. (2007)	Exposed, n=22 Not exposed, n=14	48	During pregnancy: – paroxetine (n=13) median dose: 20 – fluoxetine (n=6) median dose: 20 – sertraline (n=3) median dose: 73 At 4-year follow-up: – paroxetine (n=7) median dose: 40 – fluoxetine (n=4) median dose: 40 – sertraline (n=4) median dose: 35 – venlafaxine (n=3) median dose: 75 – citalopram (n=3) median dose: 20	Externalizing behaviours did not differ between groups using parent–teacher reports and laboratory-based observations

TCA = tricyclic antidepressant; SSRI = selective serotonin reuptake inhibitor; MAO = monoamine oxidase; CBCL = Child Behavior Checklist; BSID = Bayley Scales of Infant Development; DDST-R = Denver Developmental Screening Test, Revised.

with clonazepam (paroxetine n=16, fluoxetine n=2). A group of 23 mother–child pairs un-exposed to antidepressant or psychotropic medication and with no history of mental illness was used as a control. Most of the women began antidepressant medication during their first trimester and continued throughout their entire pregnancy. All infants were assessed between the ages of 2 and 8 months using the Bayley Scales of Infant Development. While the sample size may have been small, symptoms were self-limited, and study results showed no differences between Bayley Scales of Infant Development outcomes in children exposed and unexposed to medication, or in those with and without neonatal symptoms.

Misri et al. (2006) evaluated internalizing behaviours in 4-year-olds exposed prenatally to SSRIs alone or in combination with clonazepam, using a cohort previously assessed in the neonatal period and at 3 and 8 months of age. Internalizing behaviours, such as emotional reactivity, depression, anxiety, irritability and withdrawal, are considered behaviours that are directed internally in contrast to externalizing behaviours such as noncompliance, verbal and physical acts, disruption, emotional outbursts, etc. While externalizing behaviours often develop into externalizing disorders, such as attention deficit disorder, internalizing behaviour disorders are less obvious and more often overlooked and undertreated. Twenty-two mother–child dyads were recruited for the study, with 14 comparison pairs of healthy, non-depressed mothers unexposed to medication during pregnancy. Mothers in the exposed group were prescribed paroxetine (n=14), fluoxetine (n=5), or sertraline (n=3); 9 of these women were also administered clonazepam as well, making up the SSRI/clonazepam group. Information on the child was obtained though Child–Teacher Report Forms and the Child Behavior Checklist, specifically reporting on internalizing behaviours. Although exposed children showed significant levels of internalizing behaviour scores when compared with unexposed children, medication was not a significant predictor of this outcome, whereas maternal mood was. The same cohort was assessed for externalizing behaviour (Oberlander et al. 2007), showing no significant differences between behaviours of children in the study or control group. Increased externalizing behaviours were significantly associated with maternal depression and anxiety. Increased aggression scores were associated with a history of poor neonatal adaptation. Both poor neonatal adaptation and parental stress were suggested as "important" predictors of child behaviour, although not reaching statistical significance. Mean aggressiveness (negativity with mother + interaction with mother + roughness with toys) composite scores were significantly higher in children with a history of poor neonatal adaptation compared with children without such a history. Bayley Scales of Infant Development scores at 8 months were not predictive of subsequent child behaviour. The authors acknowledge the limitations of studying children only at birth and again at 4 years of age, as this method does not account for socialization in the home and at school, which contributes to development between the observation periods. Another speculation of the study is that depressed mothers might have a lower tolerance for behavioural aggression, and may thus misreport increases in this behaviour.

Nulman and coworkers' most recent study examined the long-term neurodevelopmental outcomes of children exposed to venlafaxine (a serotonin and norepinephrine reuptake in-hibitor) in utero using a prospectively collected database at the Hospital for Sick Children, Toronto (I Nulman, preliminary data, unpublished). Venlafaxine-exposed children (n=62)

TABLE 5.2

Summary of studies describing adverse neurocognitive outcome to antidepressant exposure

Study	Participants/exposure	Age of children tested (months)	Drug and dose (mg/day)	Results
Casper et al. (2003)	Depressed + medication + psychotherapy, n=31 Depressed + psychotherapy only, n=13	6–40	Sertraline (n=15) median dose: 113.2 Fluoxetine (n=7) median dose: 20 Paroxetine (n=8) median dose: 17.2 Fluvoxamine (n=1) median dose: 50	No significant differences in mental developmental index between unexposed and exposed children. Exposed children scored significantly lower on the BSID PDI and the Motor Quality factor of the BRS than unexposed children. Exposed children were rated significantly lower than unexposed children on the PDI and the BRS
Mortensen et al. (2003)	Exposure to antidepressants, n=50 No exposure, n=755	7–10	No separation of antidepressant drugs	Higher prevalence of abnormal Boel test in exposed children (16% vs 4%)

BSID = Bayley Scales of Infant Development; PDI = Psychomotor Developmental Index; BRS = Behavioral Rating Scale.

68

were compared with two comparison groups of children, one exposed to SSRIs (n=55), the other not exposed to teratogens (n=55). Drugs of exposure in the SSRI group included citalopram (n=18, 10–40 mg/day), fluoxetine (n=11, 15–60 mg/day), paroxetine (n=20, 10–30 mg/day), sertraline (n=12, 20–125 mg/day), and fluvoxamine (n=1, 250 mg/day average dose). Groups were individually matched for maternal age at conception, child's age at testing and sex. Children were assessed using standardized psychological tests measuring cognition, behaviour and temperament. Child's Full Scale IQ (WPPSI) was the primary outcome measure. Children not exposed to teratogens achieved significantly higher Full Scale IQ scores than venlafaxine- and SSRI-exposed children [112.3, standard deviation (SD) 11 vs 104.7, SD 14, p=0.014, and 112.3, SD 11 vs 105.1, SD 13.4, p=0.02, respectively). Significant predictors for these outcomes were maternal IQ and child's sex. On the Conners Parent Rating Scales, children in the venlafaxine-exposed group achieved worse T scores than healthy controls on Emotional Lability, Total Index, Inattentive, Hyperactive and DSM Total subscales. Children exposed to SSRIs also obtained worse T scores on the Emotional Lability and Total Index subscales. Furthermore, children exposed to venlafaxine and SSRIs demonstrated significantly poorer outcomes on the Emotional Reactive, Anxious–Depressed, Somatic Complaints, DSM Anxiety Problems, Internalizing Problems and Total Problems subscales of the Child Behavior Checklist. Significant predictors for these outcomes were group, severity of maternal depression during pregnancy and at time of child testing, and number of depressive episodes after delivery. Genetic and environmental factors are both strongly associated with children's intelligence and behaviour. Children of mothers with depression may be at increased risk for future psychopathology.

While the results of the aforementioned studies were reassuring in reporting no differences between exposed and unexposed children in neurodevelopmental outcomes, two studies found undesirable neurodevelopmental outcomes in exposed children (Table 5.2). Casper et al. (2003) compared 31 children between the ages of 6 and 40 months whose mothers took SSRIs (sertraline n=15, fluoxetine n=7, paroxetine n=8, and fluvoxamine n=1) during pregnancy with 13 children whose mothers elected not to treat their depression. Average doses of sertraline, fluoxetine and paroxetine were approximated to 113 mg/day, 20 mg/day and 17 mg/day respectively. All children were assessed using the Bayley Scales of Infant Development. Although no differences in the Mental Development Index were observed between the groups, children exposed to SSRIs achieved lower scores on the Psychomotor Developmental Index and Behavioral Rating Scale. The study was limited by the small sample size and insufficient statistical power, as well as the use of a self-rating scale to control for depressive symptoms, self-report of drug and alcohol abuse, and a lack of age matching for children being tested.

Mortensen et al. (2003) examined children whose mothers redeemed prescriptions for antidepressants, neuroleptics, antiepileptics and benzodiazepines during pregnancy. Children were assessed using a Boel test, a psychomotor development test that includes screening tests for hearing, sight and motor attention (Junker et al. 1982). Exposed children between the ages of 7 and 10 months had a higher prevalence of abnormal Boel test scores. Out of the 50 children exposed in utero to antidepressants, 8 showed abnormal Boel test results. However, the association between drug exposure and abnormal test results may be explained by uncontrolled confounders, such as the mother's underlying disease or psychological disorder, and postnatal social environment. Since the test was not administered in a standardized setting, unequal testing circumstances may easily account for differences in test results.

Although some studies assessing neurocognitive outcome present contradictory results showing motor and behavioural impairments in a small number of children, the results from a majority of studies with better design and methodology are reassuring. Approximately 400 children over the age of 8 months exposed to SSRIs and over 650 exposed to various reuptake inhibitors exhibited no differences in neurodevelopment when compared with their controls. During fetal development, many neuroactive molecules may change their functional role in the CNS and affect differentiation, neuronal growth and the establishment of a neuronal network in the immature CNS, while switching to a more modulatory role in the ongoing traffic of the mature CNS. Monoamine neurotransmitters develop early in embryogenesis mediating differentiation and neuronal growth. Their circuitry, maturation and functioning may be altered by substances that are toxic to their receptors (Durig and Hornung 2000). Pharmacological blocking of endogenous activity of neurotransmitters was found to be associated with fetal respiration suppression, and death, and impaired wiring of neural network in early life and in neonatal adaptation. Prenatal or neonatal stress as well as different medications may interfere with the wiring and cause long-term behavioural effects (Herlenius and Lagercrantz 2001). Changes in receptor subunits may impact the plasticity of the immature brain and subsequent memory storage and preservation in the adult brain (Fox et al. 1992). If the synthesis of some of these neurotransmitters or modulators is blocked pharmacologically, it does not seem to affect survival or even important physiological function, illustrating the plasticity of the brain during early development. Other neuroactive agents seem to be able to take over (Herlenius and Lagercrantz 2001).

More studies on the long-term neurocognitive effects of these drugs are necessary to corroborate current findings.

Psychosis in women
Psychosis has a higher incidence rate in women of childbearing years, and when untreated in pregnancy is associated with adverse immediate and long-term pregnancy outcomes (Kirkbride et al. 2006, MacCabe et al. 2007). Pharmacotherapy is often indicated and unavoidable. The potential teratogenic risk associated with exposure to antipsychotic medications should be weighed against the risks of untreated psychosis for both mother and child. Optimization of mothers' mental health is a critical public concern.

Psychosis is characterized by severe disturbances in emotion, thought and perception of reality. Although antipsychotic medications were primarily designed to treat schizophrenia, their clinical use is quickly expanding to other disorders with CNS involvement, including systemic diseases, drug-induced psychosis, and bipolar, major depressive and schizoaffective disorders (Baldessarini and Tarazi 2006, Gentile 2007, Newport et al. 2007). Estimates of the lifetime prevalence of psychotic disorder range from 1.5% to 3.1% (Bland 1984, van Os et al. 2001, Perälä et al. 2007); however, 4.2–17.5% of the general population may require treatment for psychotic symptoms (van Os et al. 2000). The epidemiology of psychosis in pregnancy is currently unknown, although it is documented that affective psychosis occurs more frequently in females than males (Bland 1984).

UNTREATED PSYCHOSIS

It is evident that the hazards associated with untreated psychosis during pregnancy cannot be overlooked, as they pose a significant threat to the well-being of both mother and child. Discontinuation of effective pharmacotherapy often results in relapse (Casiano and Hawkins 1987, Carpenter et al. 1990, Altshuler and Szuba 1994), and in turn may lead to increased morbidity, chronicity and mortality (Tohen et al. 1990, Post 1992, Oates 2003). The sudden termination of treatment can result in serious withdrawal and may worsen the symptoms of psychosis (Kinon et al. 2000). Active psychosis can impair the mother's ability to take care of herself and her fetus. Evidence suggests that women with psychotic disorders are more likely to suffer from malnutrition (Gjere 2001), and fail to initiate and adhere to pre-natal care regimens (Rudolph et al. 1990, Goodman and Emory 1992, Miller and Finnerty 1996). The stress induced by psychosis may also increase the likelihood that the mother will resort to using substances in an effort to cope (Pinkofsky 2000), as this population of women have a relatively high risk of both substance and alcohol abuse (Menezes et al. 1996). A mother who is out of touch with reality can form a dangerously delusional perception of the pregnancy (Miller 1990, Rudolph et al. 1990), and may even fail to recognize that she is going into labour, and attempt to prematurely deliver the baby herself (Miller 1997). A psychotic episode post partum can lead to suicide, neglect, child maltreatment and even infanticide (D'Orban 1979, Miller 1990, Gjere 2001, Gentile 2004). In the first year post partum, approximately 68% of suicides appear to be attributed to psychosis or major de-pressive disorder (Oates 1996). Uncontrolled psychosis during the postpartum period poses additional threats to mother–infant bonding, and may impair the mother's ability to parent (Mortola 1989, Rudolph et al. 1990). As a result, many of these women inevitably lose custody of their children (Coverdale et al. 1997).

Psychosis during pregnancy is also associated with adverse outcomes for the fetus and neonate. A number of studies suggest that maternal schizophrenia is correlated with a variety of adverse pregnancy outcomes including higher rates of obstetric complications, stillbirths, congenital malformations, and fetal and neonatal deaths (Rieder et al. 1975; Wrede et al. 1980; Sacker et al. 1996; Bennedsen et al. 1999, 2001a,b). Nilsson et al. (2002) reported that women who experience active psychosis during pregnancy are twice as likely to have offspring who are born preterm, are small for gestational age and die during infancy. These adverse birth outcomes were found even when other variables such as smoking, education, parity, age and single motherhood were controlled for, which suggests that psychosis itself poses risks to the fetus.

PSYCHOSIS AND PHARMACOTHERAPY

The high risk of relapse, combined with the adverse impact of uncontrolled psychosis on the mother and fetus, often leads psychiatrists to recommend maintenance of treatment with pharmacotherapy throughout pregnancy (Yaeger et al. 2006). Antipsychotic medications can be broadly divided into two classes: first generation, typical antipsychotics (consisting of three groups: butyrophenones, phenothiazines and thioxanthenes); and second generation, atypical antipsychotics (including amisulpride, aripiprazole, clozapine, olanzapine, quetiapine, risperidone and ziprasidone). Both classes of antipsychotics act as dopamine antagonists. Dopamine is a classic neurotransmitter, but also plays a critical role in brain development (Williams et al. 1992, Holson et al. 1994, Costa et al. 2004). Dopamine receptors fall into two major subtypes: D1-like (D1, D5) and D2-like (D2, D3, D4) (Jones and Pilowsky 2002). Antipsychotic drugs are thought to be effective mainly because they block the action of D2 receptors in the brain.

When typical antipsychotics were first introduced in the 1950s, they revolutionized the treatment of psychosis; however, these medications did not come without costs. This group of drugs are associated with substantial risk of adverse side-effects including extrapyramidal effects (secondary to striatal D2 receptor blockage) and hyperprolactinaemia (secondary to pituitary D2 blockage) (Jones and Pilowsky 2002). The increased release of prolactin may cause hypogonadism and menstrual dysfunction, leading to infertility (Baldessarini and Tarazi 2006, O'Keane 2008). The severity of the adverse side-effects was the impetus for the later development of atypical antipsychotics, which are differentiated by their substantially improved side-effect profile. Atypical antipsychotics emerged as the preferable treatment, consequently increasing fertility rates and decreasing institutionalization (Odegard 1980, Miller et al. 1992, Gentile 2010). As a result, approximately 60% of women with a psychotic disorder have a child, which is roughly equivalent to the birth rate for the general population (Howard et al. 2001, Seeman 2004). Accordingly, a significant number of children will inevitably be exposed to antipsychotic medications during gestation. Considering that atypical antipsychotics cross the placenta and thus are potentially teratogenic (Hammond and Toseland 1970, Newport et al. 2007), the lack of knowledge regarding the reproductive safety of these drugs may pose a serious public health concern.

Neonatal effects
Long-term CNS sequelae may result from exposure to pharmacotherapy at any time during pregnancy (Austin and Mitchell 1998, Yaeger et al. 2006). It is well documented that neonates exposed to antipsychotic drugs in utero may experience extrapyramidal symptoms for up to 10 months, primarily when exposed to typical antipsychotics (Tamer et al. 1969, Levy and Wisniewski 1974, Cleary 1977, O'Connor et al. 1981). Furthermore, exposure to these drugs in the third trimester increases tremulousness, hypertonicity and poor motor maturity in neonates (Auerbach et al. 1992).

Long-term neurodevelopment of infants and children exposed to antipsychotics
(see Tables 5.2, 5.3)
Kris (1961) described the neurodevelopment of children exposed to 50–150mg/day of chlorpromazine during gestation (n=17). Although the author states that all children underwent psychological testing, only qualitative data on three selected children are presented. The children, who were aged between 4 and 5 years, were described as "seeming normal" with "at least average" to "somewhat above-average intelligence". The development of all the other children in the group was said to be similar to the three reported cases. In a

follow-up study, Kris (1965) reported on the neurodevelopmental progress of the same group of children. Two of the children were re-tested at the age of 9, and a brief qualitative description indicating normal intellectual and behavioural development is provided. Once again, the author states that the findings for all the other children in the group are fundamentally similar to the two reported cases.

Ayd (1964) described the development of children exposed to chlorpromazine from conception to birth (n=16) or after the first trimester (n=11). The author conducted intermittent follow-ups with parents, family doctors or paediatricians. At the time of publication, all children were between 1 and 7 years of age. Although no formal testing was conducted, all children seemed to display average intelligence, and no child displayed problematic emotional or behavioural development.

In a study of 28 358 mother–child pairs, the IQ scores of children exposed to phenothiazines in utero (n=2141) were compared with those of children with no history of exposure (n=26 217) (Slone et al. 1977). IQ scores were measured at 4 years of age using the Stanford–Binet Intelligence Scale. Scores were standardized by analysis of covariance for a variety of factors including socioeconomic status and maternal education. Analysis of the adjusted mean IQ scores showed no significant difference between groups.

Kato and Arai (1990) published a case series of five women who began treatment with haloperidol between 11 and 34 weeks of gestation. The dosage of haloperidol ranged from 2 to 25 mg/day, and three of the five women required polytherapy with either carbamazepine or levomepromazine. Children were tested between the ages of 2 months and 2 years, using Enjoji's Infant Analysis Development Test, which is a standardized test used to assess language, social and motor development. For two children who were lost to follow-up, information on developmental outcome was obtained by reviewing the child's most recent medical charts. The overall development of all children was described as normal; however, all children displayed similar strengths and weaknesses in their developmental profile.

Stika et al. (1990) investigated the effects of in utero exposure to phenothiazines on the academic behaviour of children. Sixty-eight children between the ages of 9 and 10, who were exposed to either chlorpromazine or chlorprothixene during gestation, were included in the study. The control group consisted of randomly selected children matched to the exposed group for child's age at testing and maternal age at parturition. The names of both the exposed and control students were sent to their teachers; however, the teachers were blinded to the exposure status of the student. Teachers were then asked to select another student in the same class as the study student, to serve as an additional control group. The neuroleptic-exposed children and controls were compared with their teacher-selected controls in six domains: disobedient vs obedient, awkward vs handy, untalented vs very bright, apathetic vs diligent, unconcentrated vs attentive, and restless vs inhibited. No significant differences were found between the neuroleptic-exposed children and either of the two control groups.

Mortensen et al. (2003) assessed the psychomotor development of infants who were prenatally exposed to antidepressants, antiepileptics, benzodiazepines or neuroleptics (n=340). A total of 63 infants were exposed to neuroleptics. Infants whose mothers had not redeemed prescriptions for any of the above medications were randomly selected as controls (n=755). A registered nurse assessed the psychomotor development of all infants between

TABLE 5.3

Summary of studies describing long-term outcome following prenatal exposure to antipsychotics

Study	Participants/exposure	Age of children tested	Drug and dose (mg/day)	Results
Kris (1961)	Mothers exposed to chlorpromazine during pregnancy, following their release from hospitalization due to a psychotic breakdown (n=17)	4–5 years	Chlorpromazine, dose range: 50–150	All children underwent psychological testing, yet the Stanford–Binet Form L is the only test mentioned. All children were described as normal; "at least average intelligence" to "somewhat above-average intelligence"
Ayd (1964)	Women exposed to chlorpromazine from conception to birth (n=16), and mothers who began treatment after the first trimester (n=11)	1–7 years	Chlorpromazine, dose range: 150–900 (n=16) Chlorpromazine, average dose: 200 (n=11)	Intermittent follow-ups with parents, family doctors or paediatricians revealed normal development; "average intelligence" and no behavioural concerns
Kris (1965)	Mothers exposed to chlorpromazine during pregnancy (n=52)	9 years	Chlorpromazine, dose range: 50–150	All children underwent psychological testing, yet the Stanford–Binet Form L is the only test mentioned. All children were described as normal; "average intelligence" to "somewhat above-average intelligence"
Slone et al. (1977)	Mothers exposed to phenothiazines during pregnancy (n=2141), and a control group of mothers with no history of exposure (n=26 217)	4 years	No separation of phenothiazines	IQ scores were measured using the Stanford-Binet Intelligence Scale. Analysis of the adjusted mean IQ scores showed no significant difference between groups
Kato and Arai (1990)	Women exposed to haloperidol during pregnancy, after being hospitalized due to a psychotic breakdown (n=5)	2 months –2 years	Haloperidol, dose range: 2–25 (n=5) Carbamazepine, 300 (n=1) Levomepromazine, dose range: 10–50 (n=2)	Children were assessed using Enjoji's Infant Analysis Development Test, which is widely used in Japan to evaluate children's developmental age. Development was described as normal; however, a pattern of strengths and weakness emerged

Study	Sample	Age	Drug exposure	Findings
Stika et al. (1990)	Women who filled prescriptions for neuroleptics after week 20 of their pregnancy (n=68). Two control groups: one selected randomly from a group of mothers who received other prescriptions during pregnancy (n=68), and one consisting of teacher selected controls (n=68)	9–10 years	Chlorpromazine, 25 (n=3) Chlorpromazine, 10 (n=63) Chlorprothixene, 5 (n=2)	Exposed children were compared with teacher-selected controls in six domains: obedience, handiness, intelligence, diligence, attentiveness and inhibition. No significant differences were found between the exposed children and both controls groups
Mortensen et al. (2003)	Mothers exposed to neuroleptics during pregnancy (n=63), and a control group of mothers with no history of exposure (n=755)	7–10 months	No separation of neuroleptics	All children were administered the Boel test to assess psychomotor development. Results were abnormal in 4% of the control group compared to 16% of the exposed group. The crude odds ratio for an abnormal Boel test was 3.9 for neuroleptics
Yaris et al. (2005)	Women exposed to psychotropic drugs during pregnancy for depression, anxiety and psychotic disorders. Women exposed to antipsychotics (n=53), and women with no exposure (n=248)	1 year	Trifluoperazine (n=17) Thioridazine (n=14) Mesoridazine (n=6) Haloperidol (n=3) Sulpiride (n=6) Zuclopenthixol (n=3) Quetiapine (n=2) Risperidone (n=2)	All children were assessed using the Denver Developmental Screening Test. No mental or motor developmental abnormalities were found

the ages of 7 and 10 months, using the Boel test. The authors defined a score as abnormal when the infant failed one or more of the 14 items. The Boel test was abnormal in 4% of the control group compared with 16% of the exposed group. The crude odds ratio for an abnormal Boel test was 3.9 for neuroleptics.

Yaris et al. (2005) investigated the developmental outcomes of children following in utero exposure to psychotropic drugs (n=124). Fifty-three (43%) children were exposed to antipsychotics (49 typical and 4 atypical). Polytherapy was used in 85% of the women. A total of 248 controls who were not exposed to any medication during gestation were selected using random-sampling procedures. All women taking psychotropic medication for depression or anxiety (but not psychosis) discontinued pharmacotherapy after learning of their pregnancy. Mental and motor development of children was assessed at 12 months, using the Denver Developmental Screening Test. No abnormalities were found in all children exposed to psychotropic drugs during gestation.

The majority of atypical antipsychotics were introduced in the last two decades, and, as a result, the only available data regarding the neurobehavioural outcome of children exposed to this class of medication are gleaned from case reports. Three case reports have been published to date, documenting the developmental outcomes of four children exposed to 2–6mg/day of risperidone throughout pregnancy. No developmental abnormalities were reported up to 1 year of age in three of the four children (Ratnayake and Libretto 2002, McCauley-Elsom and Kulkarni 2007); one child, however, displayed minor delays in motor development at age 2 years, although overall development was still within normal range (Dabbert and Heinze 2006). Two case reports have described child development following prenatal exposure to aripiprazole. One mother discontinued her therapy at the eighth week of gestation but agreed to reinstitute treatment with 10mg/day of aripiprazole after a psychotic relapse at 20 weeks (Mendhekar et al. 2006). The second mother continued treatment with 20mg/day of aripiprazole from the eighth week of pregnancy until birth (Mervak et al. 2008). Both authors reported age-appropriate development, at 6 months and 1 year respectively. Aichhorn et al. (2008) described a woman who continued treatment with 15mg/day of olanzapine throughout pregnancy; her infant's development was reported to be normal at 6 months of age. Four case reports have been published documenting exposure to quetiapine throughout pregnancy. Doses ranged from 50 to 1200mg/day, and polytherapy was required in two of the four cases: fluvoxamine in one case, haloperidol in the other. All four children achieved normal developmental milestones at 1, 2.5, 3 and 6 months of age respectively (Tényi et al. 2002, Taylor et al. 2003, Gentile 2006, Cabuk et al. 2007). Mendhekar (2007) documented delayed speech acquisition in one child following exposure to 100mg/day clozapine throughout gestation. At 1 year of age, the child had normal developmental milestones in all areas except speech; he did not begin to speak fluently until the end of his fifth year.

The majority of the case reports outlined above describe age-appropriate neurodevelopment of children prenatally exposed to atypical antipsychotics; however, data extracted from case reports must be interpreted with caution. A major limitation of all the case reports described is that no specific testing procedures or standardized tests were used to assess child development. In addition, the majority of follow-ups took place between three months and one year after delivery, which may be too early to observe more subtle developmental delays. Interestingly, the only two case reports that continued to follow the child's development beyond 1 year of age found signs of possible delays in development (Dabbert and Heinze 2006, Mendhekar 2007).

The long-term risks associated with in utero exposure to antipsychotic medication have not been elucidated. Although the reports available to date are reassuring, as they do not suggest any significant long-term adverse neurodevelopmental impairments associated with exposure, methodologically sound research is needed to confirm these results. At this point, the benefits of treatment should be weighed carefully against the potential risks for each individual woman.

Summary

Mental health disorders in women represent a major public health concern. With rates of both mental health disorders and unplanned pregnancies in society being extremely high, we expect increasing numbers of children to be exposed to psychotropic medication during gestation.

Untreated mental health disorders in pregnancy are associated with a number of adverse outcomes for both mother and child, including an increased risk for postpartum relapse. Importantly, an association between antidepressant and antipsychotic medications and increased rates of teratology domains (miscarriages, growth impairments, birth defects and impaired functioning) above the baseline for general population in immediate pregnancy outcome was not substantiated by the studies reviewed.

With respect to long-term neurodevelopmental outcomes, child neurodevelopment may be explained by a wide variety of factors other than prenatal medication exposure. Although results in over 1000 children tested were reassuring, future research in behavioural teratology of psychotropic medications should confirm these findings. Studies should consider novel designs, acknowledge the issues of power, control for genetic factors, polytherapy, maternal stress, mental comorbidity, drug doses, time and duration of exposure, and perinatal maternal and neonatal complications.

Presently, concern also centres on the long-term neurodevelopmental outcome of infants exhibiting poor neonatal adaptation. It was reported that the degree of psychiatric comorbidity was a more significant predictor of poor transient neonatal signs than the use of SSRIs. Results of two studies testing a small number of children showed that the long-term neurodevelopment of these neonates did not differ from their unexposed controls. Moreover, thought should be given to the fact that, although about 30% of the 1000 antidepressant- and antipsychotic-exposed children studied are predicted to exhibit poor neonatal adaptation after birth, this impact was not discernable in the long-term neurocognitive test results. What remains unanswered is the incidence and nature of these neonatal signs, as well as the long-term effect on children's behavioural, cognitive and mental health. A prospective longitudinal study following and assessing the neonates presenting with postnatal signs may help to answer many of these questions.

Antidepressant and antipsychotic drugs should not be discontinued if indicated, and the safest medication option should be selected. Adjunctive interpersonal or cognitive–behavioural therapy should be recommended, and psychotherapy should always be incorporated into management, as it may prevent or minimize fetal exposure. Appropriate criteria for treatment algorithms include the course and severity of the disorder, and the safety of the medication indicated. Accurate, evidence-based, up-to-date information on reproductive safety will enable women to select the most appropriate treatment strategy. In understanding the benefits and possible risks of pharmacotherapy and the deleterious effects of untreated mental health disorders both on the mother and on her developing child, the management goal is to minimize the risk to the fetus while limiting maternal morbidity. A careful prenatal assessment (pregnancy planning) allows the best treatment choice. Since none of the decisions are free of risk, it is obligatory that the decision be made in collaboration with the patient, her family and her caring physicians.

Close follow-up should be provided to neonates exposed to antidepressants and anti-psychotics in late pregnancy according to clinical presentation and the pharmacokinetic properties of these drugs. Proper guidelines for optimal management of mental health disorders before conception, during pregnancy and post partum will lead to more favourable pregnancy outcomes for both the mother and her child.

REFERENCES

Achenbach TM (1991) *Manual for the Child Behavior Checklist/4–18 and 1991 Profile.* Burlington, VT: Burlington University of Vermont, Department of Psychiatry.

Achenbach TM, Rescorla LA (2001) *Manual for the ASEBA Preschool Forms and Profiles.* Burlington, VT: University of Vermont, Research Center for Children, Youth, and Families.

Aichhorn W, Yazdi K, Kralovec K, et al. (2008) Olanzapine plasma concentration in a newborn. *J Psycho-pharmacol* **22**: 923–924.

Altshuler LL, Szuba MP (1994) Course of psychiatric disorders in pregnancy. *Neurol Clin* **12**: 613–635.

Altshuler LL, Cohen L, Szuba MP, et al. (1996) Pharmacologic management of psychiatric illness during pregnancy: dilemmas and guidelines. *Am J Psychiatry* **153**: 592–606.

Auerbach JG, Hans SL, Marcus J, Maeir S (1992) Maternal psychotropic medication and neonatal behaviour. *Neurotoxicol Teratol* **14**: 399–406.

Austin MV, Mitchell PB (1998) Psychotropic medications in pregnant women: treatment dilemmas. *Med J Aust* **169**: 428–431.

Ayd FJ (1964) Children born to mothers treated with chlorpromazine during pregnancy. *Clin Med* **71**: 1758–1763.

Bayley N (1993) *Bayley Scales of Infant Development, 2nd edn.* New York: Psychological Corporation.

Baldessarini RJ, Tarazi FI (2006) Pharmacotherapy of psychosis and mania. In: Brunton LL, Lazo JS, Parker KL, eds. *Goodman & Gilman's The Pharmacological Basis of Therapeutics. 11th edn.* New York: McGraw-Hill, pp 461–500.

Beardslee WR, Bemporad J, Keller MB, Klerman GL (1983) Children of parents with a major affective disorder: a review. *Am J Psychiatry* **140**: 825–832.

Beardslee WR, Versage EM, Gladstone TRG. (1998) Children of affectively ill parents: a review of the past 10 years. *J Am Acad Child Adolesc Psychiatry* **37**: 1134–1141.

Bennedsen BE, Mortensen PB, Olesen AV, Henriksen TB (1999) Preterm birth and intra-uterine growth retardation among children of women with schizophrenia. *Br J Psychiatry* **175**: 239–245.

Bennedsen BE, Mortensen PB, Olesen AV, Henriksen TB (2001a) Congenital malformations, stillbirths, and infant deaths among children of women with schizophrenia. *Arch Gen Psychiatry* **58**: 674–679.

Bennedsen BE, Mortensen PB, Olesen AV, et al. (2001b) Obstetric complications in women with schizophrenia. *Schizophr Res* **47**: 167–175.

Bernstein PS (2000) Autumn in New York – confronting preterm delivery in the 21st century: from molecular intervention to community action. Conference report. *Medscape Ob/Gyn Womens Health* **5** (2).

Bland RC (1984) Long term mental illness in Canada: an epidemiological perspective on schizophrenia and affective disorders. *Can J Psychiatry* **29**: 242–246.

Bolton HL, Hughes PM, Turton P, Sedgwick P (1998) Incidence and demographic correlates of depressive symptoms during pregnancy in an inner London population. *J Psychosom Obstet Gynaecol* **19**: 202–209.

Bostwick JM, Pankratz VC (2000) Affective disorders and suicide risk: a re-examination. *Am J Psychiatry* **157**: 1925–1932.

Bromiker R, Kaplan M (1994) Apparent intrauterine fetal withdrawal from clomipramine hydrochloride. *JAMA* **272**: 1722–1723 (letter).

Burke KC, Burke JD, Rae DS, Regier DA (1991) Comparing age at onset of major depression and other psychiatric disorders by birth cohorts in five US community populations. *Arch Gen Psychiatry* **48**: 789–795.

Cabuk D, Sayin A, Derinöz O, Biri A. (2007) Quetiapine use for the treatment of manic episode during pregnancy. *Arch Womens Ment Health* **10**: 235–236.

Carey WB, McDevitt SC (1978) Revision of the Infant Temperament Questionnaire. *Pediatrics* **61**: 735–739.

Carpenter WT, Hanlon TE, Heinrichs DW, et al. (1990) Continuous versus targeted medication in schizophrenic outpatients: outcome results. *Am J Psychiatry* **147**: 1138–1148.

Casiano ME, Hawkins DR (1987) Major mental illness and child bearing: a role for the consultation–liaison psychiatrist in obstetrics. *Psychiatric Clin North Am* **10**: 35–51.

Casper RC, Fleischer BE, Lee Ancajas JC, et al. (2003) Follow-up of children of depressed mothers exposed or not exposed to antidepressant drugs during pregnancy. *J Pediatr* **4**: 402–408.

Chambers CD, Johnson KA, Dick LM, et al. (1996) Birth outcomes in pregnant women taking fluoxetine. *N Engl J Med* **335**: 1010–1015.

Cleary MF (1977) Fluphenazine decanoate during pregnancy. *Am J Psychiatry* **134**: 815–816.

Cohen LS, Altshuler LL, Harlow BL, et al. (2006) Relapse of major depression during pregnancy in women who maintain or discontinue antidepressant treatment. *JAMA* **295**: 499–507.

Costa LG, Steardo L, Cuomo V (2004) Structural effects and neurofunctional sequelae of developmental exposure to psychotherapeutic drugs: experimental and clinical aspects. *Pharmacol Rev* **56**: 103–147.

Coull JT (1998) Neural correlates of attention and arousal: insights from electrophysiology, functional neuroimaging and psychopharmacology. *Prog Neurobiol* **55**: 343–361.

Coverdale JH, Bayer TL, McCullough LB, Chervenak FA (1993) Respecting the autonomy of chronic mentally ill women in decision about contraception. *Hosp Community Psychiatry* **44**: 671–674.

Coverdale JH, Turbott SH, Roberts H (1997) Family planning needs and STD risk behaviours of female psychiatric outpatients. *Br J Psychiatry* **171**: 69–72.

Cowe L, Lloyd DJ, Dawling S (1982) Neonatal convulsions caused by withdrawal from maternal clomipramine. *BMJ (Clin Res Ed)* **284**: 1837–1838.

Dabbert D, Heinze M (2006) Follow-up of a pregnancy with risperidone microspheres. *Pharmacopsychiatry* **39**: 235.

Davies A, McIvor R, Kumar R (1995) Impact of childbirth on a series of schizophrenic mothers; possible influence of oestrogen on schizophrenia. *Schizophr Res* **16**: 25–31.

Dean C, Kendell RE (1981) The symptomatology of puerperal illness. *Br J Psychiatry* **139**: 128–133.

Deave T, Heron J, Evans J, Emond A (2008) The impact of maternal depression in pregnancy on early child development. *Br J Obstet Gynaecol* **115**: 1043–1051.

D'Orban PT (1979) Women who kill their children. *Br J Psychiatry* **134**: 560–571.

Durig J, Hornung, JP (2000) Neonatal serotonin depletion affects developing and mature mouse cortical neurons. *Neuroreport* **20**: 833–837.

Einarson A, Selby P, Koren G (2001) Abrupt discontinuation of psychotropic drugs during pregnancy: fear of teratogenic risk and impact of counseling. *J Psychiatry Neurosci* **26**: 44–48.

Ellman LM, Huttunen M, Lönqvist J, Cannon D (2007) The effects of genetic liability for schizophrenia and maternal smoking during pregnancy on obstetric complications. *Schizophr Res* **93**: 229–236.

Evans J, Heron J, Francomb H, et al. (2001) Cohort study of depressed mood during pregnancy and after childbirth. *BMJ* **323**: 257–260.

Falterman CG, Richardson CJ (1980) Small left colon syndrome associated with maternal ingestion of psychotropic drugs. *J Pediatr* **97**: 308–310.

Ferguson J (2001) SSRI antidepressant medications: adverse effects and tolerability. *Prim Care Companion J Clin Psychiatry* **3**: 22–27.

Field T (1995) Infants of depressed mothers. *Infant Behav Dev* **18**: 1–13.

Field T, Diego M, Dieter J, et al. (2004) Prenatal depression effects on the fetus and the newborn. *Infant Behav Dev* **27**: 216–229.

Fox K, Henley J, Isaac J (1992) Experience-dependent development of NMDA receptor transmission. *Nat Neurosci* **2**: 297–299.

79

Frankenburg WK, Dodds JB, Fandal A (1970) *The Revised Denver Developmental Screening Test Manual.* Denver: University of Colorado Press.

Fullard W, McDevitt S, Carey W (1978) *The Toddler Temperament Scale.* Philadelphia: Temple University Press.

Gentile S (2004) Clinical utilization of atypical antipsychotics in pregnancy and lactation. *Ann Pharmacother* **38**: 1265–1271.

Gentile S (2006) Quetiapine–fluvoxamine combination during pregnancy and while breastfeeding. *Arch Womens Ment Health* **9**: 158–159 (letter).

Gentile S (2007) Atypical antipsychotics in the treatment of bipolar disorder. More shadow that lights. *CNS Drugs* **21**: 367–387.

Gentile S (2010) Antipsychotic therapy during early and late pregnancy: a systematic review. *Schizophr Bull* **36**: 518–544.

Gesell AJ, Amatruda CS (1941) *Developmental Diagnosis. 2nd edn.* New York: Paul B Hoeber.

Gjere NA. (2001) Psychopharmacology in pregnancy. *J Perinat Neonatal Nurs* **14**: 12–25.

Goodman SH, Emory EK (1992) Perinatal complications in births to low socioeconomic status schizophrenic and depressed women. *J Abnorm Psychol* **101**: 225–229.

Gotlib IH, Whiffen VE, Mount JH, et al. (1989) Prevalence rates and demographic characteristics associated with depression in pregnancy and the postpartum. *J Consult Clin Psychol* **57**: 269–274.

Halbreich U (2004) Prevalence of mood symptoms and depressions during pregnancy: implications for clinical practice and research. *CNS Spectr* **9**: 177–184.

Halligan SL, Herbert J, Goodyer I, Murray L (2004) Exposure to postnatal depression predicts elevated cortisol in adolescent offspring. *Biol Psychiatry* **55**: 376–381.

Hammond JE, Toseland PA (1970) Placental transfer of chlorpromazine. Case report. *Arch Dis Child* **45**: 139–140.

Hansen D, Lou HC, Olsen J (2000) Serious life events and congenital malformations: a national study with complete follow-up. *Lancet* **356**: 875–880.

Hay DF, Kumar R (1995) Interpreting the effects of mothers' postnatal depression on children's intelligence: a critique and reanalysis. *Child Psychiatry Hum Dev* **25**: 165–181.

Heikkinen T, Ekblad U, Kero P, et al. (2002) Citalopram in pregnancy and lactation. *Clin Pharmacol Ther* **72**: 184–191.

Heikkinen T, Ekblad U, Pertti P, Laine K (2003) Pharmacokinetics of fluoxetine and norfluoxetine in pregnancy and lactation. *Clin Pharmacol Ther* **73**: 330–337.

Herlenius E, Lagercrantz H (2001) Neurotransmitters and neuromodulators during early human development. *Early Hum Dev* **65**: 21–37.

Hirschfeld RM, Keller MB, Panico S, et al. (1997) The National Depressive and Manic–Depressive Association consensus statement on the undertreatment of depression. *JAMA* **277**: 333–340.

Hobel CJ, Dunkel-Schtter C, Roesch SC, et al. (1999) Maternal plasma corticotrophin releasing hormone associated with stress at 20 weeks' gestation in pregnancies ending in preterm delivery. *Am J Obstet Gynecol* **180**: S257–S263.

Holson RR, Webb PJ, Grafton TF, Hansen DK (1994) Prenatal neuroleptic exposure and growth stunting in the rat: an in vivo and in vitro examination of sensitive periods and possible mechanisms. *Teratology* **50**: 125–136.

Howard LM, Kumar R, Thornicroft G (2001) Psychosocial characteristics and needs of mothers with psychotic disorders. *Br J Psychiatry* **178**: 427–432.

Huizink A, Robles de Medina PG, Mulder EJH, et al. (2003) Stress during pregnancy is associated with developmental outcome in infancy. *J Child Psychol Psychiatry* **44**: 810–818.

Jameson PB, Gelfand DM, Kulcsar E, Teti D (1997) Mother–toddler interaction patterns associated with maternal depression. *Dev Psychopathol* **9**: 537–550.

Jones HM, Pilowsky LS (2002) Dopamine and antipsychotic drug action revisited. *Br J Psychiatry* **181**: 271–275.

Junker KS, Barr B, Maliniemi S, Wasz-Hockert O (1982) BOEL – a screening program to enlarge the concept of infant health. *Paediatrician* **11**: 85–89.

Kato T, Arai M (1990) Maternal haloperidol effects on pregnancy and development of the children. *Seishin Shinkeigaku Zasshi* **92**: 277–293.

Kinon BJ, Basson RR, Gilmore JA, et al. (2000) Strategies for switching from conventional antipsychotic drugs or risperidone to olanzapine. *J Clin Psychiatry* **61**: 833–840.

Kirkbride JB, Fearon P, Morgan C, et al. (2006) Heterogeneity in incidence rates of schizophrenia and other psychotic syndromes: findings from the 3-center AeSOP study. *Arch Gen Psychiatry* **63**: 250–258.

Kuczynski L, Kochanska G (1990) Development of children's noncompliant strategies from toddlerhood to age five. *Dev Psychol* **26**: 398–408.

Kris EB (1961) Children born to mothers maintained on pharmacotherapy during pregnancy and postpartum. *Recent Adv Biol Psychiatry* **4**: 180–187.

Kris EB (1965) Children of mothers maintained on pharmacotherapy during pregnancy and postpartum. *Curr Ther Res Clin Exp* **7**: 785–789.

Kumar R, Robson MK (1984) A prospective study of emotional disorders of childbearing women. *Br J Psychiatry* **144**: 35–47.

Lappin J (2001) Depressed mood during pregnancy and after childbirth: Time points for assessing perinatal mood must be optimized. *BMJ* **323**: 1367 (letter).

Lazinsky M, Shea A, Steiner M (2008) Effects of maternal prenatal stress on offspring development: a commentary. *Arch Womens Ment Health* **11**: 363–375.

Levy W, Wisniewski K (1974) Chlorpromazine causing extrapyramidal dysfunction. *N Y State J Med* **74**: 684–685.

Lyons-Ruth K, Zoll D, Connell D, Grunebaum HU (1986) The depressed mother and her one-year-old infant: environment, interaction, attachment, and infant development. *New Dir Child Dev* **34**: 61–82.

Lyons-Ruth K, Wolfe R, Lyubchik A (2000) Depression and the parenting of young children: making the case for early preventive mental health services. *Harvard Rev Psychiatry* **8**: 148–153.

MacCabe JH, Martinsson L, Lichtenstein P, et al. (2007) Adverse pregnancy outcomes in mothers with affective psychosis. *Bipolar Disord* **9**: 305–309.

Maschi S, Clavenna A, Campi R, et al. (2008) Neonatal outcome following pregnancy exposure to antidepressants: a prospective controlled cohort study. *BJOG* **115**: 283–289.

McCarthy D (1972) *McCarthy Scales of Children's Abilities.* New York: Psychological Corporation.

McCauley-Elsom K, Kulkarni J (2007) Managing psychosis in pregnancy. *Aust N Z J Psychiatry* **41**: 289–292.

McDevitt SC, Carey WB (1978) The measurement of temperament in 3–7 year old children. *J Child Psychol Psychiatry* **19**: 245–253.

McElhatton PR, Garbis HM, Elefant E, et al. (1996) The outcome of pregnancy in 689 women exposed to therapeutic doses of antidepressants: a collaborative study of the European Network of Teratology Information Services (ENTIS). *Reprod Toxicol* **10**: 285–294.

McLean M, Bisits A, Davies J, et al. (1995) A placental clock controlling the length of human pregnancy. *Nat Med* **1**: 460–463.

Meaney M, Tannenbaum B, Francis D, et al. (1994) Early environmental programming hypothalamic–pituitary–adrenal responses to stress. *Semin Neurosci* **6**: 247–259.

Mendhekar DN (2007) Possible delayed speech acquisition with clozapine therapy during pregnancy and lactation. *J Neuropsychiatry Clin Neurosci* **19**: 196–197 (letter).

Mendhekar DN, Sunder KR, Andrade C (2006) Aripiprazole use in a pregnant schizoaffective woman. *Bipolar Disord* **8**: 299–300.

Menezes PR, Johnson S, Thornicroft G, et al. (1996) Drug and alcohol problems among individuals with severe mental illnesses in south London. *Br J Psychiatry* **168**: 612–619.

Mervak B, Collins J, Valenstein M (2008) Case report of aripiprazole usage during pregnancy. *Arch Womens Ment Health* **11**: 249–250.

Miller LJ (1990) Psychotic denial of pregnancy: phenomenology and clinical management. *Hosp Community Psychiatry* **41**: 1233–1237.

Miller LJ (1997) Sexuality, reproduction and family planning in women with schizophrenia. *Schizophr Bull* **23**: 623–635.

Miller LJ, Finnerty M (1996) Sexuality, pregnancy, and childrearing among women with schizophrenia-spectrum disorders. *Psychiatr Serv* **47**: 502–506.

Miller WH, Bloom JD, Resnick MP (1992) Prenatal care for pregnant chronic mental ill patients. *Hosp Community Psychiatry* **43**: 942–943.

Misri S, Sivertz K (1991) Tricyclic drugs in pregnancy and lactation: a preliminary report. *Int J Psychiatry Med* **21**: 157–171.

Misri S, Reebye P, Kendrick K, et al. (2006) Internalizing behaviors in 4-year-old children exposed in utero to psychotropic medications. *Am J Psychiatry* **163**: 1026–1032.

Morse CA, Buist A, Durkin S (2000) First-time parenthood: influences on pre and postnatal adjustment in fathers and mothers. *J Psychosom Obstet Gynaecol* **21**: 109–120.

81

Mortensen JT, Olsen J, Larsen H, et al. (2003) Psychomotor development in children exposed in utero to benzodiazepines, antidepressants, neuroleptics, and anti-epileptics. *Eur J Epidemiol* **18**: 769–771.

Mortola JF (1989) The use of psychotropic agents in pregnancy and lactation. *Psychiatr Clin North Am* **12**: 69–87.

Murray L (1992) The impact of postnatal depression on infant development. *J Child Psychol Psychiatry* **33**: 543–561.

Murray L, Cooper P (1997) Effects of postnatal depression on infant development. *Arch Dis Child* **77**: 99–101.

Murray L, Hipwell A, Hooper R, et al. (1996) The cognitive development of 5 year old children of postnatally depressed mothers. *J Child Psychol Psychiatry* **37**: 927–935.

Netter P, Hennig J, Roed IS (1996) Serotonin and dopamine as mediators of sensation seeking behaviour. *Neuropsychobiology* **34**: 155–165.

Newport DJ, Wilcox MM, Stowe ZN (2001) Antidepressants during pregnancy and lactation: defining exposure and treatment issues. *Semin Perinatol* **25**: 177–190.

Newport D, Calamaras MR, DeVane CL, et al. (2007) Atypical antipsychotics administration during late pregnancy: placental passage and obstetrical outcomes. *Am J Psychiatry* **164**: 1214–1220.

Nilsson E, Lichtenstein P, Cnattingius S, et al. (2002) Women with schizophrenia: pregnancy outcome and infant death among their offspring. *Schizophr Res* **58**: 221–229.

Nordeng H, Spigset O (2005) Treatment with selective serotonin reuptake inhibitors in the third trimester of pregnancy: effects on the infant. *Drug Safety* **28**: 565–581.

Nulman I, Rovet J, Stewart D, et al. (1997) Neurodevelopment of children exposed in utero to antidepressant drugs. *N Engl J Med* **336**: 258–262.

Nulman I, Rovet J, Stewart D, et al. (2002) Child development following exposure to tricyclic antidepressants or fluoxetine througout fetal life: a prospective, controlled study. *Am J Psychiatry* **159**: 1889–1895.

Oates M (1996) Psychiatric services for women following childbirth. *Int Rev Psychiatry* **8**: 87–98.

Oates M (2003) Perinatal psychiatric disorders: a leading cause of maternal morbidity and mortality. *Br Med Bull* 67: 219–229.

Oberlander T, Grunau RE, Fitzgerald C, et al. (2002) Prolonged prenatal psychotropic medication exposure alters neonatal acute pain response. *Pediatr Res* **51**: 443–453.

Oberlander T, Misri S, Fitzgerald C, et al. (2004) Pharmocologic factors associated with transient neonatal symptoms following prenatal psychotropic medication exposure. *J Clin Psychiatry* **65**: 230–237.

Oberlander T, Grunau RE, Fitzgerald C, et al. (2005) Pain reactivity in 2-month-old infants after prenatal and postnatal selective serotonin reuptake inhibitor medication exposure. *Pediatrics* **115**: 411–425.

Oberlander T, Reebye P, Misri S, et al. (2007) Externalizing and attentional behaviours in children of depressed mothers treated with a selective serotonin reuptake inhibitor antidepressant during pregnancy. *Arch Pediatr Adolesc Med* **161**: 22–29.

O'Connor M, Johnson GH, James DI (1981) Intrauterine effect of phenothiazines. *Med J Aust* **1**: 416–417.

O'Connor TG, Ben-Shlomo Y, Heron J, et al. (2005) Prenatal anxiety predicts individual differences in cortisol in pre-adolescent children. *Biol Psychiatry* **58**: 211–217.

Odegard O (1980) Fertility of psychiatric first admission in Norway 1936–1975. *Act Psychiatr Scand* **62**: 212–220.

O'Hara MW (1986) Social support, life events, and depression during pregnancy and the puerperium. *Arch Gen Psychiatry* **43**: 569–573.

O'Hara MW (1994) Depression during pregnancy. In: *Postpartum Depression: Causes and Consequences.* New York: Springer-Verlag, pp 110–120.

O'Keane V (2008) Antipsychotic-induced hyperprolactinaemia, hypogonadism and osteoporosis in the treatment of schizophrenia. *J Psychopharmacol* **22S**: 70–75.

O'Keane V, Marsh M (2007) Depression during pregnancy. *BMJ* **334**: 1003–1005.

Orr S, Miller CA (1995) Maternal depressive symptoms and the risk of poor pregnancy outcome. *Epidemiol Rev* **15**: 165–171.

Owens MJ, Morgan WN, Plott SJ, Nemeroff CB (1997) Neurotransmitter receptor and transporter binding profile of antidepressants and their metabolites. *J Pharmacol Exp Ther* **283**: 1305–1322.

Pastuszak A, Schick-Boshcetto B, Zuber C, et al. (1993) Pregnancy outcome following first trimester exposure to fluoxetine. *JAMA* **269**: 2246–2248.

Perälä J, Suvisaari J, Saarni SI, et al. (2007) Lifetime prevalence of psychotic and bipolar I disorders in a general population. *Arch Gen Psychiatry* **64**: 19–28.

Pincus HA, Tanielian TL, Marcus SC, et al. (1998) Prescribing trends in psychotropic medications. *JAMA* **279**: 526–531.

Pinkofsky HB (2000) Effects of antipsychotics on the unborn child: what is known and how should this influence prescribing? *Paediatr Drugs* **2**: 83–90.

Pliszka SR, McCracken JT, Maas JW (1996) Catecholamines in attention deficit hyperactivity disorder: current perspectives. *J Am Acad Child Adolesc Psychiatry* **35**: 264–272.

Post RM (1992) Transduction of psychosocial stress into the neurobiology of recurrent affective disorder. *Am J Psychiatry* **149**: 999–1010.

Preskorn SH (1999) *Outpatient Management of Depression: A Guide for the Practitioner. 2nd edn.* Caddo, OK: Professional Communications.

Ratnayake T, Libretto SE (2002) No complications with risperidone treatment before and throughout pregnancy and during the nursing period. *J Clin Psychiatry* **63**: 76–77.

Reebye P, Morison SJ, Panikkar H, Misri et al. (2002) Affect expression in prenatally psychotropic exposed and nonexposed mother–infant dyads. *Infant Ment Health J* **234**: 403–416.

Reynell JK (1977) *The Reynell Developmental Language Scales (Revised).* Windsor: National Foundation for Educational Research.

Rice D, Barone S (2000) Critical periods of vulnerability for the developing nervous system: evidence from human and animal models. *Environ Health Perspect* **108**: 511–528.

Rieder RO, Rosenthal D, Wender P, Blumenthal H (1975) The offspring of schizophrenics. Fetal and neonatal deaths. *Arch Gen Psychiatry* **32**: 200–211.

Roid GH (2003) *Stanford–Binet Intelligence Scales, 5th edn. Examiner's Manual.* Itaska, IL: Riverside Publishing.

Rosenfeld JA, Everett KD (1996) Factors related to planned and unplanned pregnancies. *J Fam Pract* **43**: 161–166.

Rudolph B, Larson GL, Sweeny S, et al. (1990) Hospitalized pregnancy psychotic women: characteristics and treatment issues. *Hosp Community Psychiatry* **41**: 159–163.

Sacker A, Done DJ, Crow TJ (1996) Obstetric complications in children born to parents with schizophrenia: a meta-analysis of case–control studies. *Psychol Med* **26**: 279–287.

Schimmell MS, Katz EZ, Shaag Y, et al. (1991) Toxic neonatal effects following maternal clomipramine therapy. *J Toxicol Clin Toxicol* **29**: 479–484.

Schore AN (1994) *Affect Regulation and the Origin of the Self: The Neurobiology of Emotional Development.* Hillsdale, NJ: Lawrence Erlbaum.

Seeman MV (2004) Schizophrenia and motherhood. In: Gopfert M, Webster J, Seeman MV, eds. *Parental Psychiatric Disorders, 2nd edn.* Cambridge: Cambridge University Press, pp 161–171.

Sharp D, Hay DF, Pawlby S, et al. (1995) The impact of postnatal depression on boys' intellectual development. *J Child Psychol Psychiatry* **36**: 1315–1336.

Shearer WT, Schreiner RL, Marshall RE (1972) Urinary retention in a neonate secondary to maternal ingestion of nortriptyline. *J Pediatr* **81**: 570–572.

Simon GE, Cunningham ML, Davis RL (2002) Outcomes of prenatal antidepressant exposure. *Am J Psychiatry* **159**: 2055–2061.

Sivojelezova A, Shuhaiber S, Sarkissian L, et al. (2005) Citalopram use in pregnancy: prospective comparative evaluation of pregnancy and fetal outcome. *Am J Obstet Gynecol* **193**: 2004–2009.

Slone D, Siskind V, Heinonen OP, et al. (1977) Antenatal exposure to the phenothiazines in relation to congenital malformations, perinatal mortality rate, birth weight, and intelligence quotient score. *Am J Obstet Gynecol* **128**: 486–488.

Stika L, Elisová K, Honzáková L, et al. (1990) Effects of drug administration in pregnancy on children's school behaviour. *Pharm Weekbl Sci* **12**: 252–255.

Stokes AH, Hastings TG, Vrana KE (1999) Cytotoxic and genotoxic potential of dopamine. *J Neurosci Res* **55**: 659–665.

Stowe ZN, Nemeroff CB (1995) Women at risk for postpartum-onset major depression. *Am J Obstet Gynecol* **173**: 639–645.

Susman E, Schmeelk K, Ponirakis A, Gariepy JL (2001) Maternal prenatal, postpartum, and concurrent stressors and temperament in 3-year-olds: a person and variable analysis. *Dev Psychopathol* **13**: 629–652.

Tamer A, McKey R, Arias D, et al. (1969) Phenothiazine-induced extrapyramidal dysfunction in the neonate. *J Pediatr* **75**: 479–480.

Tatsumi M, Groshan K, Blakely RD, Richelson E (1997) Pharmacological profile of antidepressants and related compounds at human monoamine transporters. *Eur J Pharmacol* **340**: 249–258.

Taylor A, Fisk NM, Glover V (2000) Mode of delivery and subsequent stress response. *Lancet* **355**: 120 (letter).

Taylor TM, O'Toole MS, Ohlsen RI, et al. (2003) Safety of during pregnancy. *Am J Psychiatry* **160**: 588–589 (letter).

Tényi T, Trixler M, Keresztes Z (2002) Quetiapine and pregnancy. *Am J Psychiatry* **159**: 674 (letter).

Teti DM, Gelfand DM (1991) Behavioural competence among mothers of infants in the first year: the mediational role of maternal self-efficacy. *Child Dev* **62**: 918–929.

Tohen M, Waternaux CM, Tsuang MT (1990) Outcome in mania. A 4-year prospective follow-up of 75 patients utilizing survival analysis. *Arch Gen Psychiatry* **47**: 1106–1111.

Troutman B, Cutrona C (1990) Nonpsychotic postpartum depression among adolescent mothers. *J Abnorm Psychol* **99**: 69–78.

Vallone D, Picetti R, Borrelli E (2000) Structure and function of dopamine receptors. *Neurosci Biobehav Rev* **24**: 125–132.

van Os J, Hanssen M, Bijl RV, Ravelli A (2000) Strauss (1969) revisited: a psychosis continuum in the general population? *Schizophr Res* **45**: 11–25.

van Os J, Hanssen M, Bijl RV, Vollebergh W (2001) Prevalence of psychotic disorder and community level of psychotic symptoms: an urban–rural comparison. *Arch Gen Psychiatry* **58**: 663–668.

Webster PA (1973) Withdrawal symptoms in neonates associated with maternal antidepressant therapy. *Lancet* **2**: 318–319.

Weissman MM, Olfson M (1995) Depression in women: implications for health care research. *Science* **269**: 799–801.

Weissman MM, Warner V, Wickramaratne P, et al. (1997) Offspring of depressed parents: Ten years later. *Arch Gen Psychiatry* **54**: 932–940.

Wisborg K, Barklin A, Hedegaard M, Henriksen TB (2008) Psychological stress during pregnancy and stillbirth: prospective study. *Brit J Obstet Gynaecol* **115**: 882–885.

Williams R, Ali SF, Scalzo FM, et al. (1992) Prenatal haloperidol exposure: effects on brain weights and caudate neurotransmitter levels in rats. *Brain Res Bull* **29**: 449–458.

Wrede G, Mednick SA, Huttunen MO, Nilsson CG (1980) Pregnancy and delievery complications in births of an unselected series of Finnish children with schizophrenic mothers. *Acta Psychiatr Scand* **62**: 369–381.

Yaeger D, Smith HG, Altshuler LL (2006) Atypical antipsychotics in the treatment of schizophrenia during pregnancy and the postpartum. *Am J Psychiatry* **163**: 2064–2070.

Yaris F, Kadioglu M, Kesim M, et al. (2004) Newer antidepressants in pregnancy: a prospective outcome of a case series. *Reprod Toxicol* **19**: 235–238.

Yaris F, Ulku C, Kesim M, et al. (2005) Psychotropic drugs in pregnancy: a case–control study. *Prog Neuro-psychopharmacol Biol Psychiatry* **29**: 333–338.

Yim I, Glynn L, Schetter CD, et al. (2009) Risk of postpartum depressive symptoms with elevated corticotropin-releasing hormone in human pregnancy. *Arch Gen Psychiatry* **66**: 162–169.

Zilberman M, Tavares H, Blume S, el-Guebaly N (2003) Substance use disorders: sex differences and psychiatric comorbidities. *Can J Psychiatry* **48**: 5–13.

Zuckerman B, Amaro H, Bauchner H, Cabral H (1989) Depressive symptoms during pregnancy: Relationship to poor health behaviours. *Am J Obstet Gynecol* **160**: 1107–1111.

6
DIAGNOSIS OF FETAL ALCOHOL SYNDROME: EMPHASIS ON EARLY DETECTION

Margaret Barrow and Edward P Riley

Recognition of the fetal alcohol syndrome (FAS) dates to two landmark papers published in 1973 (Jones et al. 1973, Jones and Smith 1973). In those papers the offspring of 11 women who were heavy alcohol abusers were described as having growth deficiency, a similar pattern of craniofacial anomalies, and evidence of central nervous system (CNS) dysfunction. These are basically the same criteria that are still used today to make a diagnosis of FAS. While several different schemata for diagnosing FAS have been suggested (Astley and Clarren 2000, Bertrand et al. 2004, Chudley et al. 2005, Hoyme et al. 2005), and additional diagnostic terms have been added to encompass a broader range of outcomes, in reality, all of these diagnostic guides use similar criteria for the diagnosis of FAS. The differences between them are in terms of cut-offs for centiles for growth retardation or palpebral fissure size, the number of facial anomalies required for a diagnosis, or how CNS dysfunctions are defined.

Facial features

The cardinal diagnostic facial features of FAS have been clarified in several reviews, and schemata for diagnosis have been presented by several authors. For example, in *The Fetal Alcohol Syndrome: Guidelines for Referral and Diagnosis* published by the Centers for Disease Control and Prevention (CDC) (Bertrand et al. 2004) the following three facial characteristics are required for a diagnosis of FAS: smooth philtrum (ridge running from under the nose to the top of the upper lip), thin vermilion border (upper lip), and small palpebral fissures (at or below the 10th centile – Hall et al. 1989) (Fig. 6.1). In contrast, Hoyme et al. (2005), in their proposed clarification of the Institute of Medicine recommendations (Stratton et al. 1996) for diagnosing fetal alcohol spectrum disorder, require just two out of the same three facial features. A commonly used diagnostic schema, the '4-digit code' (Astley 2004) (Table 6.1), has a simple formula to compute facial dysmorphology based upon the same three standard facial characteristics, but has a more stringent requirement for palpebral fissure size (3rd centile) and requires all three facial features. The Canadian guidelines (Chudley et al. 2005) are similar to those proposed in the 4-digit code. A cartoon of the characteristic face of FAS is presented in Figure 6.2, and the guide typically used to

TABLE 6.1
The 4-Digit Code for diagnosing fetal alcohol syndrome (FAS)

Score	Growth	Facial phenotype	CNS rank	Alcohol exposure
4	Severe – height and weight below 3rd centile	Severe – lip and philtrum ranked 4 or 5 on lip/philtrum guide and palpebral fissure <2 SD	Definite – structural and/or neurological anomalies	High risk –confirmed exposure and exposure places the fetus at 'high risk' on a regular basis during early gestation
3	Moderate – either height or weight below 3rd centile	Moderate – two of the three facial features as in Severe, and the other one either ranked a 3 (lip/ philtrum) or 1–2 SD (palpebral fissure)	Probable – significant dysfunction	Some risk – confirmed exposure but amount is unknown or less than required for a 4
2	Mild – height and/or weight between 10th and 3rd centiles	Mild	Possible – mild or moderate delay or dysfunction	Exposure is unknown
1	None	None	Unlikely	Alcohol exposure is confirmed to be absent

The 4-Digit Code rates growth, facial characteristics, CNS anomalies and alcohol exposure, each on a 1–4 scale. A diagnosis of 'FAS alcohol exposed' would be obtained with any of the following codes.
    2433   3433   4433   2434   3434   4434
    2443   3443   4443   2444   3444   4444
A diagnosis of 'FAS alcohol exposure unknown' would be obtained with any of the following codes.
    2432   3432   4432   2442   3442   4442
Other diagnostic labels would be applied to other codes including 'partial FAS', 'static encephalopathy' and 'neurobehavioural disorder' – see Astley (2004).
Table adapted from Canadian FASD Guidelines: http://www.faslink.org/CanadianFASDdiagnosisGuidelines.pdf.

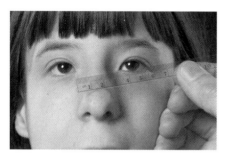

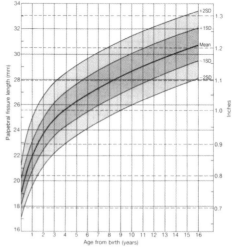

Fig. 6.1. *(Above)* Measuring palpebral fissure length. The child is asked to look upwards, and a transparent ruler is rested on the nasal bridge, measuring endocanthion to endocanthion.*(Right)* Graph showing palpebral fissure length (both sexes), from birth to 16 years. (Reproduced by permission from Hall et al. 1989.)

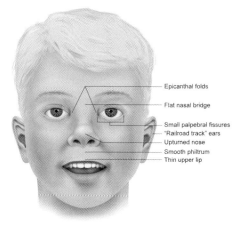

Fig. 6.2. Facial features in a child diagnosed with fetal alcohol syndrome, illustrating the key features used in the diagnosis: smooth philtrum, thin upper lip, small palpebral fissures. (Reproduced by permission from Wattendorf and Muenke 2005.)

Epicanthal folds

Flat nasal bridge

Small palpebral fissures
"Railroad track" ears
Upturned nose
Smooth philtrum
Thin upper lip

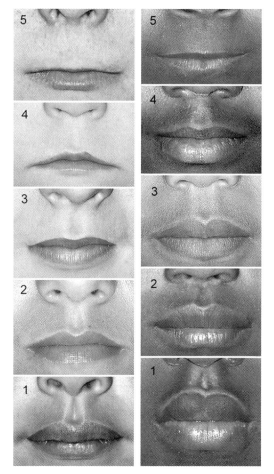

Fig. 6.3. Caucasian (left) and African-American (right) lip–philtrum guides used to rank upper lip thinness and philtrum smoothness, where 1 = unaffected and 5 = most severe. Numerical ranks 4 and 5 would be consistent with a diagnosis of fetal alcohol syndrome. (Reproduced by permission from Astley 2004.)

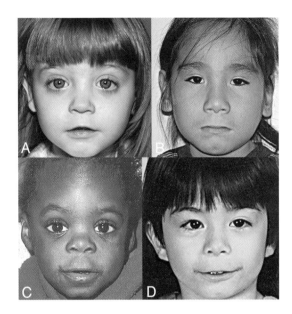

Fig. 6.4. Examples of fetal alcohol syndrome in various ethnicities. (A) Child of Northern European descent. (B) Native American child. (C). Black child. (D) Biracial (white, black) child. (Reproduced by permission from Wattendorf and Muenke 2005.)

determine the smoothness of the philtrum and the thinness of the upper lip is shown in Figure 6.3. All of the proposed diagnostic schemata require a 4 or a 5 ranking for vermilion thinness and philtrum smoothness. Besides these cardinal features, other facial features are often observed in children with FAS. Among the most frequently reported are anteverted nares, midface hypoplasia, flat nasal bridge, ptosis and strabismus. Pictures of children of various ethnic backgrounds with FAS are shown in Figure 6.4.

Growth retardation

According to the CDC guidelines, growth retardation is defined as "confirmed prenatal or postnatal height or weight, or both, at or below the 10th percentile, documented at any one point in time (adjusted for age, sex, gestational age, and race or ethnicity)." The revised Institute of Medicine criteria also use the 10th centile, adjusted for racial norms if possible. The 4-digit code again uses a simple method to compute the height and weight deficit, but includes a more stringent criterion of the 3rd centile to achieve the maximum score, although growth retardation between the 3rd and 10th centiles also qualifies for a ranking consistent with an FAS diagnosis. The Canadian guidelines also use the 10th centile and also include a disproportionately low weight-to-height ratio. Thus, all of the schemata appear to agree that the 10th centile is a reasonable cut-off for growth retardation in the diagnosis of FAS.

Central nervous system anomalies

Anomalies of the CNS are in reality the primary concern in dealing with clients with FAS, since they can cause life-long debilitating issues. However, these are probably the hardest to discern and then to attribute to the effects of gestational alcohol exposure. In determining the CNS involvement, the different diagnostic schemata take somewhat different approaches. The revised Institute of Medicine criteria take the simplest approach, requiring evidence of structural brain abnormality or a head circumference ≤10th centile. However, the revised Institute of Medicine criteria also have a diagnostic category labelled partial FAS (pFAS), described later, that has more functionally based criteria for measuring CNS dysfunction. The CDC define a CNS anomaly as being structural, neurological or functional, or a combination thereof. Structural changes can be a head circumference ≤10th centile but disproportionately small relative to overall size in a growth-retarded child, or changes noted using brain imaging techniques. Neurological evidence, such as seizures, or soft signs outside normal limits, would also meet criteria for a CNS defect. Perhaps the most difficult assessment to try to meet this criterion is one based upon functional attributes. Here, there must be evidence of a global cognitive deficit or, in young children, significant developmental delays or deficits in three or more specific functional domains. These could include problems in executive functioning, specific learning deficits (particularly in numeracy and/or visuo-spatial ability), motor functional domains, attention, hyperactivity and social skills. One would expect to see deficits relative to norms of at least one standard deviation (SD) in any particular domain. Importantly, other potential causes of these functional deficits have to be excluded, since functional deficits that might be attributed to prenatal alcohol exposure could result from many other factors (e.g. home environment, familial intellectual disabilities). Coexisting disorders (e.g. autism, affective disorders) must also be considered. The 4-digit code utilizes both structural and functional deficits in defining this CNS criterion. Functional deficits include deficits (>2 SD) in three or more domains. The Canadian guidelines detail evidence of impairment in at least three of the following CNS domains: hard and soft neurological signs; brain structure; cognition; communication; academic achievement; memory; executive functioning and abstract reasoning; attention deficit/hyperactivity; adaptive behaviour; social skills, social communication. The nature and degree of functional deficits related to prenatal alcohol exposure will probably continue to be of concern in the diagnosis of FAS until relatively specific behavioural profile or profiles are determined.

Partial fetal alcohol syndrome

Following the identification of FAS, it became clear that many children exposed to significant levels of alcohol during gestation did not meet all of the criteria to qualify for an FAS diagnosis. Frequently, they may have had only two of the facial characteristics or did not demonstrate growth retardation. Initially, these children were often labelled as demonstrating 'fetal alcohol effects'. However, this classification probably brought more confusion than assistance and it is no longer used. Today, several of the diagnostic schemata include a category labelled partial FAS (pFAS). Table 6.2 provides an overview of the differences between FAS and pFAS based on the Canadian guidelines. Other terminologies that are frequently used are 'alcohol-related neurodevelopmental disorder' and 'alcohol-related birth defect'. The fomer is used to describe cognitive, behavioural, emotional or motor problems that are felt to be the result of in utero alcohol exposure (see Chapter 7), while the latter is occasionally used to describe a specific birth defect that may to be attributed to such exposure, as described later.

TABLE 6.2
Fetal alcohol syndrome (FAS) vs partial FAS (pFAS): diagnostic criteria

Criterion	FAS	pFAS
Growth impairment	Yes	No
Facial features – Short palpebral fissures – Thin upper lip – Indistinct philtrum	All 3 present	2 of 3 present
Brain injury	Minimum of 3 CNS domains impaired	Minimum of 3 CNS domains impaired
Alcohol exposure	Confirmed or unconfirmed	Confirmed

Alcohol exposure

Alcohol exposure histories during gestation are often unavailable (for example in the case of a foreign adoption) or inaccurate (there is a great deal of underreporting for a variety of reasons); see below and other chapters within this volume for a discussion of these issues. With experience it has been possible to discern that the characteristics of FAS are sufficiently specific that a diagnosis of FAS can be given if potential phenocopies can be eliminated as causes, even if there is no firm evidence of maternal drinking. However, for a diagnosis of pFAS, some schemata (e.g. Canadian guidelines) require confirmation of maternal drinking.

Differential diagnosis

Given the subtle phenotype of FAS, it is not surprising that it shares features with other syndromes, and thus FAS should probably best be thought of as a diagnosis of exclusion. For example, FAS shares many common features with velocardiofacial syndrome, which is caused by a microdeletion of chromosome 22q11. Specific chromosomal fluorescence in situ hybridization studies should therefore be performed to rule out this possibility. In particular, children with velocardiofacial syndrome can show short palpebral fissures, malar hypoplasia and microcephaly. Other conditions that may present in the neonatal period include Williams syndrome (a microdeletion of chromosome 7q11), which features irritability due to hypercal-caemia, microcephaly, short palpebral fissures, very long philtrum and aortic stenosis. The de Lange syndrome has facial features that include microcephaly, synophrys (fusion of the eyebrows), thin upper lip and flat philtrum, with downturned mouth corners and a variety of limb and hand abnormalities. Specific genetic testing for de Lange syndrome is now avail-able. In addition, familial facial features, particularly a long philtrum and thin upper lip, may not necessarily be related to alcohol exposure; the infant's facial features should there-fore be assessed in the context of the parental face. Other teratogens in pregnancy, including some antiepileptic drugs, can also produce a long philtrum and thin upper lip. Lists of syn-dromes sharing similar characteristics with FAS are presented in Tables 6.3 and 6.4. Ideally, a full pedigree with all syndromic diagnoses, required to encompass three generations, should be acquired, paying particular attention to other individuals with learning disability, behavioural problems, growth disorders, alcohol dependency and hearing abnormality.

TABLE 6.3
Syndromes with constellations of features that overlap with those of fetal alcohol syndrome (FAS)

Syndrome	Overlapping features	Features of this syndrome that differentiate it from FAS
Aarskog syndrome	Widely spaced eyes, small nose with anteverted nares, broad philtrum, mid-facial recession	Round face, downslanted palpebral fissures, widow's peak, prominent 'lop' ears, specific contracture of digits on extension. Inherited as an X-linked trait. Molecular defect identified
Brachman–de Lange or Cornelia de Lange syndrome	Long philtrum, thin vermilion border of upper lip, depressed nasal bridge, anteverted nares, microcephaly	Single eyebrow across eyes and forehead (synophrys), long eyelashes, downturned corners of mouth, short upper limbs particularly involving ulnar side, very short stature. Molecular defect identified
Dubowitz syndrome	Short palpebral fissures, widely spaced eyes, epicanthal folds, variable ptosis (droopy eyes) and blepharophimosis, microcephaly	Shallow supraorbital ridges, broad nasal tip, clinodactyly
Fetal anticonvulsant syndrome (includes fetal hydantoin and fetal valproate syndromes)	Widely spaced eyes, depressed nasal bridge, mid-facial recession, epicanthal folds, long philtrum, thin vermilion border of upper lip	Bowed upper lip, high forehead, small mouth
Maternal phenylketonuria, fetal effects	Epicanthal folds, short palpebral fissures, long poorly formed philtrum, thin vermilion border of upper lip, microcephaly	Prominent glabella, small upturned nose, round face
Noonan syndrome	Low nasal bridge, epicanthal folds, widely spaced eyes, long philtrum	Downslanted palpebral fissures, wide mouth with well-formed philtrum, protruding upper lip. Molecular defect identified
Williams syndrome	Short palpebral fissures, anteverted nares, broad long philtrum, maxillary hypoplasia, depressed nasal bridge, epicanthal folds, microcephaly	Wide mouth with full lips and pouting lower lip, stellate pattern of iris, periorbital fullness, connective tissue dysplasia, specific cardiac defect of supravalvar aortic stenosis in many. Chromosome deletion on fluorescence in situ hybridization probe analysis of 7q
Other chromosome deletion and duplication syndromes	Many have short palpebral fissures, mid-facial hypoplasia, smooth philtrum	Chromosomal analysis by standard analysis and some select syndromes by specific fluorescence in situ hybridization probe analysis

Adapted by permission from Chudley et al. (2005).

TABLE 6.4
**Differential diagnosis of individual features associated with fetal
alcohol syndrome**

Feature	Syndromes
Smooth philtrum	Cornelia de Lange syndrome
	Floating–Harbor syndrome
	Geleophysic dysplasia
	Opitz syndrome
Thin vermilion border	Miller–Dieker (lissencephaly) syndrome
	Fetal valproate syndrome
	Geleophysic dysplasia
	Cornelia de Lange syndrome
Small palpebral fissures	Campomelic dysplasia
	DiGeorge sequence
	Dubowitz syndrome
	Duplication 10q sequence
	Duplication 15q sequence
	FG syndrome
	Maternal phenylketonuria, fetal effects
	Oculodentodigital syndrome
	Opitz syndrome
	Trisomy 18 syndrome
	Williams syndrome
	Velocardiofacial syndrome
	Toluene embryopathy

Adapted by permission from Bertrand et al. (2004).

Early detection of fetal alcohol syndrome

One of the protective factors identified in the secondary disabilities study of FAS (Streissguth et al. 2004) was early identification, yet diagnosis of this condition in the newborn infant is often not attempted (Little et al. 1990) or is described as 'problematic' (Hoyme et al. 2005). Most children with FAS obtain their diagnosis in early childhood or after they start school and behavioural problems become more obvious. For example, in a recent prospective national surveillance study in Australia (Elliott et al. 2008) the median age at diagnosis was 3.3 years (range, newborn to 11.9 years); 6.5% were diagnosed at birth and 63% by 5 years of age. While the situation is improving, and attempts are being made to use technologically more sophisticated methods to assist in the early diagnosis of FAS (Astley and Clarren 1996, Bookstein et al. 2007, Kfir et al. 2010), obviously more work needs to be done in this area. This is especially important since the outcome of the child may be improved by early intervention, or if a child is considered at risk they can be followed more closely for issues related to alcohol exposure. Early identification must involve better tools for identifying high-risk mothers, developing biomarkers for alcohol exposure, and better training for paediatricians and paediatric nurses in the identification of the range of outcomes resulting from prenatal alcohol exposure. Fetal alcohol spectrum disorder (FASD) is a new non-diagnostic umbrella term to describe the range of effects resulting from prenatal alcohol

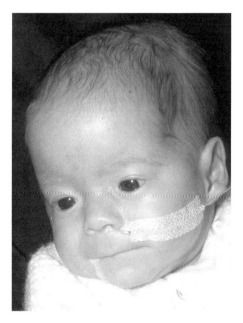

Fig. 6.5. Neonatal presentation of fetal alcohol syndrome.

exposure. It can encompass perinatal death and FAS, at the severe end, to subtle behavioural changes at the less severe end.

The diagnosis of FAS in the newborn and infant period currently is based upon the same criteria as used for children. Despite these guidelines for diagnosing FAS, the unique timing of newborn presentation provides challenges in each of the diagnostic areas and has major health implications for both mother and baby.

Neonatal features of fetal alcohol syndrome (Fig. 6.5)
PRETERM BIRTH
Alcohol consumption in pregnancy has been linked with both preterm birth and low birthweight. Heavy drinking (defined as one or more drinks per day in pregnancy) doubles the risk of preterm birth and is also associated with extreme preterm delivery (<32 weeks) (Floyd et al. 2005). For every unit increase in alcohol consumption, the risk of extreme preterm delivery increased significantly (odds radio 34.8) (Chudley et al. 2005, Bailey and Sokol 2008). The Australian surveillance study (Elliott et al. 2008) reported that of the 92 children referred for their study, 35.7% were born preterm (<37 weeks' gestation).

LOW BIRTHWEIGHT
There is a strong association between alcohol consumption during pregnancy and low birthweight (Floyd et al. 2005). Heavy drinking is associated with an almost five-fold increase in the likelihood of low birthweight (Chudley et al. 2005, Bailey and Sokol 2008). Furthermore, in a study of over 1000 infants, consumption of three or more drinks per week during pregnancy more than doubled the risk of low birthweight in the offspring, with an average

reduction in birthweight of 143 g (Bailey and Sokol 2008). As noted above, growth retardation (low birthweight for gestational age, pre- or postnatal height or weight reductions below the 10th centile or both) is one of the key diagnostic features of FAS. While there are many other causes of intrauterine growth retardation, in the face of known alcohol exposure it is a significant finding and one that needs to be carefully considered by the paediatrician. However, there are reports that cigarette smoking often occurs among women who are drinking and that this may contribute significantly to the low birthweights in these children (Abel and Hannigan 1995).

FACIAL FEATURES

The cardinal diagnostic facial features of FAS have been reviewed above and are similar in the neonate and infant (see Fig. 6.5), although certain measures may be more difficult to obtain. For example, neither palpebral fissure measurement nor use of the lip philtrum guide (Astley and Clarren 2000; see Fig. 6.3) may be of much help in the neonatal period. The neonate's eyes may be swollen and are unlikely to be open long enough for measuring palpebral fissure size, which is difficult even under the best of circumstances. Stoler and Holmes (2004) devised a facial score for use in the neonatal period, giving one point for the presence of each of the following six features: depressed nasal bridge, wide nasal bridge, anteverted nares, long philtrum, hypoplastic philtrum, and thin upper vermilion border. Babies with four or more of these features were considered to have a positive facial score. This facial score was found to correlate with the infant exposure status as measured by maternal self-report from an in-depth interview and an alcoholism screening questionnaire. Interestingly, Sokol et al. (1991) had some success using a computerized landmark-based system for identifying FAS in neonates. Landmarks corresponded to short palpebral fissure, a scooping out of the nasal bridge and a thin vermilion border. Other investigators are currently pursuing both computerized and photographic assessment of FAS in neonates, and this strategy may help in facilitating the diagnosis during this period.

CNS ABNORMALITIES/MICROCEPHALY

Head circumference at or below the 10th centile or structural brain abnormalities are evidence of the deficient brain growth or abnormal morphogenesis associated with FAS. Unlike growth retardation, which may improve during childhood, small head size often remains a constant feature of this condition throughout life and is universally a poor prognostic indicator in terms of developmental delay and behavioural outcomes. The microcephaly in FAS is symmetrical and frequently in proportion with a reduction in height and weight, leading to a symmetrical and proportionately growth-retarded phenotype. However, severe types of microcephaly may also be apparent postnatally. Babies at high risk for FAS should undergo head ultrasonography postnatally to check for recognizable structural brain abnormalities. However, such scans will detect only the more obvious structural malformations, as more subtle abnormalities, for example neuronal migration defects and volume reductions, will be detected only by detailed brain magnetic resonance imaging at a slightly later stage. Many paediatric radiologists prefer to defer postnatal brain magnetic resonance imaging until 6 months of age, thus allowing for greater clarity and interpretation.

The following brain alterations have been described as a consequence of heavy alcohol exposure (Spadoni et al. 2007) and are reviewed elsewhere in this volume in more detail (Chapter 7).

1. *Overall reduction in brain size – microcephaly.* Hypoplasia of all of the lobes of the brain, with reductions beyond those predicted by the degree of microcephaly in the parietal and frontal lobes.

2. *Grey and white matter differences.* White matter hypoplasia throughout the brain, but most prevalent in the perisylvian and inferior parietal regions. Conversely, increased grey matter density corresponds to the white matter hypoplasia in these areas. Several more recent diffusion tensor imaging studies support a decrease is the integrity of white matter in neuronal tracts.

3. *Cerebellum.* Reduced surface area and volume of the cerebellum is often reported in FAS, in addition to specific reduction in the volume of the anterior cerebellar vermis.

4. *Corpus callosum.* A higher rate of agenesis of the corpus callosum has been reported in individuals with FAS. Also, corpus callosum agenesis is commonly accompanied by ventricular abnormalities, as midline structures typically adjoining the corpus callosum are displaced. Hypoplasia of the corpus callosum has been frequently reported, with significant reductions in the anterior and posterior callosal regions. The splenium of the corpus callosum is significantly reduced and displaced. Alcohol-exposed individuals also exhibit increased variability in the shape of the corpus callosum, raising the possibility that shape-based analyses of the corpus callosum may prove to be an important diagnostic tool.

5. *Basal ganglia.* Evidence of reduced volume of the basal ganglia in prenatally alcohol exposed individuals has been reported. The basal ganglia are composed of five principal nuclei: caudate, nucleus accumbens, putamen, globus pallidus and subthalamic nucleus. The caudate appears to be particularly affected.

6. *Other brain abnormalities.* At a lesser frequency, midline brain defects such as varying degrees of holoprosencephaly are found. Migration errors have also been reported, and most recently a thicker cortex in certain brain regions has been reported in FAS.

ORGAN MALFORMATIONS AND ALCOHOL-RELATED BIRTH DEFECTS

Congenital heart defects are among the most significant abnormalities in FASD, second to brain malformation. A recent paper (Burd et al. 2007) that surveyed the available literature located 29 studies of FASD that met their inclusionary criteria. The proportion of congenital heart defects varied according to the study type: in 12 case series reports, 67% were reported to have a congenital heart defect, with 56.3% having a ventricular or atrial septal defect. In 14 retrospective studies, the rate of ventricular septal defects was 21%. However, as mortality rates are increased in FASD, under-ascertainment due to deaths from comorbid congenital heart defects and FASD is likely. Other cardiac malformations described in this condition include aberrant great vessels and conotruncal heart defects.

Congenital malformations can also occur in other organ systems. Baumann et al. (2006) performed an analysis of a perinatal database of over 170 000 women and found an increased rate of respiratory, genital, integumental and other limb and musculoskeletal anomalies among the offspring of women who admitted to drinking during pregnancy. Interestingly, many of these anomalies were more prominent in children born to women over the age of 30. Most recently, Hofer (2009) reviewed anomalies of the kidney, liver and gastrointestinal tract in FASD. While they did not identify any specific pattern of anomalies, they did find numerous reports of structural and functional impairments in the liver and kidney. Renal malformations consisted of aplasia, hypoplasia and dysplasia of the kidneys, horseshoe kidneys and ureteral duplications.

Skeletal anomalies have also been noted in FAS. For example, Habbick et al. (1998) reported a delay in bone growth, more prominent in males than females, in a large number of children with FAS. Fusion of the carpal bones has also been reported, as have joint contractures.

EXAMINATION OF THE ALCOHOL-EXPOSED NEONATE

The dysmorphologist's approach to risk assessment for FAS in the neonate is complicated and compounded by several factors.

1. *Condition of infant.* If the infant is preterm and of low birthweight, there may be ensuing aspects of intensive care that mitigate against full examination. It is not easy to access a tiny baby in an incubator, especially if the child is ventilated, because of the plethora of equipment that surrounds them. The postnatal course for an infant with FAS can include irritability, hyper- or hypotonia, opisthotonus, tremors, poor feeding, poor state regulation, poor habituation and EEG changes (Welch-Carre 2005). There may be differences in the threshold, latency and pitch of the cry of exposed infants. Infants withdrawing from alcohol may also have seizures.

2. *Growth parameters and head circumference.* These should be carefully noted and plotted according to gestation and racial norms. A cut-off below the 10th centile for height and weight and head circumference is stipulated in the diagnostic criteria for FAS. As noted, there is a strong association between gestational alcohol exposure and low birthweight. Similarly there is an increased risk of preterm birth among the offspring of heavy drinkers (Chudley et al. 2005, Bailey and Sokol 2008). Prenatal alcohol exposure was also associated with an increased risk of extreme preterm delivery (<32 weeks gestation).

3. *Examination.* The presence of the cardinal facial features, namely short palpebral fissures, long philtrum and thin upper lip, can be noted if the neonate is tube-free around the face. Oral and palatal clefting are not common in FAS but have been reported, so the palate should be checked. Eye examination should be carried out, by an ophthalmologist, to check for subtle ocular findings of FAS, including optic nerve hypoplasia, ptosis and retinal vascular abnormalities (Strömland 2004).

Examination of cardiac murmurs, to include echocardiography, is indicated. Examination of the hands may show short fifth digits, clinodactyly of the fifth fingers, hypoplastic nails or camptodactyly. A 'hockey stick' palmar crease (Fig. 6.6a) may be found. Skeletal malformations may include pectus carinatum or excavatum, scoliosis and joint contractures. The 'railroad track ear' (Fig. 6.6b) described in Native North American populations is not typically seen in northern European ones. Full notes of thorough physical examination should be recorded, as neonates with FAS can, on occasion, present with multiple congenital anomalies that are not characteristic of this disorder. For example, the first author has seen

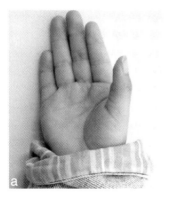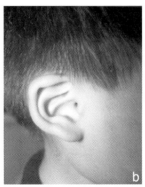

Fig. 6.6. (a) Example of a 'hockey stick' crease showing the widening of the upper palmar crease ending between the index and middle fingers. (b) Example of a 'railroad track' ear. (Reproduced by permission from Hoyme et al. 2005.)

an affected neonate from a severely alcohol-dependent mother with a diaphragmatic defect. Whilst causality cannot be assumed, a vigorous search for other, hitherto unrelated, birth defects must take place.

4. *Investigations specific to the diagnosis of FAS*. Infants suspected of heavy alcohol exposure should have the following investigations: (1) brain imaging including cerebral ultrasound and, later, brain magnetic resonance imaging; (2) renal scan; (3) ophthalmological evaluation; (4) cardiac evaluation, including echocardiography; (5) chromosomal analysis to include fluorescence in situ hybridization 22q11 studies; (6) hearing tests, including neonatal hearing screening, since hearing deficits are common in these children, but often overlooked (Church and Kaltenbach 1997).

Presentation in the older child and adult
As previously stated, the diagnosis of FAS is typically made in the young child, rather than in the neonate. The presentation in the child, however, is similar to that described above (Fig. 6.7), although as the child ages, better indications of CNS involvement are available. Typically, the child is referred for diagnosis, not because of his/her facial features, but rather because of some developmental delay or behavioural issues. These behavioural factors are discussed in Chapter 7. As the child ages into adolescence, the facial characteristics of FAS may change, and it may become more difficult to diagnosis FAS in the young adult, simply because the facial features become less apparent. However, CNS problems may become more prominent and secondary disabilities may develop. FAS is a lifelong condition, even if the facial characteristics upon which the diagnosis is dependent diminish with increasing age. This is one reason why good maternal alcohol histories are imperative in the paediatric records.

Maternal risk factors (see also Chapter 13)
Numerous maternal risk factors have been identified for giving birth to a child with FAS

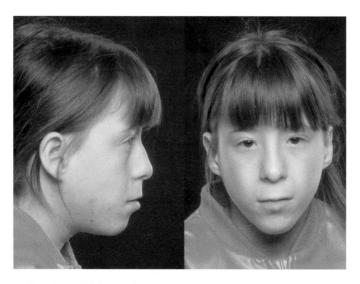

Fig. 6.7. Facial features in a 12-year-old with fetal alcohol syndrome.

(Welch-Carre 2005), including age >25 years; documented high blood-alcohol concentrations or intoxication in pregnancy; history of alcohol abuse and/or other substance abuse; history of living with an alcohol abuser; low socio-economic status; low self-esteem; loss of children to foster care system; single status; more than three children; a previous child with FAS; unemployment and social transience.

Involvement with community alcohol teams prior to pregnancy is a risk factor even if the woman maintains that she has stopped drinking during pregnancy. The timing of alcohol cessation is important as women may tell their physician or midwife that they are not drinking alcohol at their booking or first appointment, when in fact they have only recently become abstinent and there has been significant alcohol exposure early in gestation, during critical periods of organogenesis. The primary care provider (e.g. general practitioner) may often be uniquely placed to comment on maternal drinking habits as they will be ultimately involved with community management of such cases and be in a position to comment as to whether there is ongoing compliance with intervention programmes. Specific examples are given in Chapter 13.

Women who have babies with classic FAS are likely to be highly vulnerable alcohol abusers. Their close families are often very aware of their problem drinking, but that does not necessarily mean that all appropriate agencies have been involved. The mortality in mothers whose babies present in the neonatal period with FAS is high, and there may be a family history of alcoholism and alcohol-related deaths in other relatives. Identifying such women and allowing for appropriate and urgent health-care intervention is a primary challenge for healthcare professionals in prenatal, perinatal, neonatal and paediatric settings. Another issue in this regard is sibling mortality. Recently, Burd et al. (2008) examined the mortality rates in individuals with FASD and their siblings. The rate in the FASD group was 2.4%, but more surprisingly, for the siblings it was 4.5%. There are also preliminary reports of an association between sudden infant death and prenatal alcohol exposure (e.g. Burd et al. 2004).

Identifying problem drinkers in pregnancy

Identifying women who are at high risk for an alcohol-exposed pregnancy and intervening with them is an essential strategy for preventing alcohol-exposed pregnancies. If 2.5% of women are drinking frequently in pregnancy (Caprara et al. 2007), how can they be identified and helped?

Pregnant women are not likely to volunteer information about their drug or alcohol consumption given the likely stigmatization of such behaviours. In fact, they tend to hide such behaviours because of fears of being deemed unfit to bring up their baby, and possibly other older siblings, if there are child protection issues. As such, self-reporting of alcohol consumption is notoriously unreliable, even in the non-pregnant population. As discussed in Chapter 2, this is partly due to real confusion over alcohol labelling, strengths and volumes. While many individuals equate a 'glass' with a UK unit of alcohol, in fact, a standard glass of 125 mL is now rarely available in UK drinking establishments with the tendency to increasing glass sizes and concentrations of table wines. Drink size is also an issue in other countries as well, where rarely is a standard drink poured (for a recent discussion of the assessment of drink size, see Kaskutas and Kerr 2008).

Despite these limitations, a number of tools have been developed to try to assess at-risk drinking among pregnant women. Some of these have simply been 'borrowed' from the alcohol field in general. Commonly used screening tools are questionnaires such as TWEAK, T-ACE and the Timeline Followback Calendar. These questionnaires have been shown to be effective in primary care in distinguishing risky from non-risky drinkers (Bailey and Sokol 2008).

These brief screening interventions can improve identification of women with alcohol misuse problems in clinical settings better than clinician questioning alone, and have been validated in pregnant and non-pregnant women. The four-item T-ACE has sensitivity and specificity of 76% and 89% respectively, in identifying risky drinkers during gestation (Caprara et al. 2007).

The five-item TWEAK performs with similar accuracy and may also be used to assess moderate-risk drinking (sensitivity and specificity ranging from 70% to 79% and from 63% to 83% respectively). The Canadian guidelines for FASD (Chudley et al. 2005) recommend that all pregnant women should be screened for alcohol use with a validated screening tool and should receive early intervention if the results are positive. These instruments, however, tend to assess the alcohol dependence of the mother and fail to identify women who are not, strictly speaking, alcohol dependent. The Timeline Followback Calendar is a calendar that includes the date of conception and date of pregnancy recognition and may be useful in accurately assessing timing, frequency and amount of alcohol consumed. A combination of these two methods may increase accuracy. However, the use of such screening instruments in maternal settings is not widespread. For example, in the UK midwife's 'booking in form', usually completed in the first trimester, there is a small section relating to alcohol, asking the question, "Do you drink alcohol? (Yes/No)"; and identifying only the number of units in those who admit to drinking. This section also includes questions on exposure to cigarettes and other drugs, but these are 'tick box' sections that can easily be passed over. Thus an important opportunity for interventions to reduce maternal drinking can be missed. Most recently, the 4P's Plus, a general screening tool for alcohol and substance abuse, has gained some attention (Chasnoff et al. 2007). It is a short questionnaire asking about one's parents' and partner's substance use, as well as the individual's own use during pregnancy. While the test shows good sensitivity and specificity, and a very high negative predictive validity, its positive predictive validity is low. However, it does provide an opportunity for opening a discussion about the use of alcohol and drugs during pregnancy. Further training of health-care professionals including midwives and clinicians in this aspect of pregnancy management is now well overdue, particularly in the context of the increasing numbers of at-risk women of childbearing age.

Intervention to reduce or eliminate alcohol use in pregnancy

Alcohol-dependent women in the antenatal setting need referrals to specialized treatment agencies including multidisciplinary alcohol abuse teams. In the UK, access to such teams is often facilitated by primary care professionals, midwives or obstetricians (US experience is outlined in Chapter 13). Many alcohol-dependent women will already be known to these agencies, but sadly not all will be compliant with treatment. For non-dependent women who are consuming alcohol in pregnancy, brief interventions have been documented as effective in reducing alcohol use (Bailey and Sokol 2008). Such brief interventions include motivational interviewing, a directive patient-centred counselling style intended to minimize resistance to change. Motivational interviewing involves the expression of empathy, management of resistance without confrontation and support of patient self-efficacy.

Successful interventions follow the FRAMES approach summarized below.

F – *feedback of personal risk:* compare the patient's level of drinking with pregnancy recommended abstinence

R – *responsibility:* stress upon patient's responsibility to stop drinking for the health of her baby

A – *advice:* give direct advice to change drinking behaviour

M – *menu of ways to reduce/stop drinking*

E – *empathy:* remain positive and encouraging and avoid being judgemental or preaching

S – *self-efficacy:* elicit and reinforce self-motivation.

In one randomized controlled trial of 255 pregnant women who reported alcohol consumption in a community-based setting, assigned to receive either intervention or assessment only, the women who received intervention were five times more likely to report abstinence by the end of the pregnancy. Their babies had significantly higher birthweights and lengths, and a fetal mortality three times lower than the assessment controls (O'Connor and Whaley 2007). Another highly successful programme for dealing with high-risk women is the Parent–Child Assistance Program developed at the University of Washington (see Chapter 13). In this programme, paraprofessional case managers work with families enrolled into the programme during pregnancy or post partum. Advocates help these families connect with community services, coordinate services and deal with the range of problems typically faced by these high-risk women. As an example of its success, among 156 mothers enrolled, 88% completed a substance abuse programme, 73% were using contraception, and of those who became pregnant, 41% were sober throughout pregnancy and another 37% became sober after pregnancy recognition. Many of these interventions are discussed elsewhere in this volume.

Retrospective alcohol history in the alcohol-dependent mother in a postnatal setting
The diagnosis of FAS should, in the neonatal context, include confirmation of maternal alcohol exposure if at all possible. Ready access to maternity notes, and close links with primary care midwives and health visitors around the time of delivery make this one of the few times that such corroboration can be successfully pursued. This is in contrast to the older child with FAS who is more likely to be in care, often without access to key maternal records, alcohol history or pedigree details. Such confirmation, if obtained, must be clearly documented in the neonatal notes as this may be the only unequivocal documentation of maternal alcohol exposure in years to come.

Direct questioning of an alcohol-dependent mother after delivery will probably be met with a hostile response, and maternal denial will be an understandable reaction to avoid perceived opprobrium or questions as to her ability to look after the baby after discharge. Very few clinicians or nurses feel able to ask questions about alcohol intake in pregnancy. The questionnaires described above (TWEAK and T-ACE) are less likely to be of use in the postnatal setting. However, empathy, kindness, understanding and a knowledge of alcohol abuse and dependency are still key to eliciting this sensitive information. If a baby has a prolonged neonatal stay, it is likely that neonatal staff will be taken into confidence by the parents. Neonatal teams are also very experienced observers of parental behaviour and notice patterns of attachment with older siblings, and may detect intoxication or may elicit information from, for example, other family members about maternal drinking habits. Known alcohol abusers, including fathers, may act erratically on the ward. Alcohol-dependent mothers may self-discharge against medical advice to return to a home base where alcohol is available. Anger and denial over a possible FAS diagnosis is common, with a real potential for breakdown between parents and health-care professionals in this context. Neonatologists may, in extreme circumstances of maternal alcohol dependency, feel that it is not in the best interests of the baby to go home with the mother, giving rise to a child protection investigation and (in England and Wales) usually initiate a strategy meeting under section 47 of the Children Act 1989.

Admission of alcohol exposure during pregnancy by mothers who may not currently be alcohol dependent is more likely in the context of a trusting working relationship, often with the infant's paediatrician, and may occur over a period of time. Later maternal acknowledgement of the alcohol-exposed pregnancy is often the 'missing link' in the clinician's understanding of a complex or hitherto unexplained pattern of abnormality in the dysmorphic infant.

BIOMARKERS FOR IN UTERO ALCOHOL EXPOSURE
Self-report of alcohol use is fairly unreliable as to the amount consumed, yet this information

is critical for establishing public health policy and linking exposure data to outcome. Furthermore, early detection of infants with significant exposure histories is critical so that they can be monitored for possible developmental problems. This would allow the implementation of intervention at the earliest possible time. The presence of biomarkers of exposure in the fetus or of alcohol use in the mother would be a tremendous asset to assist in this linkage. To date, there are few potential biological markers to identify prenatal alcohol exposure (Caprara et al. 2007). Measuring ethanol itself is not sufficient evidence to support long-term fetal exposure to alcohol, because alcohol is a highly hydrophilic molecule that is rapidly eliminated in vivo. The association between gestational alcohol consumption and maternal serum biochemical markers such as gamma-glutamyl transferase, mean corpuscular volume, haemoglobin-associated acetyldehyde and carbohydrate-deficient transferrin is still under evaluation as a means of identifying heavy drinking in pregnancy.

Fatty acid ethyl esters (FAEEs) are products of the non-oxidative metabolism of alcohol. Elevated FAEEs can persist in the blood for hours to days after the consumption of alcohol. Fetal FAEEs do not cross the human placenta and thus have been established as the first direct biomarker of fetal exposure to ethanol, being produced by the fetus from ethanol transferred via the placenta. Meconium comprises the neonate's first bowel movements, identified by its dark green colour and lack of odour. Fetal meconium formation begins at approximately 12 weeks of gestation, making it an optimal static matrix once deposited in the fetal intestines for assessing prenatal exposure to alcohol (Caprara et al. 2007). However, a limitation is that it only provides information about exposure after 12 weeks of gestation, while most heavy drinking has been reported in the first trimester.

An application of this biomarker to a population-based sample in Canada (Gareri et al. 2008) showed that 17 of 682 meconium samples tested positive for significant prenatal alcohol exposure (>2.0 nmol/g). This analysis compared FAEE analysis with standard postpartum questionnaires regarding alcohol consumption and detected five-fold more ethanol-exposed pregnancies (2.5% vs 0.5%). The prevalence of ethanol-exposed pregnancies was consistent with CDC estimates of 'frequent' prenatal drinking (>7 drinks per week) and previously published estimates of FASD prevalence in the general North American population. Cumulative FAEE levels above 2.0 nmol/g are indicative of heavy (>2 drinks per day) or binge (>5–6 drinks per occasion) ethanol use during pregnancy, but may also be capable of detecting ethanol exposure at the 'frequent' level. The study concluded that identification of 2.5% of pregnancies as ethanol exposed was consistent with the 1% disease prevalence of FASD taking into account that approximately 40% of exposed fetuses are affected. Such studies have shown that a cut-off of total cumulative FAEE of 2 nmol/g of meconium demonstrates 100% sensitivity and 98% specificity in distinguishing neonates born to non-drinking mothers from offspring of heavy drinkers (Caprara et al. 2007).

Whilst there are clearly ethical considerations surrounding the adoption of meconium screening to detect in utero alcohol exposure (the samples in this study were anonymously collected), the development of a reliable neonatal marker would help target resources not only to the at-risk neonate, but also allow beneficial intervention for the at-risk alcohol-consuming mother. Appropriate support services and intervention programmes would be mandated prior to the adoption of such a neonatal screening tool in line with the agreed criteria for introduction of a screening programme, and effective health-care interventions in ascertained cases will be available. However, the aims of such screening, the nature of informed consent and national targets for the percentage of neonates screened would not be dissimilar to those for current antenatal screening programmes for other conditions such as human immunodeficiency virus in pregnancy, which also might result in stigmatization, but in which treatment has been shown to be efficacious.

A more recent finding is that FAEE can be measured in hair samples, from both the mother and infant. Unlike meconium, neonatal hair collection can occur up to three months after birth, when it typically sheds. Drugs are deposited in the cortex of the hair and thus exposures during the last trimester of pregnancy might be found in neonatal hair after birth. Animal studies indicate that FAEEs are present in higher amounts in hair of neonates exposed to excessive amounts of alcohol in utero. Caprara et al. (2007) confirmed in guinea pigs that chronic exposure to alcohol during pregnancy leads to increased levels of FAEE in both maternal and neonatal hair. While there are some case reports involving FASD and the measurement of FAEE in hair samples, there are no significant human studies validating this measure.

Prenatal presentation of fetal alcohol syndrome

Modern obstetric care allows antenatal detection of a wide variety of birth defects. The advent of routine detailed fetal ultrasonography and standardization of fetal growth charts allows attention to be focused on the abnormal fetus, even in the absence of a previously volunteered history of maternal alcohol exposure. Structural brain anomalies including microcephaly, cerebellar abnormalities with hypoplasia of the anterior vermis, and hypoplasia of the corpus callosum, may be detectable by fetal ultrasonography or fetal brain magnetic resonance imaging. Recent work has shown that a shortened frontal thalamic distance can be detected via prenatal ultrasonography during the second and third trimesters (Kfir et al. 2010).

AETIOLOGICAL FACTORS

Numerous controlled experimental studies with animals have demonstrated the teratogenicity of alcohol. Ethanol freely crosses the placenta, thus directly affecting developing embryonic and fetal tissue (Goodlett et al. 2005). The mechanisms for alcohol-induced teratogenesis are not yet fully elucidated, being complicated by the complex cellular influences exerted by ethanol. Some of the postulated mechanisms by which alcohol exerts its effects are induction of apoptosis, cell adhesion defects, accumulation of free radicals, effects on growth factors and antagonism of retinoic acid biosynthesis (Gemma et al. 2007). As with most other teratogens, the mechanisms of ethanol damage may vary according to the stage of embryological development. At the time of conception and during the first weeks of pre-natal development, ethanol may act as a cytotoxic or mutagenic agent, causing cell death or lethal chromosome abnormalities. Evidence for this comes from the increased risk of miscarriage in alcohol-exposed pregnancies (Kesmodel et al. 2002).

During the period from four to 10 weeks after conception, alcohol can cause excessive cell death in the CNS and abnormalities in neuronal migration. Abnormal migration leads to disorganization of tissue structures and cell loss to microcephaly. Early shortening of the anterior cranial base due to alcohol-induced deficiency of brain growth may help to explain the alterations in the shape of the mid-face (Niccols 2007).

The disorganization and delay of cell migration with cell death all contribute to a diverse pattern of fetal malformation, with the developing brain and heart particularly vulnerable. The cerebellum and prefrontal cortex can be subject to damage in the third trimester. Exactly how alcohol impairs neuronal migration is still under research. Kumada et al. (2007) suggest that calcium signalling and cyclic nucleotides signalling are the central targets of action of alcohol in neuronal cell migration. Parnell et al. (2007) suggest that it is not cerebral hypoxia that is the mechanism of brain damage but rather elevation in brain blood flow. In the ovine (sheep) model, they concluded that exposure to moderate doses of ethanol during the third trimester alters fetal cerebral vascular function and increases blood flow in brain regions, including the cerebellum, that are vulnerable to ethanol in the presence of acidaemia and hypercapnia, and in the absence of hypoxia.

A recent study (Vangipuram et al. 2008) looked at the effects of alcohol upon fetal human brain-derived neural progenital cells, which did not show an increase in apoptosis but demonstrated more rapid coalescence and increased volume of neurospheres. In addition, the expression of genes associated with cell adhesion was significantly altered, leading the authors to hypothesize that changes in surface adhesion interactions between neural progenital cells may underlie aspects of neurodevelopmental abnormalities in FAS.

Alcohol interferes with neurotransmitter production in the CNS leading to neuroendocrine abnormalities. These include suppression of growth hormone release by the hypothalamus, which may account for the postnatal growth deficits observed in FAS. Alcohol consumption increases maternal and fetal hypothalamic–pituitary–adrenal activity, affecting the development of fetal endocrine functions.

As only 10–40% of women who consume alcohol to excess in pregnancy have babies with FAS, other factors must be involved. These include patterns and dose of consumption, age, parity and nutritional status. There is also an increasing amount of information suggesting that allelic variants encoding for the enzymes involved in ethanol metabolism may put some ethnic populations at higher risk of having an affected child. One of the major factors determining peak blood exposure to the fetus is the metabolic activity of the mother, in addition to placental and fetal metabolism (Gemma et al. 2007).

Polymorphisms of the alcohol metabolizing enzymes ADH (acetyl dehydrogenase) and CYP2E1 [hepatic CYP2E1 is responsible for a limited (10%) amount of ethanol oxidation but is inducible when ADH is saturated] and their frequency in different populations and affected FAS offspring are the subject of research into the possible protective roles of some of these allelic variants. For example, the ADH2 polymorphism in a mixed ancestry population in the Western Cape province of South Africa showed the ADH2*2 allele to be more common in unaffected individuals (Viljoen et al. 2001).

Child protection issues

In the case of a known alcohol-dependent mother, social services and care proceedings are likely to be put into place. Assessing the capability of an alcoholic mother to care for her baby is complex and takes time: this is explored in more detail in Chapters 12 and 13. Agencies need to be aware that the infant with possible or definite FAS will, after discharge, have an increased risk of mortality (May et al. 2000). A recent study of mortality rates in infants and children with FASD and their siblings found an FAS case mortality rate of 3.5% with a sibling mortality rate of 4.7%. The overall mortality for the 304 linked FASD registry children was 2.4%. The case mortality for pFAS was 1.4%, and for alcohol-related neuro-developmental disorder was 1.7%. Infants were found to be at increased risk of mortality compared to older children. The diagnosis of an FASD is also an under-appreciated risk marker for mortality in their siblings. Therefore mother, infant and siblings are candidates for increased surveillance for a wide range of adverse outcomes.

Failure to attend follow-up clinics, paediatric or specialist review, and lack of accessibility for community health-care professionals to the home are all signs of an at-risk domestic situation.

For the mother of an alcohol-exposed neonate with FAS, a wide range of interventions should be in place including alcohol reduction strategies and periconceptional counselling. The sibling recurrence risk in FAS is 75%, underlying the need for careful counselling and assessment of maternal dependency prior to any future pregnancy.

Long-term paediatric follow-up

The newborn infant with FAS should have multidisciplinary paediatric follow-up focusing on growth and development, with assessment of hearing, ophthalmological and cardiac status. Prior to school entry, developmental assessment should be carefully undertaken to identify specific cognitive or behavioural deficits so that these can be addressed in the education system. A high degree of awareness needs to be maintained to identify later difficulties not apparent at school entry (see Chapter 7).

Finally, FAS is rarely a 'pure' syndrome of alcohol teratogenesis alone. It is rather a multifactorial disorder with component aspects of genetics, environment, ethnicity, social and nutritional status and often involves other drugs of abuse than alcohol alone. In the light of increasing levels of alcohol consumption in young women, this condition has become a major public health issue. Detection of alcohol-exposed neonates and early and prompt diagnosis can improve the future potential of infants with FAS, given the development of specific educational and behavioural strategies to improve long-term outcomes.

There is a need for effective strategies for prevention of this condition, education to facilitate earlier diagnosis, referral and reporting of cases. An infrastructure for the referral, diagnosis and management of FAS and FASD should be readily available.

REFERENCES

Abel EL, Hannigan JH (1995) Maternal risk factors in fetal alcohol syndrome: provocative and permissive inluences. *Neurotoxicol Teratol* **17**: 445–462.

Astley SJ (2004) *Diagnostic Guide for Fetal Alcohol Spectrum Disorders: The 4-Digit Diagnostic Code.* Seattle: University of Washington.

Astley SJ, Clarren SK (1996) A case definition and photographic screening tool for the facial phenotype of fetal alcohol syndrome. *J Pediatr* **129**: 33–41.

Astley SJ, Clarren SK (2000) Diagnosing the full spectrum of fetal alcohol-exposed individuals: introducing the 4-digit diagnostic code. *Alcohol Alcohol* **35**: 400–410.

Bailey BA, Sokol RJ (2008) Pregnancy and alcohol use: evidence and recommendations for prenatal care. *Clin Obstet Gynecol* **51**: 436–444.

Baumann P, Schild C, Hume RF, Sokol RJ (2006) Alcohol abuse—a persistent preventable risk for congenital anomalies. *Int J Gynaecol Obstet* **95**: 66–72.

Bertrand J, Floyd RL, Weber MK, et al. (2004) *Fetal Alcohol Syndrome: Guidelines for Referral and Diagnosis.* Atlanta, GA: US Department of Health and Human Services, Centers for Disease Control and Prevention.

Bookstein FL, Connor PD, Huggins JE, et al. (2007) Many infants prenatally exposed to high levels of alcohol show one particular anomaly of the corpus callosum. *Alcohol Clin Exp Res* **31**: 868–879.

Burd L, Klug MG, Martsolf J (2004) Increased sibling mortality in children with fetal alcohol syndrome. *Addiction Biol* **9**: 179–186.

Burd L, Deal E, Rios R, et al. (2007) Congenital heart defects and fetal alcohol spectrum disorders. *Congenit Heart Dis* **2**: 250–255.

Burd L, Klug MG, Bueling R, et al. (2008) Mortality rates in subjects with fetal alcohol spectrum disorders and their siblings. *Birth Defects Res A Clin Mol Teratol* **82**: 217–223.

Caprara DL, Nash K, Greenbaum R, et al. (2007) Novel approaches to the diagnosis of fetal alcohol spectrum disorder. *Neurosci Biobehav Rev* **31**: 254–260.

Chasnoff IJ, Wells AM, McGourty RF, Bailey LK (2007) Validation of the 4P's Plus screen for substance use in pregnancy validation of the 4P's Plus. *J Perinatol* **27**: 744–748.

Chudley AE, Conry J, Cook JL, et al. (2005) Fetal alcohol spectrum disorder: Canadian guidelines for diagnosis. *CMAJ* **172**: S1–S21.

Church MW, Kaltenbach JA (1997) Hearing, speech, language, and vestibular disorders in the fetal alcohol syndrome: A literature review. *Alcohol Clin Exp Res* **21**: 495–512.

Elliott EJ, Payne J, Morris A, et al. (2008) Fetal alcohol syndrome: a prospective national surveillance study. *Arch Dis Child* **93**: 732–737.

Floyd RL, O'Connor MJ, Sokol RJ, et al. (2005) Recognition and prevention of fetal alcohol syndrome. *Obstet Gynecol* **106**: 1059–1064.

Gareri JLH, Lynn H, Handley M, et al. (2008) Prevalence of fetal ethanol exposure in a regional population-based sample by meconium analysis of fatty acid ethyl esters. *Ther Drug Monit* **30**: 239–245.

Gemma S, Vichi S, Testai E (2007) Metabolic and genetic factors contributing to alcohol induced effects and fetal alcohol syndrome. *Neurosci Biobehav Rev* **31**: 221–229.

Goodlett CR, Horn KH, Zhou FC (2005) Alcohol teratogenesis: mechanisms of damage and strategies for intervention. *Exp Biol Med* **230**: 394–406.

Habbick BF, Blakley PM, Houston CS, et al. (1998) Bone age and growth in fetal alcohol syndrome. *Alcohol Clin Exp Res* **22**: 1312–1316.

Hall JG, Froster-Iskenius UG, Allanson JE (1989) *Handbook of Normal Physical Measurements.* Oxford: Oxford University Press.

Hofer RBL (2009) Review of published studies of kidney, liver, and gastrointestinal birth defects in fetal alcohol spectrum disorders. *Birth Defects Res A Clin Mol Teratol* **85**: 179–183.

Hoyme HE, May PA, Kalberg WO, et al. (2005) A practical clinical approach to diagnosis of fetal alcohol spectrum disorders: clarification of the 1996 Institute of Medicine criteria. *Pediatrics* **115**: 39–47.

Jones KL, Smith DW (1973) Recognition of the fetal alcohol syndrome in early infancy. *Lancet* **ii**: 999–1001.

Jones KL, Smith DW, Ulleland CN, Streissguth AP (1973) Pattern of malformation in offspring of chronic alcoholic mothers. *Lancet* **i**: 1267–1271.

Kaskutas LA, Kerr WC (2008) Accuracy of photographs to capture respondent-defined drink size. *J Stud Alcohol Drugs* **69**: 605–610.

Kessmodel U, Wisborg K, Olsen SF, et al. (2002) Moderate alcohol intake in pregnancy and the risk of spontaneous abortion. *Alcohol* **37**: 87–92.

Kfir M, Yevtushok L, Onishchenko S, et al. (2010) Can prenatal ultrasound detect the effects of in-utero alcohol exposure? A pilot study. *Ultrasound Obstet Gynecol* **33**: 683–689.

Kumada T, Jiang Y, Cameron DB, Komuro H (2007) How does alcohol impair neuronal migration? *J Neurosci Res* **85**: 465–470.

Little BB, Snell LM, Rosenfeld CR, et al. (1990) Failure to recognize fetal alcohol syndrome in newborn infants. *Am J Dis Child* **144**: 1142–1146.

May PA, Brooke L, Gossage JP, et al. (2000) Epidemiology of fetal alcohol syndrome in a South African community in the Western Cape Province. *Am J Pub Health* **90**: 1905–1912.

Niccols A (2007) Fetal alcohol syndrome and the developing socio-emotional brain. *Brain Cogn* **65**: 135–142.

O'Connor MJ, Whaley SE (2007) Brief intervention for alcohol use by pregnant women. *Am J Public Health* **97**: 252–258

Parnell SE, Ramadoss J, Delp MD, et al. (2007) Chronic ethanol increases fetal cerebral blood flow specific to the ethanol-sensitive cerebellum under normoxaemic, hypercapnic and acidaemic conditions: ovine model. *Exp Physiol* **92**: 933–943.

Sokol RJ, Chik L, Martier SS, Salari V (1991) Morphometry of the neonatal fetal alcohol syndrome face from 'snapshots'. *Alcohol Alcohol Suppl* **1**: 531–534.

Spadoni AD, McGee CL, Fryer SL, Riley EP (2007) Neuroimaging and fetal alcohol spectrum disorders. *Neurosci Biobehav Rev* **31**: 239–245.

Stoler JM, Holmes LB (2004) Recognition of facial features of fetal alcohol syndrome in the newborn. *Am J Med Genet C Semin Med Genet* **127C**: 21–27.

Stratton K, Howe C, Battaglia F (1996) *Fetal Alcohol Syndrome: Diagnosis, Epidemiology, Prevention, and Treatment.* Washington, DC: National Academy Press.

Streissguth AP, Bookstein FL, Barr HM, et al. (2004) Risk factors for adverse life outcomes in fetal alcohol syndrome and fetal alcohol effects. *J Dev Behav Pediatr* **25**: 228–238.

Strömland K (2004) Visual impairment and ocular abnormalities in children with fetal alcohol syndrome. *Addict Biol* **9**: 153–157; discussion 159–160.

Thomas IT, Gaitantzis YA, Frias JL (1987) Palpebral fissure length from 29 weeks gestation to 14 years. *J Pediatr* **111**: 267–268.

Vangipuram SD, Grever WE, Parker GC, Lyman WD (2008) Ethanol increases fetal human neurosphere size and alters adhesion molecule gene expression. *Alcohol Clin Exp Res* **32**: 339–347.

Viljoen DL, Carr LG, Foroud TM, et al. (2001) Alcohol dehydrogenase-2*2 allele is associated with decreased prevalence of fetal alcohol syndrome in the mixed-ancestry population of the Western Cape Province, South Africa. *Alcohol Clin Exp Res* **25**: 1719–1722.

Wattendorf DJ, Muenke M (2005) Fetal alcohol spectrum disorders. *Am Fam Physician* **72**: 279–282; 285.

Welch-Carre E (2005) The neurodevelopmental consequences of prenatal alcohol exposure. *Adv Neonat Care* **5**: 217–229.

7

THE EFFECTS OF PRENATAL ALCOHOL EXPOSURE ON BRAIN AND BEHAVIOUR

Christie L McGee Petrenko and Edward P Riley

The devastating consequences of prenatal alcohol exposure have been alluded to for centuries (Calhoun and Warren 2007). However, it was not until the late 1960s and early '70s that fetal alcohol syndrome (FAS) was first identified by the medical community (Lemoine et al. 1968, Jones and Smith 1973, Jones et al. 1973). Diagnostic criteria for FAS have not changed dramatically in the last 30 years, and include characteristic facial features, growth retardation and central nervous system (CNS) dysfunction (Bertrand et al. 2004, Hoyme et al. 2005). It is clear from the scientific and clinical literature that FAS is not the only consequence of prenatal alcohol exposure. Recently, the non-diagnostic term fetal alcohol spectrum disorders (FASDs) was proposed to encompass the full spectrum of effects ranging from FAS to more subtle physical, cognitive and behavioural effects resulting from prenatal alcohol exposure (Bertrand et al. 2004, Hoyme et al. 2005). More detailed information on the diagnosis, epidemiology and embryology of FAS and related conditions can be found in Chapters 3 and 6. This chapter reviews the CNS dysfunctions associated with prenatal alcohol exposure beginning with a discussion of changes in various brain structures and how the function of these structures is altered by prenatal alcohol exposure. The cognitive and behavioural impairments identified in alcohol-exposed individuals are then reviewed.

Methodological considerations

Before discussing the research findings, it is important to consider differences in recruitment methodology in the field as this often aids in reconciling discrepancies between studies. Typically in prospective designs, detailed information on alcohol consumption is gathered from women during pregnancy, and their children are followed longitudinally from birth. These studies often represent population-based research, and the exposures are mostly at moderate or 'social drinking' levels [a mean of 0.31 ounces (8.8 g or 1.1 British units) per day and 2.17 drinks (approximately 26 g or 3.3 British units) per occasion] during pregnancy (Streissguth 2007). Advantages of this design include more accurate measurement of alcohol consumption, greater control of confounding factors, stronger conclusions regarding changes over time, and the ability to examine dose–response relationships. Disadvantages include the expense and time it takes to conduct such studies, the often small numbers of heavily exposed individuals sampled, and the large number of participants that must be recruited to detect effects related to the exposure. In retrospective designs, individuals are identified

TABLE 7.1
Cognitive functions commonly associated with brain structures

Brain structure	Functions
Cerebral cortex	
Frontal lobe	Executive functions, motor skills, language production, attention, personality
Temporal lobe	Hearing, object and face recognition, language comprehension
Parietal lobe	Somatosensory perception, visuospatial processing, attention
Occipital lobe	Visual perception
Cerebellum	Balance, motor coordination, attention, eye blink conditioning, executive functions, classical conditioning
Corpus callosum	Interhemispheric transfer, bimanual coordination
Basal ganglia	Motor coordination, executive functions
Hippocampus	Memory

at some time after the alcohol exposure occurred, often during childhood or adolescence. Accurate measurement of alcohol consumption is difficult in such designs, and therefore studies place more emphasis on alcohol-related diagnoses (i.e. FAS) in prenatally exposed children. Confirmed maternal alcohol consumption is typically required for diagnosis and is defined as a pattern of excessive intake characterized by substantial regular intake (e.g. two 'drinks' per day, see Chapter 2) or heavy episodic or binge drinking (e.g. four or more drinks per occasion; Hoyme et al. 2005). Retrospective samples frequently contain a large number of 'clinically referred' participants who come to the study because of some clinically significant manifestation of the exposure. The advantages of this methodology include increased sampling of more severe cases, smaller overall sample size required to detect effects, reduced time and cost to conduct the study, and the ability to include distinct control or comparison groups. Reporting and ascertainment biases are disadvantages of retrospective designs. Each type of study provides a different perspective for the researcher.

Brain abnormalities

Early autopsy studies of individuals with prenatal alcohol exposure revealed widespread CNS disorganization, including microcephaly (small head size), neuroglial heterotopias (abnormal migration of neuronal and glial cells), and anomalies of the ventricles, corpus callosum, basal ganglia and cerebellum (for a review, see Clarren 1986). However, material available for autopsy is usually the most severely affected and may not be typical of the brain changes that occur in the majority of individuals with prenatal alcohol exposure. More recently, structural and functional neuroimaging techniques have allowed for identification of specific alterations in brains of living individuals exposed prenatally to a range of alcohol levels. Findings from neuroimaging studies reveal a pattern of structural and functional abnormalities consistent with the cognitive and behavioural impairments found in individuals with prenatal alcohol exposure. These findings confirm the experimental data discussed by Sulik and colleagues in Chapter 3. Table 7.1 lists cognitive functions commonly associated with specific brain structures, while Figure 7.1 illustrates brain

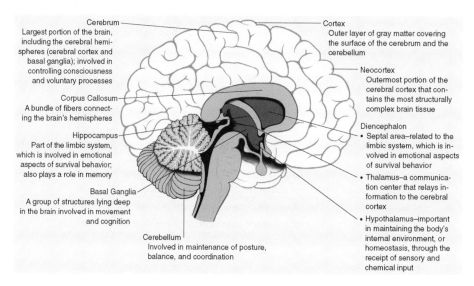

Cerebrum
Largest portion of the brain, including the cerebral hemispheres (cerebral cortex and basal ganglia); involved in controlling consciousness and voluntary processes

Corpus Callosum
A bundle of fibers connecting the brain's hemispheres

Hippocampus
Part of the limbic system, which is involved in emotional aspects of survival behavior; also plays a role in memory

Basal Ganglia
A group of structures lying deep in the brain involved in movement and cognition

Cerebellum
Involved in maintenance of posture, balance, and coordination

Cortex
Outer layer of gray matter covering the surface of the cerebrum and the cerebellum

Neocortex
Outermost portion of the cerebral cortex that contains the most structurally complex brain tissue

Diencephalon
• Septal area–related to the limbic system, which is involved in emotional aspects of survival behavior
• Thalamus–a communication center that relays information to the cerebral cortex
• Hypothalamus–important in maintaining the body's internal environment, or homeostasis, through the receipt of sensory and chemical input

Fig. 7.1. Areas of the brain that can be damaged in utero by maternal alcohol consumption. (Reproduced by permission from Mattson et al. 1994.) For colour version of this figure, see plate section at end of book.

structures often affected by prenatal alcohol exposure. A summary of the brain changes discussed below is presented in Table 7.2.

STRUCTURAL CHANGES
Cerebral volume and shape abnormalities
A reduction in the overall size of the brain is consistently found in individuals with heavy prenatal alcohol exposure (Mattson et al. 1992, 1994, 1996c; Johnson et al. 1996; Swayze et al. 1997; Archibald et al. 2001; Sowell et al. 2001b, 2002a; Autti-Rämö et al. 2002). An analysis of the different parts of the cerebrum (the various lobes) reveals reductions in the parietal, frontal and temporal lobe volumes (Sowell et al. 2002a); however, when the reduction in overall brain size is considered, only the parietal and frontal lobes are disproportionately reduced (Archibald et al. 2001, Sowell et al. 2002a). Thus, the frontal and parietal lobes are smaller than one would expect based on the overall volume reduction of the brain, and these lobes appear to be especially susceptible to the effects of prenatal alcohol exposure. Detailed regional analyses find local reductions in brain growth in inferior parietal and orbito-frontal cortices resulting in changes to the overall shape of the brain, such that alcohol-exposed children have smaller and narrower brains with some blunting in frontal areas when compared with typically developing children (Fig. 7.2) (Sowell et al. 2002a). Prenatal ultrasonography also reveals reductions in frontal lobe size in fetuses exposed to alcohol prenatally (Wass et al. 2001, Kfir et al. 2009). These changes in the frontal lobe are consistent with findings of executive functioning deficits in this population (Rasmussen 2005). Alterations to the parietal lobe may relate to impairments seen in individuals with prenatal alcohol exposure in spatial working memory, object and face recognition, and arithmetic and language

110

TABLE 7.2
Summary of brain changes found in individuals with prenatal alcohol exposure

Brain structure	Changes
Cerebrum	
Volume	Reductions in overall brain volume; disproportionate reductions in parietal and frontal lobes
Shape	Smaller and narrower brains with blunting in frontal areas
Grey and white matter	White matter reduced more than grey matter, especially in the parietal lobe; increased cortical thickness and grey matter volumes at the junction of parietal and temporal lobes and frontal regions
Cerebellum	
Volume	Reduced cerebellar volume
Vermis	Anterior vermis reduced more than posterior vermis; anterior vermis shape alterations
Corpus callosum	
Gross abnormalities	Complete or partial absence of the structure, thinning
Volume	Reductions in overall volume; disproportionate reductions in posterior regions, especially the splenium
Shape	Abnormal curvature of splenium; excess variability in shape
Microstructure	Altered microstructure in white matter fibres in posterior regions
Basal ganglia	
Volume	Reduced overall volume; disproportionate reductions in the caudate
Hippocampus	
Volume	Reduced volume, thinning, asymmetry

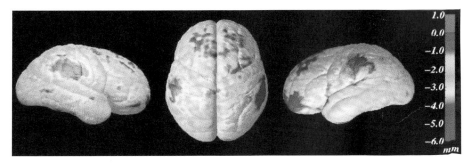

Fig. 7.2. Structural magnetic resonance imaging study that measured the difference in shape of the cerebrum in alcohol-exposed individuals and controls. Shape was quantified by measuring the distance from the centre of the brain to the surface (DFC) in millimeters. Areas highlighted in red reflect average differences of 4–6 mm in cortical thickness between alcohol-exposed individuals and controls. Negative values indicate that alcohol-exposed individuals have smaller DFC values than controls. Results illustrate that alcohol-exposed individuals have smaller brains than typically developing children, with narrowing in the inferior parietal region and some blunting in frontal areas. (Reproduced by permission from Sowell et al. 2002a.) For colour version of this figure, see plate section at end of book.

111

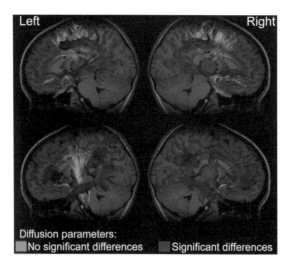

Fig. 7.3. Integrity of 10 white matter tracts in the cerebrum of children with prenatal alcohol exposure using diffusion tensor imaging tractography techniques. Diffusion tensor imaging allows measurement of white matter microstructure, which can be recreated in three dimensions through tractography. Of the 10 tracts studied, seven showed significant abnormalities in the alcohol-exposed group. These tracts included the genu and splenium of the corpus callosum, cingulum, corticospinal tracts, inferior fronto-occipital fasciculus, and inferior and superior longitudinal fasciculus. (Adapted by permission from Lebel et al. 2008.) For colour version of this figure, see plate section at end of book.

processing (Mattson and Riley 1998, Sowell et al. 2002b). These behavioural changes will be discussed later.

Differences in grey and white matter
Grey matter is composed of neuron cell bodies that make up the cortex and deep subcortical structures (e.g. basal ganglia, thalamus). White matter, on the other hand, is composed primarily of myelinated axons carrying information away from the cell. Myelin increases the speed at which impulses move along the axon and is primarily composed of lipids, giving it a white colour. In individuals with prenatal alcohol exposure the amounts of both grey and white matter tissues are reduced (Archibald et al. 2001, Sowell et al. 2001b). However, white matter appears more affected and is disproportionately reduced, and the reduction is more severe than in grey matter, especially in the parietal lobe (Archibald et al. 2001). There is also an increase in the proportional grey matter and reductions in white matter at the junction of the left temporal and parietal lobes in alcohol-exposed individuals when compared with controls (Sowell et al. 2001b). Consistent with findings of proportional increases in grey matter, measures of cortical thickness are higher in this region, as well as in right frontal areas (Sowell et al. 2008b). Increased cortical thickness in frontal regions is related to poorer verbal recall in individuals with prenatal alcohol exposure. The increases in grey matter and cortical thickness observed through magnetic resonance imaging may actually be unmyelinated axon fibres, reflecting abnormal and decreased myelination, which is

112

consistent with diffusion tensor imaging studies looking at white matter microstructure in these regions (Fig. 7.3) (Lebel et al. 2008, Sowell et al. 2008a).

Cerebellum

The cerebellum consists of two hemispheres joined by the vermis and is located below the occipital lobe and directly connects to the brainstem. Similar to the volume reductions in the cerebrum, the size of the cerebellum is also reduced in individuals prenatally exposed to alcohol (Mattson et al. 1992, 1994; Riikonen et al. 1999; Archibald et al. 2001; Autti-Rämö et al. 2002; Bookstein et al. 2006). Prenatal ultrasonography also shows reductions in cerebellar width in heavily exposed fetuses (Handmaker et al. 2006). In addition to the overall size reduction of the cerebellum, disproportionate reductions are found in the anterior, or older, portion of the vermis, whereas the later-developing posterior regions are relatively spared (Sowell et al. 1996, O'Hare et al. 2005). The anterior vermis is also displaced more than other regions of the vermis in alcohol-exposed individuals compared with non-exposed controls (O'Hare et al. 2005). Vermal displacement is correlated with deficits in verbal learning and memory in alcohol-exposed individuals (O'Hare et al. 2005). In addition, alterations to the cerebellum may be related to the deficits in postural balance (Roebuck et al. 1998a), temporal processing (Wass et al. 2002), eye-blink conditioning (Coffin et al. 2005, Jacobson et al. 2008) and attention (Streissguth et al. 1995; Coles et al. 1997, 2002) commonly seen in individuals with prenatal alcohol exposure.

Corpus callosum

The corpus callosum is a major white matter tract that connects the two cerebral hemispheres and facilitates interhemispheric communication. Reports of agenesis or complete absence of the corpus callosum have been noted in children and adolescents prenatally exposed to alcohol, as well as less severe alterations such as thinning, hypoplasia or partial agenesis (Mattson et al. 1992, Riley et al. 1995, Johnson et al. 1996, Swayze et al. 1997, Riikonen et al. 1999, Clark et al. 2000, Sowell et al. 2001a, Autti-Rämö et al. 2002, Bhatara et al. 2002). Detailed analyses reveal disproportionate reductions in select regions of the corpus callosum, most notably in the splenium, or most posterior area (Riley et al. 1995, Sowell et al. 2001a). In addition, the splenium is displaced downward, and displacement is a significant predictor of verbal learning deficits in alcohol-exposed individuals (Fig. 7.4) (Sowell et al. 2001a). In a study utilizing paediatric ultrasonography of infants in the first three months of life, half of the sample of alcohol-exposed infants showed a change in the angle of curvature of the splenium (Bookstein et al. 2007). Other studies find an excess variability of callosal shape (Bookstein et al. 2001, 2002a), which relates to differential performance on motor or executive functioning tasks (Bookstein et al. 2002b). Finally, portions of the corpus callosum in children and young adults with prenatal alcohol exposure exhibit abnormal microstructure, especially in posterior regions (see Fig. 7.3) (Ma et al. 2005, Wozniak et al. 2006, Lebel et al. 2008, Sowell et al. 2008a). In one study, abnormal microstructure in the splenium correlated with visuomotor performance in children with prenatal alcohol exposure (Sowell et al. 2008a). In addition to the directly measured brain–behaviour correlates discussed above, alterations to the corpus callosum may relate to alcohol-related

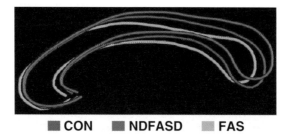

CON **NDFASD** **FAS**

Fig. 7.4. Displacement of the corpus callosum, the major fibre tract between the two cerebral hemispheres, in children with prenatal alcohol exposure. The figure displays contours of the corpus callosum generated from structural magnetic resonance imaging. The area outlined in red is the shape and location of the corpus callosum of the control (non-alcohol-exposed) group; the contour in green represents that of the FAS group; and the contour in blue represents that of the alcohol-exposed children who did not meet criteria for FAS. Results illustrate the displacement of the isthmus and splenium (most posterior regions) in the inferior and anterior direction for alcohol-exposed children relative to non-exposed controls. (Adapted by permission from Sowell et al. 2001a.)
CON = control group (typically developing children with no history of alcohol exposure).
NDFASD = non-dysmorphic fetal alcohol spectrum disorder (children exposed to significant levels of alcohol in utero, but who did not meet full criteria for a diagnosis of FAS).
FAS = fetal alcohol syndrome (children who met full clinical criteria for FAS).
For colour version of this figure, see plate section at end of book.

impairments found in bimanual coordination (Roebuck-Spencer et al. 2004), interhemispheric transfer (Roebuck et al. 2002), attention (Streissguth et al. 1995; Coles et al. 1997, 2002) and executive functioning (Rasmussen 2005).

Basal ganglia
The basal ganglia are a group of subcortical nuclei, including the caudate, nucleus accumbens and lenticular nucleus, that are located just below the corpus callosum. The basal ganglia of alcohol-exposed individuals are reduced in volume, compared with controls (Mattson et al. 1992, 1994, 1996c). However, when overall brain size is taken into account, dispro-portionate reductions are evident only in the caudate, a structure more heavily involved in cognitive functions, while the volumes of the lenticular nucleus and nucleus accumbens remain relatively spared (Mattson et al. 1992, 1996c; Archibald et al. 2001). In fact, the reduction in the volume of the caudate may be the most severe of any brain structure. The basal ganglia maintain many connections with other regions of the brain and may be in-volved in a number of critical functions such as motor coordination, executive functioning, spatial memory, perseveration and set shifting, all of which are impaired in individuals with prenatal alcohol exposure (Mattson and Riley 1998, Rasmussen 2005).

Hippocampus
The hippocampus is located inside the medial temporal lobe and is part of the limbic system. Hippocampal abnormalities including volumetric reductions, hypoplasia, regional thinning and asymmetry are noted in some studies (Riikonen et al. 1999, Autti-Rämö et al. 2002,

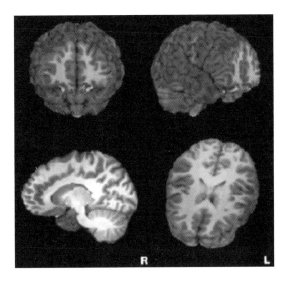

Fig. 7.5. Functional magnetic resonance imaging during a response inhibition task. Areas highlighted in blue indicate greater brain activation for alcohol-exposed children, whereas areas in orange reflect greater activation for control children during the task. During performance of the inhibition task, alcohol-exposed children showed greater activation in the right middle frontal and left superior frontal gyri (top views) and less activation in the right caudate nucleus (bottom views) relative to controls. (Reproduced by permission from Fryer et al. 2007b.) For colour version of this figure, see plate section at end of book.

Willoughby et al. 2008), whereas another study failed to find disproportionate reductions in hippocampal volume (Archibald et al. 2001). One study found that hippocampal volumes were correlated with verbal memory performance in children with FASD (Willoughby et al. 2008).

FUNCTIONAL CHANGES
Alterations in brain metabolism have been identified in individuals with prenatal alcohol exposure using functional imaging techniques (e.g. single photon emission computerized tomography, positron emission tomography, magnetic resonance spectroscopy) in areas consistent with structural changes (Riikonen et al. 1999, 2005; Clark et al. 2000; Bhatara et al. 2002; Cortese et al. 2006; Fagerlund et al. 2006). Hypoperfusion or reduced cerebral blood flow have been noticed. Other functional imaging studies utilizing functional magnetic resonance imaging techniques have examined brain response while participants complete specific cognitive tasks. Functional magnetic resonance imaging measures blood oxygen utilization to assess what brain areas are activated during the performance of various tasks. During a verbal paired-associate memory task, alcohol-exposed children showed less activation in left medial and posterior temporal regions and more activation in the frontal cortex, suggesting a compensatory mechanism for dysfunctional medial temporal memory systems (Sowell et al. 2007). On a response inhibition task, alcohol-exposed children exhibited increased frontal and decreased caudate activation, indicating that frontal–subcortical

circuits are sensitive to prenatal alcohol exposure (Fig. 7.5) (Fryer et al. 2007b). Finally, a third study examining working memory found increased activation in the inferior and middle frontal cortices in alcohol-exposed participants but not in controls, although no between-group comparisons were conducted (Malisza et al. 2005). Although further functional studies are needed, these early studies are consistent with structural findings and provide more direct evidence for altered brain–behaviour relationships in individuals with prenatal alcohol exposure.

Cognitive impairments

A summary of cognitive and behavioural impairments found in individuals with prenatal alcohol exposure is presented in Table 7.3.

GENERAL INTELLECTUAL FUNCTIONING

The effect of prenatal alcohol exposure on intellectual functioning has received considerable attention, and FAS is frequently cited as the leading known cause of intellectual disability (mental retardation) in the developed world (Pulsifer 1996). However, only about 25% of individuals with FAS have intellectual disability (Streissguth et al. 2004), as defined by an IQ <70, and IQ scores vary widely, ranging from as low as 20 to a high of at least 120 (Mattson and Riley 1998). The average IQ of individuals with FAS is estimated to be around 65–75 (Mattson and Riley 1998), and estimates for individuals without FAS, but with histories of heavy prenatal alcohol exposure, average from the low to mid 80s (Mattson et al. 1997). Prospective studies of children with low to moderate levels of exposure are more variable, with reductions in IQ relating more to the pattern of exposure and other maternal and environmental characteristics than to average alcohol consumption across pregnancy. Specifically, reductions in IQ are seen with children exposed to a binge pattern of drinking (Streissguth et al. 1989, Bailey et al. 2004), born to older mothers, and receiving less optimal cognitive stimulation in the home environment (Jacobson et al. 2004).

INFORMATION PROCESSING

Deficits in information processing – the process of acquiring, retaining and using information – occur in both infants and children with histories of prenatal alcohol exposure (Sampson et al. 1997, Jacobson 1998, Simmons et al. 2002, Kable and Coles 2004, Burden et al. 2005a, Streissguth 2007). In general, increased or more variable response time on cognitive tasks is found, suggesting that individuals prenatally exposed to alcohol suffer from inefficient cognitive processing systems. A generalized deficit in complex information processing may help explain many of the cognitive difficulties seen in children with prenatal alcohol exposure (Kodituwakku 2007, Aragon et al. 2008). Consistent with this hypothesis, one study found that alcohol-exposed children demonstrated deficits in peripheral processing speed (i.e. time involved in transmitting the impulse along the motor pathway and executing movement), but not central processing speed (i.e. time involved in processing information in the cortex prior to initiating movement) when cognitive demands were low (the task is simple), but showed deficits in both central and peripheral processing during more complex, harder tasks (Simmons et al. 2002).

TABLE 7.3
Summary of cognitive and behavioural deficits found in individuals with prenatal alcohol exposure

Deficits	Features
Cognitive deficits	
Intelligence	Average IQ is between 65 and 75 for fetal alcohol syndrome, and in the 80s for the full spectrum; individual scores vary widely
Information processing	Deficits in information processing are common, especially on more complex tasks; response times tend to be longer or more variable
Attention	Many receive diagnoses of attention-deficit–hyperactivity disorder; have difficulties encoding and shifting attention, and deficits in sustained attention also commonly found
Language	Both receptive and expressive deficits, which are consistent with IQ
Visuopatial	Visuospatial deficits; more difficulty with perception of local features than global features
Learning and memory	Active recall of learned information impaired, whereas automatic or habitual processing largely intact
– Verbal	Impaired verbal learning but generally intact recall for learned information
– Nonverbal	Both encoding and retrieval deficits; spatial learning impaired whereas object recall is generally intact
Motor	Fine and gross motor deficits; difficulties with postural balance and bimanual coordination
Executive functioning	Deficits in planning, set shifting and flexibility, inhibition, fluency, working memory, concept formation, problem solving, abstract reasoning
Academic skills	Poor academic achievement, especially in mathematics
Behavioural deficits	
Adaptive and social skills	Mean adaptive age of 7 years; greatest difficulties in socialization; have greater difficulty meeting age expectations in socialization as they get older; normal frequency of social interactions and adequate nonverbal behaviours but poor and inappropriate quality of interactions; impaired social problem solving
Behavioural and emotional functioning	Most significant difficulties in the areas of attention, disruptive and delinquent behaviour, and social problems; lower moral maturity
Psychopathology	High rates of psychopathology; most common diagnoses in children include attention-deficit–hyperactivity disorder, mood disorders and disruptive behaviour problems. Common diagnoses in adults include alcohol and drug dependence, depressive disorders and anxiety disorders
Quality of life	Likely to be in a dependent living environment and have difficulty with employment; difficulty managing finances, making decisions, and obtaining services; parenting problems and separation from children

ATTENTION

Attention is an important domain of study in FASD given the characteristic attention deficits exhibited by individuals with prenatal alcohol exposure. In fact, many children with FASD receive diagnoses of attention-deficit–hyperactivity disorder (ADHD) (Steinhausen and Spohr 1998, Burd et al. 2003, Fryer et al. 2007a). Studies comparing attention measures in

FASD and ADHD populations support somewhat different patterns of impairment (Nanson and Hiscock 1990, Coles et al. 1997). For example, in one study, children with FASD had the most difficulty with encoding and shifting attention, whereas children with ADHD demonstrated greater difficulty focusing and sustaining attention (Coles et al. 1997). Children with prenatal alcohol exposure exhibit greater impairments in sustained visual attention, while auditory attention is less affected (Coles et al. 2002, Mattson et al. 2006); however, a study with adults found the opposite pattern (Connor et al. 1999). The Seattle 500 prospective study, which has been studying the same individuals since the mid-1970s, has consistently documented difficulties with attention across age (Streissguth 2007). However, other prospective studies have failed to find a relationship between prenatal alcohol exposure and sustained attention performance with children aged 7 or younger (Boyd et al. 1991, Brown et al. 1991, Fried et al. 1992b, Coles et al. 1997, Burden et al. 2005b).

LANGUAGE
Retrospective studies report consistent deficits in receptive and expressive language in children with prenatal alcohol exposure (Conry 1990, Carney and Chermak 1991, Janzen et al. 1995, Church et al. 1997, Mattson et al. 1998, McGee et al. 2009), and these deficits tend to be commensurate with estimates of IQ (Becker et al. 1990, McGee et al. 2008a). Prospective studies, which tend to focus on children with lower alcohol exposures [i.e. a mean of 0.18–0.61 ounces (5.1–17.3 g) or 0.6–2.2 British units of alcohol per day], are less consistent and results are variable in young children (Gusella and Fried 1984; Fried and Watkinson 1988, 1990; Greene et al. 1990; Fried et al. 1992a). However, one large study with adolescents found a moderate dose–response relationship between alcohol exposure and phonological processing, which underlies basic reading skills (Streissguth et al. 1994a). In addition to age and level of exposure, task complexity may also account for the differences among studies (Kodituwakku 2007).

VISUOSPATIAL SKILLS
Impairments in visuospatial skills are consistently found in alcohol-exposed children (Conry 1990, Janzen et al. 1995, Mattson et al. 1998, Streissguth 2007), although one study suggested that deficits on some tests may be due to motor rather than perceptual problems (Janzen et al. 1995). With hierarchical stimuli consisting of larger forms made from smaller forms, alcohol-exposed children display difficulties recalling local features (the smaller forms), but show little to no impairment in recalling the global features when compared with controls (Mattson et al. 1996a).

LEARNING AND MEMORY
A number of studies demonstrate significant learning and memory impairments in individuals with prenatal alcohol exposure, with later work attempting to discern specific patterns of strengths and weaknesses in this domain. Explicit memory, or the active storage and retrieval of learned information (e.g. recalling mathematical facts or what happened at the baseball game), is impaired in alcohol-exposed individuals, whereas implicit memory, or more automatic and habitual processing (e.g. knowing how to ride a bike), appears largely intact,

although only limited data are available (Mattson and Riley 1999). Within the domain of explicit memory, individuals prenatally exposed to alcohol display deficits in both encoding (i.e. learning new information such as mathematical facts) (Mattson et al. 1996b, Mattson and Roebuck 2002, Kaemingk et al. 2003) and retrieval (i.e. active recall of learned information) (Mattson and Riley 1999, Roebuck-Spencer and Mattson 2004). Studies have also examined the type of information to be encoded and retrieved. Several studies have demonstrated that children with heavy prenatal alcohol exposure show impaired verbal learning (encoding) but are able to retain and retrieve information once learned (Mattson et al. 1996b, Mattson and Roebuck 2002, Kaemingk et al. 2003). However, when an inferred learning strategy (e.g. words to be recalled belong to several specific categories such as fruits or furniture) is not included, alcohol-exposed children have difficulty retaining and retrieving information above and beyond what is expected due to poor encoding or initial learning (Roebuck-Spencer and Mattson 2004). Similarly, children with light to moderate levels of prenatal alcohol exposure, especially those exposed to binge patterns of drinking, demonstrate impaired learning of verbal information that accounts for the observed memory deficits (Willford et al. 2004).

For material presented nonverbally, children with heavy prenatal alcohol exposure show impairment of both encoding and retrieval (Mattson and Roebuck 2002, Kaemingk et al. 2003). Prospective studies are more variable, with some finding a relationship between prenatal alcohol exposure and difficulty with nonverbal memory (Streissguth 2007), in contrast to others that found no such link (Willford et al. 2004). These differences may be a result of level and pattern of exposure, task complexity and type of stimuli used. Individuals with prenatal alcohol exposure exhibit spatial learning and recall deficits, whereas object recall is generally intact (Streissguth et al. 1994c; Uecker and Nadel 1996, 1998; Hamilton et al. 2003). However, the amount of information initially learned was not controlled for in these studies and therefore it is unknown if spatial recall deficits are due to learning (encoding) impairments or retrieval deficits.

MOTOR ABILITIES
The majority of studies of motor abilities report fine and gross motor deficits in children and adolescents with prenatal alcohol exposure (Jones et al. 1973, Barr et al. 1990, Conry 1990, Streissguth et al. 1994b, Mattson et al. 1998, Adnams et al. 2001, Korkman et al. 2003, Kalberg et al. 2006). In addition, impairments in postural balance are well characterized (Roebuck et al. 1998a,b). Specifically, children with prenatal alcohol exposure show greater body sway when somatosensory information is unreliable, and balance impairments are related to CNS dysfunction rather than problems with peripheral sensory or motor function. Alcohol-exposed children also are slower and less accurate on bimanual coordination tasks, where information has to cross the corpus callosum, especially with increased task complexity (Roebuck-Spencer et al. 2004). Findings with retrospectively identified adults with heavy alcohol exposure suggest that these motor deficits are persistent. However, a longitudinal prospective study failed to find the same dose-dependent relationship between motor performance and alcohol exposure at age 25 (Connor et al. 2006) that was present at age 4 (Barr et al. 1990), suggesting developmental compensation.

EXECUTIVE FUNCTIONING

Executive functioning is a complex construct that has been broadly defined as "the ability to maintain an appropriate problem solving set for the attainment of a goal" (Welsh and Pennington 1988). A variety of cognitive domains are subsumed under this general definition, including inhibition (i.e. stopping a highly practised response), set shifting and set maintenance (e.g. to maintain or shift between tasks when necessary), planning (i.e. generating and modifying a plan for problem solving), working memory (e.g. manipulating information in the mind to solve a problem), and the ability to integrate information across time and space (Pennington and Ozonoff 1996). Executive functions are essential for adaptive responses to novel situations and are the basis of many cognitive, emotional regulation and social interaction skills (Lezak et al. 2004). Individuals prenatally exposed to alcohol have deficits on measures of planning, set shifting and flexibility, some aspects of inhibition, fluency (i.e. quickly generating information such as words that start with a specific letter), working memory, concept formation, problem solving and abstract reasoning (e.g. understanding how concepts are related) (Kodituwakku et al. 1995, 2001, 2006b; Kopera-Frye et al. 1996; Carmichael Olson et al. 1998; Mattson et al. 1998, 1999; Connor et al. 2000; Schonfeld et al. 2001; Burden et al. 2005b; Green et al. 2007; McGee et al. 2008b). Deficits in verbal fluency are greater when children have to quickly generate words beginning with the same letter versus words belonging to the same category (e.g. animals) (Schonfeld et al. 2001, Kodituwakku et al. 2006a). On measures of planning and problem solving, children with prenatal alcohol exposure have difficulty inhibiting responses and developing effective strategies to solve problems within given task constraints (Kodituwakku et al. 1995, Mattson et al. 1999). Research demonstrates that deficits in executive functioning are above and beyond deficits on more basic component processes. For example, on a common measure of set-shifting, the Trail Making Test, individuals are asked to switch between connecting numbers and letters in order. Alcohol-exposed individuals show deficits on this task even after taking into account their performance on similar conditions in which they only have to connect numbers or letters in order, or trace a line as fast as possible (Mattson et al. 1999).

ACADEMIC PERFORMANCE

Children and adolescents with histories of prenatal alcohol exposure often have difficulty in school, and many require remedial placements or educational resources and support (Streissguth et al. 1990, 2004; Spohr et al. 2007). Standardized testing reflects significant impairments in academic achievement for most samples, with arithmetic performance being especially poor (Coles et al. 1991, Goldschmidt et al. 1996, Kopera-Frye et al. 1996, Mattson et al. 1998, Howell et al. 2006, Streissguth 2007). For example, one US study found mean achievement scores in a retrospective sample of older adolescents and adults in reading, spelling and arithmetic at the fourth (9 years), third (8 years) and second grade levels (6–7 years), respectively (Streissguth et al. 1991). Prenatal alcohol exposure and arithmetic performance exhibit a linear dose–response relationship, whereas reading and spelling performance are affected only after a threshold of exposure of greater than one drink per day during the second trimester (Goldschmidt et al. 1996). Numeracy and reading scores are also negatively correlated to teacher-rated inattentive symptoms (Kodituwakku et al. 2006b).

120

The deficits seen in numeracy may be related to the changes seen in the parietal lobe. Academic interventions have also been studied in children with prenatal alcohol exposure. Two randomly controlled trials targeting specific interventions in either mathematics or language and early literacy skills in children with prenatal alcohol exposure demonstrated improvements in academic performance in comparison to alcohol-exposed children in control treatments (Adnams et al. 2007, Kable et al. 2007).

Behavioural changes (see Table 7.3)
ADAPTIVE AND SOCIAL FUNCTIONING
Adaptive functioning is one of the most important aspects of behaviour because it involves being able to perform daily activities and adapt to changes in one's environment. Without effective adaptive skills, an individual would have difficulty coping with everyday stressors and completing even basic tasks of daily living. Studies with retrospectively identified alcohol-exposed children and adults demonstrate significantly poorer adaptive functioning in comparison with non-exposed controls, especially in the domain of social functioning (Streissguth et al. 1991, Whaley et al. 2001). For example, one study found that although the mean chronological age of the sample was 17 years, the mean adaptive age was only approximately 7 years. In this sample, alcohol-exposed individuals showed the highest scores in the domain of daily living (mean age equivalent of 9 years) and the lowest scores in socialization (mean age equivalent of 6 years), with no individual meeting age expectations in the domains of communication or socialization (Streissguth et al. 1991). In contrast, a longitudinal prospective study found no significant differences in adaptive functioning with respect to level of alcohol exposure at ages 6 or 15, with scores falling in the average range (Coles et al. 1991, Howell et al. 2006). Possible explanations for this discrepancy between studies include differences in ascertainment method (e.g. lower exposures, fewer children with FAS), the demographics of populations sampled (e.g. African–American children from low socio-economic backgrounds), and differences in caregiver expectations.

Additional studies with retrospectively identified children with prenatal alcohol exposure have found that socialization skills plateau with age, suggesting that as expectations increase as children get older, children with prenatal alcohol exposure have more difficulty meeting age-expected standards (Thomas et al. 1998, Whaley et al. 2001). Comparisons with specific contrast groups demonstrate that deficits in socialization are above and beyond what would be expected based on deficits in intellectual functioning (Thomas et al. 1998) or the presence of problems requiring clinical intervention (Whaley et al. 2001). Within the socialization domain, interpersonal functioning is particularly affected (Thomas et al. 1998). While children with prenatal alcohol exposure display a normal frequency of social interactions with appropriate facial expressions and nonverbal behaviours, the quality of their social interactions with others is often poor and inappropriate (Bishop et al. 2007). Several studies suggest possible mechanisms for these deficits, including poorer attachment to adult caregivers during early childhood (O'Connor et al. 2002a), which may limit exposure to and learning of appropriate social skills; deficits in executive functioning (Schonfeld et al. 2006); impairments in social problem solving (McGee et al. 2008a); and increased difficulty providing sufficient information to communicative partners (Coggins et al. 1998).

One well-designed, randomly controlled trial demonstrated the effectiveness of a structured, manualized, 12-week parent-assisted friendship training group on the social skills of alcohol-exposed children, who showed further improvement at the 3-month follow-up (O'Connor et al. 2006).

BEHAVIOURAL AND EMOTIONAL FUNCTIONING

Retrospectively identified children and young adults with prenatal alcohol exposure are generally rated by their caregivers and teachers as having more significant behavioural problems than their typically developing peers (Steinhausen and Spohr 1998, Roebuck et al. 1999, Mattson and Riley 2000, Steinhausen et al. 2003, Spohr et al. 2007). The most significant and consistent difficulties are seen in the areas of attention, disruptive and delinquent behaviour, and social problems. Prospective studies also find alcohol-related behaviour problems in children and adolescents with prenatal alcohol exposure, but results are somewhat less consistent and may be due to differences in caregiver expectations or demographic characteristics of individual samples (Brown et al. 1991, Carmichael Olson et al. 1997, Sood et al. 2001, Bailey et al. 2004). Delinquent and aggressive behaviour problems are most commonly found across prospective studies, and a binge pattern of drinking is related more strongly to delinquent behaviour problems than a steady pattern of prenatal drinking (Carmichael Olson et al. 1997, Bailey et al. 2004). High rates of delinquent behaviour are associated with a lower level of moral maturity seen in children with prenatal alcohol exposure, especially with respect to their relationships with others (Schonfeld et al. 2005).

PSYCHOPATHOLOGY

Most studies on the prevalence of psychopathology in individuals with prenatal alcohol exposure report high rates of psychiatric diagnoses across the age range, and comorbidity is common. In a large retrospective study (Streissguth et al. 1996) of alcohol-exposed individuals between the ages of 6 and 51 (n=415), 94% of the sample had experienced at least one mental health problem and 23% had been hospitalized in an inpatient psychiatric facility for treatment. Additional studies with children find similar rates of psychopathology with 87–97% of the alcohol-exposed cohorts meeting criteria for at least one psychiatric disorder, and 62–71% of children meeting criteria for two or more comorbid disorders (O'Connor et al. 2002b, Burd et al. 2003, Fryer et al. 2007a). ADHD is one of the most prevalent conditions among children with prenatal alcohol exposure, and rates of mood disorders and other disruptive behaviour disorders are also relatively high in comparison to rates in the general population. One longitudinal retrospective investigation demonstrated the persistence of psychopathological symptoms from preschool through young adulthood and found a positive relationship between number of symptoms and severity of exposure (Steinhausen and Spohr 1998, Spohr et al. 2007).

Studies with adults also identify high rates of psychopathology. The most common diagnoses are alcohol and drug dependence, depressive disorders and anxiety disorders. Maternal binge drinking is associated with increased incidence of several adult disorders in comparison to a steady drinking pattern (Famy et al. 1998, Barr et al. 2006). Several studies find that prenatal alcohol exposure is a stronger predictor of alcohol problems in adolescence and young adulthood than a positive family history of alcoholism (Baer et al. 1998, 2003; Alati et al. 2006). High rates of suicide in adults and adolescents with histories of prenatal alcohol exposure are also commonly noted (Streissguth et al. 1996, O'Malley and Huggins 2005, Baldwin 2007).

QUALITY OF LIFE

Many individuals with prenatal alcohol exposure have a reduced quality of life, and are more likely to be in a dependent living environment and have difficulty with employment (Streissguth et al. 1996, Grant et al. 2005, Spohr et al. 2007). For example, in one sample of 90 adults with histories of prenatal alcohol exposure, 83% were in a dependent living environment (e.g. group home, with relatives) and 79% had problems with employment. A large proportion had difficulty managing finances and making decisions on their own, and many had difficulty obtaining medical and social services. Alcohol-exposed individuals had more difficulty holding down a job than obtaining one, and employment problems often included getting easily frustrated, poor task comprehension, poor judgement, social problems, unreliability, poor anger management and problems with supervisors. In addition, almost half of the adults in the sample were parents, and half of these individuals were separated from their children.

Protective factors for improved outcomes include early identification and diagnosis, a stable and nurturing home, no violence against oneself, and access to developmental disabilities services (Streissguth et al. 1996). Limited research demonstrates that, while impaired relative to their typically developing peers, children in foster placements with histories of prenatal alcohol exposure have significantly higher scores on measures of intelligence, attention and academic functioning, and relatively fewer behavioural problems than alcohol-exposed children living with their biological families (Victor et al. 2008). However, differences in cognitive and behavioural status were observed between children who had experienced one stable foster care placement and those who had had multiple placements. Alcohol-exposed children with multiple placements tended to have relatively poorer outcomes than those with one stable foster placement. Outcomes were best when children were in a stable, nurturing foster or adoptive family; less good with a history of multiple foster placements; and least good when remaining with their birth parents.

Summary

Prenatal alcohol exposure can lead to permanent brain damage and related impairments in cognition and behaviour. Brain alterations seen in these individuals include reduced brain size, alterations in shape, tissue density and symmetry, and volumetric reductions and abnormalities of the cerebellum, corpus callosum, basal ganglia and hippocampus. The shape and tissue abnormalities are consistent with functional impairments and highlight the regional nature of brain morphological differences. Many individuals with histories of prenatal alcohol exposure experience life-long impairments in cognition and behaviour. Rates of psychopathology are high across the lifespan, and adverse outcomes including disrupted school experiences, delinquency, substance use, dependency on caregivers and community services, and poor quality of life are prevalent in this population. Clearly FASDs constitute a major public health concern and affect all levels of society. FASDs are entirely preventable, and continued research is needed to enhance efforts to educate and convince women to abstain from alcohol during pregnancy. For those individuals already born with FASD, early and effective intervention is needed to prevent or reduce adverse outcomes. While several recent studies have identified effective interventions for targeted behaviours in children with FASD, much more work is needed.

REFERENCES

Adnams CM, Kodituwakku PW, Hay A, et al. (2001) Patterns of cognitive–motor development in children with fetal alcohol syndrome from a community in South Africa. *Alcohol Clin Exp Res* **25**: 557–562.

Adnams CM, Sorour P, Kalberg WO, et al. (2007) Language and literacy outcomes from a pilot intervention study for children with fetal alcohol spectrum disorders in South Africa. *Alcohol* **41**: 403–414.

Alati R, Al Mamun A, Williams GM, et al. (2006) In utero alcohol exposure and prediction of alcohol disorders in early adulthood: A birth cohort study. *Arch Gen Psychiatry* **63**: 1009–1016.

Aragon AS, Kalberg WO, Buckley D, et al. (2008) Neuropsychological study of FASD in a sample of American Indian children: Processing simple versus complex information. *Alcohol Clin Exp Res* **32**: 2136–2148.

Archibald SL, Fennema-Notestine C, Gamst A, et al. (2001) Brain dysmorphology in individuals with severe prenatal alcohol exposure. *Dev Med Child Neurol* **43**: 148–154.

Autti-Rämö I, Autti T, Korkman M, et al. (2002) MRI findings in children with school problems who had been exposed prenatally to alcohol. *Dev Med Child Neurol* **44**: 98–106.

Baer JS, Barr HM, Bookstein FL, et al. (1998) Prenatal alcohol exposure and family history of alcoholism in the etiology of adolescent alcohol problems. *J Stud Alcohol* **59**: 533–543.

Baer JS, Sampson PD, Barr HM, et al. (2003) 21-year longitudinal analysis of the effects of prenatal alcohol exposure on young adult drinking. *Arch Gen Psychiatry* **60**: 377–385.

Bailey BN, Delaney-Black V, Covington CY, et al. (2004) Prenatal exposure to binge drinking and cognitive and behavioral outcomes at age 7 years. *Am J Obstet Gynecol* **191**: 1037–1043.

Baldwin MR (2007) Fetal alcohol spectrum disorders and suicidality in a healthcare setting. *Int J Circumpolar Health* **66**: 54–60.

Barr HM, Streissguth AP, Darby BL, Sampson PD (1990) Prenatal exposure to alcohol, caffeine, tobacco, and aspirin: effects on fine and gross motor performance in 4-year-old children. *Dev Psychol* **26**: 339–348.

Barr HM, Bookstein FL, O'Malley KD, et al. (2006) Binge drinking during pregnancy as a predictor of psychiatric disorders on the structured clinical interview for DSM-IV in young adult offspring. *Am J Psychiatry* **163**: 1061–1065.

Becker M, Warr-Leeper GA, Leeper HA (1990) Fetal alcohol syndrome: a description of oral motor, articulatory, short-term memory, grammatical, and semantic abilities. *J Commun Disord* **23**: 97–124.

Bertrand J, Floyd RL, Weber MK, et al. (2004) *National Task Force on FAS/FAE: Guidelines for Referral and Diagnosis.* Atlanta, GA: Centers for Disease Control and Prevention.

Bhatara VS, Lovrein F, Kirkeby J, et al. (2002) Brain function in fetal alcohol syndrome assessed by single photon emission computed tomography. *S D J Med* **55**: 59–62.

Bishop S, Gahagan S, Lord C (2007) Re-examining the core features of autism: a comparison of autism spectrum disorder and fetal alcohol spectrum disorder. *J Child Psychol Psychiatry* **48**: 1111–1121.

Bookstein FL, Sampson PD, Streissguth AP, Connor PD (2001) Geometric morphometrics of corpus callosum and subcortical structures in the fetal-alcohol-affected brain. *Teratology* **64**: 4–32.

Bookstein FL, Sampson PD, Connor PD, Streissguth AP (2002a) Midline corpus callosum is a neuroanatomical focus of fetal alcohol damage. *Anat Rec* **269**: 162–174.

Bookstein FL, Streissguth AP, Sampson PD, et al. (2002b) Corpus callosum shape and neuropsychological deficits in adult males with heavy fetal alcohol exposure. *Neuroimage* **15**: 233–251.

Bookstein FL, Streissguth AP, Connor PD, Sampson PD (2006) Damage to the human cerebellum from prenatal alcohol exposure: the anatomy of a simple biometrical explanation. *Anat Rec B New Anat* **289B**: 195–209.

Bookstein FL, Connor PD, Huggins JE, et al. (2007) Many infants prenatally exposed to high levels of alcohol show one particular anomaly of the corpus callosum. *Alcohol Clin Exp Res* **31**: 868–879.

Boyd TA, Ernhart CB, Greene TH, et al. (1991) Prenatal alcohol exposure and sustained attention in the preschool years. *Neurotoxicol Teratol* **13**: 49–55.

Brown RT, Coles CD, Smith IE, et al. (1991) Effects of prenatal alcohol exposure at school age. II. Attention and behavior. *Neurotoxicol Teratol* **13**: 369–376.

Burd L, Klug MG, Martsolf JT, Kerbeshian J (2003) Fetal alcohol syndrome: Neuropsychiatric phenomics. *Neurotoxicol Teratol* **25**: 697–705.

Burden MJ, Jacobson SW, Jacobson JL (2005a) Relation of prenatal alcohol exposure to cognitive processing speed and efficiency in childhood. *Alcohol Clin Exp Res* **29**: 1473–1483.

Burden MJ, Jacobson SW, Sokol RJ, Jacobson JL (2005b) Effects of prenatal alcohol exposure on attention and working memory at 7.5 years of age. *Alcohol Clin Exp Res* **29**: 443–452.

Calhoun F, Warren K (2007) Fetal alcohol syndrome: historical perspectives. *Neurosci Biobehav Rev* **31**: 168–171.

Carmichael Olson H, Streissguth AP, Sampson PD, et al. (1997) Association of prenatal alcohol exposure with behavioral and learning problems in early adolescence. *J Am Acad Child Adolesc Psychiatry* **36**: 1187–1194.

Carmichael Olson H, Feldman JJ, Streissguth AP, et al. (1998) Neuropsychological deficits in adolescents with fetal alcohol syndrome: clinical findings. *Alcohol Clin Exp Res* **22**: 1998–2012.

Carney LJ, Chermak GD (1991) Performance of American Indian children with fetal alcohol syndrome on the test of language development. *J Commun Disord* **24**: 123–134.

Church MW, Eldis F, Blakley BW, Bawle EV (1997) Hearing, language, speech, vestibular, and dentofacial disorders in fetal alcohol syndrome. *Alcohol Clin Exp Res* **21**: 227–237.

Clark CM, Li D, Conry J, et al. (2000) Structural and functional brain integrity of fetal alcohol syndrome in nonretarded cases. *Pediatrics* **105** :1096–1099.

Clarren SK (1986) Neuropathology in fetal alcohol syndrome. In: West JR, ed. *Alcohol and Brain Development.* New York: Oxford University Press, pp 158–166.

Coffin JM, Baroody S, Schneider K, O'Neill J (2005) Impaired cerebellar learning in children with prenatal alcohol exposure: a comparative study of eyeblink conditioning in children with ADHD and dyslexia. *Cortex* **41**: 389–398.

Coggins TE, Friet T, Morgan T (1998) Analysing narrative productions in older school-age children and adolescents with fetal alcohol syndrome: an experimental tool for clinical applications. *Clin Linguist Phon* **12**: 221–236.

Coles CD, Brown RT, Smith IE, et al. (1991) Effects of prenatal alcohol exposure at school age. I. Physical and cognitive development. *Neurotoxicol Teratol* **13**: 357–367.

Coles CD, Platzman KA, Raskind-Hood CL, et al. (1997) A comparison of children affected by prenatal alcohol exposure and attention deficit, hyperactivity disorder. *Alcohol Clin Exp Res* **21**: 150–161.

Coles CD, Platzman KA, Lynch ME, Freides D (2002) Auditory and visual sustained attention in adolescents prenatally exposed to alcohol. *Alcohol Clin Exp Res* **26**: 263–271.

Connor PD, Streissguth AP, Sampson PD, et al. (1999) Individual differences in auditory and visual attention among fetal alcohol-affected adults. *Alcohol Clin Exp Res* **23**: 1395–1402.

Connor PD, Sampson PD, Bookstein FL, et al. (2000) Direct and indirect effects of prenatal alcohol damage on executive function. *Dev Neuropsychol* **18**: 331–354.

Connor PD, Sampson PD, Streissguth AP, et al. (2006) Effects of prenatal alcohol exposure on fine motor co-ordination and balance: a study of two adult samples. *Neuropsychologia* **44**: 744–751.

Conry J (1990) Neuropsychological deficits in fetal alcohol syndrome and fetal alcohol effects. *Alcohol Clin Exp Res* **14**: 650–655.

Cortese BM, Moore GJ, Bailey BA, et al. (2006) Magnetic resonance and spectroscopic imaging in prenatal alcohol-exposed children: preliminary findings in the caudate nucleus. *Neurotoxicol Teratol* **28**: 597–606.

Fagerlund Å, Heikkinen S, Autti-Rämö I, et al. (2006) Brain metabolic alterations in adolescents and young adults with fetal alcohol spectrum disorders. *Alcohol Clin Exp Res* **30**: 2097–2104.

Famy C, Streissguth AP, Unis AS (1998) Mental illness in adults with fetal alcohol syndrome or fetal alcohol effects. *Am J Psychiatry* **155**: 552–554.

Fried PA, Watkinson B (1988) 12- and 24-month neurobehavioural follow-up of children prenatally exposed to marihuana, cigarettes and alcohol. *Neurotoxicol Teratol* **10**: 305–313.

Fried PA, Watkinson B (1990) 36- and 48-month neurobehavioral follow-up of children prenatally exposed to marijuana, cigarettes, and alcohol. *J Dev Behav Pediatr* **11**: 49–58.

Fried PA, O'Connell CM, Watkinson B (1992a) 60- and 72-month follow-up of children prenatally exposed to marijuana, cigarettes, and alcohol: cognitive and language assessment. *J Dev Behav Pediatr* **13**: 383–391.

Fried PA, Watkinson B, Gray R (1992b) A follow-up study of attentional behavior in 6-year-old children exposed prenatally to marihuana, cigarettes, and alcohol. *Neurotoxicol Teratol* **14**: 299–311.

Fryer SL, McGee CL, Matt GE, et al. (2007a) Evaluation of psychopathological conditions in children with heavy prenatal alcohol exposure. *Pediatrics* **119**: 733–741.

Fryer SL, Tapert SF, Mattson SN, et al. (2007b) Prenatal alcohol exposure affects frontal–striatal BOLD response during inhibitory control. *Alcohol Clin Exp Res* **31**: 1415–1424.

Goldschmidt L, Richardson GA, Stoffer DS, et al. (1996) Prenatal alcohol exposure and academic achievement at age six: a nonlinear fit. *Alcohol Clin Exp Res* **20**: 763–770.

Grant T, Huggins J, Connor P, Streissguth A (2005) Quality of life and psychosocial profile among young women with fetal alcohol spectrum disorders. *Mental Health Aspects Dev Disabil* **8**: 33–39.

Green CR, Munoz DP, Nikkel SM, Reynolds JN (2007) Deficits in eye movement control in children with fetal alcohol spectrum disorders. *Alcohol Clin Exp Res* **31**: 500–511.

Greene T, Ernhart CB, Martier SS, et al. (1990) Prenatal alcohol exposure and language development. *Alcohol Clin Exp Res* **14**: 937–945.

Gusella JL, Fried PA (1984) Effects of maternal social drinking and smoking on offspring at 13 months. *Neurobehav Toxicol Teratol* **6**: 13–17.

Hamilton DA, Kodituwakku P, Sutherland RJ, Savage DD (2003) Children with fetal alcohol syndrome are impaired at place learning but not cued-navigation in a virtual Morris water task. *Behav Brain Res* **143**: 85–94.

Handmaker NS, Rayburn WF, Meng C, et al. (2006) Impact of alcohol exposure after pregnancy recognition on ultrasonographic fetal growth measures. *Alcohol Clin Exp Res* **30**: 892–898.

Howell KK, Lynch ME, Platzman KA, et al. (2006) Prenatal alcohol exposure and ability, academic achievement, and school functioning in adolescence: a longitudinal follow-up. *J Pediatr Psychol* **31**: 116–126.

Hoyme HE, May PA, Kalberg WO, et al. (2005) A practical clinical approach to diagnosis of fetal alcohol spectrum disorders: clarification of the 1996 Institute of Medicine criteria. *Pediatrics* **115**: 39–47.

Jacobson SW (1998) Specificity of neurobehavioral outcomes associated with prenatal alcohol exposure. *Alcohol Clin Exp Res* **22**: 313–320.

Jacobson SW, Jacobson JL, Sokol RJ, et al. (2004) Maternal age, alcohol abuse history, and quality of parenting as moderators of the effects of prenatal alcohol exposure on 7.5-year intellectual function. *Alcohol Clin Exp Res* **28**: 1732–1745.

Jacobson SW, Stanton ME, Molteno CD, et al. (2008) Impaired eyeblink conditioning in children with fetal alcohol syndrome. *Alcohol Clin Exp Res* **32**: 365–372.

Janzen LA, Nanson JL, Block GW (1995) Neuropsychological evaluation of preschoolers with fetal alcohol syndrome. *Neurotoxicol Teratol* **17**: 273–279.

Johnson VP, Swayze VW, Sato Y, Andreasen NC (1996) Fetal alcohol syndrome: craniofacial and central nervous system manifestations. *Am J Med Genet* **61**: 329–339.

Jones KL, Smith DW (1973) Recognition of the fetal alcohol syndrome in early infancy. Lancet 2: 999–1001.

Jones KL, Smith DW, Ulleland CN, Streissguth AP (1973) Pattern of malformation in offspring of chronic alcoholic mothers. *Lancet* **1**: 1267–1271.

Kable JA, Coles CD (2004) The impact of prenatal alcohol exposure on neurophysiological encoding of environmental events at six months. *Alcohol Clin Exp Res* **28**: 489–496.

Kable JA, Coles CD, Taddeo E (2007) Socio-cognitive habilitation using the math interactive learning experience program for alcohol-affected children. *Alcohol Clin Exp Res* **31**: 1425–1434.

Kaemingk KL, Mulvaney S, Tanner Halverson P (2003) Learning following prenatal alcohol exposure: performance on verbal and visual multitrial tasks. *Arch Clin Neuropsychol* **18**: 33–47.

Kalberg WO, Provost B, Tollison SJ, et al. (2006) Comparison of motor delays in young children with fetal alcohol syndrome to those with prenatal alcohol exposure and with no prenatal alcohol exposure. *Alcohol Clin Exp Res* **30**: 2037–2045.

Kfir M, Yevtushok L, Onishchenko S, et al. (2009) Can prenatal ultrasound detect the effects of in-utero alcohol exposure? – A pilot study. *Ultrasound Obstet Gynecol* **33**: 683–689.

Kodituwakku PW (2007) Defining the behavioral phenotype in children with fetal alcohol spectrum disorders: a review. *Neurosci Biobehav Rev* **31**: 192–201.

Kodituwakku PW, Handmaker NS, Cutler SK, et al. (1995) Specific impairments in self-regulation in children exposed to alcohol prenatally. *Alcohol Clin Exp Res* **19**: 1558–1564.

Kodituwakku PW, May PA, Clericuzio CL, Weers D (2001) Emotion-related learning in individuals prenatally exposed to alcohol: an investigation of the relation between set shifting, extinction of responses, and behavior. *Neuropsychologia* **39**: 699–708.

Kodituwakku PW, Adnams CM, Hay A, et al. (2006a) Letter and category fluency in children with fetal alcohol syndrome from a community in South Africa. *J Stud Alcohol* **67**: 502–509.

Kodituwakku P, Coriale G, Fiorentino D, et al. (2006b) Neurobehavioral characteristics of children with fetal alcohol spectrum disorders in communities from Italy: preliminary results. *Alcohol Clin Exp Res* **30**: 1551–1561.

Kopera-Frye K, Dehaene S, Streissguth AP (1996) Impairments of number processing induced by prenatal alcohol exposure. *Neuropsychologia* **34**: 1187–1196.

Korkman M, Kettunen S, Autti-Rämö I (2003) Neurocognitive impairment in early adolescence following prenatal alcohol exposure of varying duration. *Child Neuropsychol* **9**: 117–128.

Lebel C, Rasmussen C, Wyper K, et al. (2008) Brain diffusion abnormalities in children with fetal alcohol spectrum disorder. *Alcohol Clin Exp Res* **23**: 1732–1740.

Lemoine P, Harousseau H, Borteyru J-P, Menuet J-C (1968) [Children of alcoholic parents. Abnormalities observed in 127 cases.] *Ouest Med* **21**: 476–482 (French).

Lezak MD, Howieson DB, Loring DW, et al. (2004) *Neuropsychological Assessment. 4th edn.* New York: Oxford University Press.

Ma X, Coles CD, Lynch ME, et al. (2005) Evaluation of corpus callosum anisotropy in young adults with fetal alcohol syndrome according to diffusion tensor imaging. *Alcohol Clin Exp Res* **29**: 1214–1222.

Malisza KL, Allman A-A, Shiloff D, et al. (2005) Evaluation of spatial working memory function in children and adults with fetal alcohol spectrum disorders: a functional magnetic resonance imaging study. *Pediatr Res* **58**: 1150–1157.

Mattson SN, Riley EP (1998) A review of the neurobehavioral deficits in children with fetal alcohol syndrome or prenatal exposure to alcohol. *Alcohol Clin Exp Res* **22**: 279–294.

Mattson SN, Riley EP (1999) Implicit and explicit memory functioning in children with heavy prenatal alcohol exposure. *J Int Neuropsychol Soc* **5**: 462–471.

Mattson SN, Riley EP (2000) Parent ratings of behavior in children with heavy prenatal alcohol exposure and IQ-matched controls. *Alcohol Clin Exp Res* **24**: 226–231.

Mattson SN, Roebuck TM (2002) Acquisition and retention of verbal and nonverbal information in children with heavy prenatal alcohol exposure. *Alcohol Clin Exp Res* **26**: 875–882.

Mattson SN, Riley EP, Jernigan TL, et al. (1992) Fetal alcohol syndrome: a case report of neuropsychological, MRI and EEG assessment of two children. *Alcohol Clin Exp Res* **16**: 1001–1003.

Mattson SN, Riley EP, Jernigan TL, et al. (1994) A decrease in the size of the basal ganglia following prenatal alcohol exposure: a preliminary report. *Neurotoxicol Teratol* **16**: 283–289.

Mattson SN, Gramling L, Delis D, et al. (1996a) Global-local processing in children prenatally exposed to alcohol. *Child Neuropsychol* **2**: 165–175.

Mattson SN, Riley EP, Delis DC, et al. (1996b) Verbal learning and memory in children with fetal alcohol syndrome. *Alcohol Clin Exp Res* **20**: 810–816.

Mattson SN, Riley EP, Sowell ER, et al. (1996c) A decrease in the size of the basal ganglia in children with fetal alcohol syndrome. *Alcohol Clin Exp Res* **20**: 1088–1093.

Mattson SN, Riley EP, Gramling LJ, et al. (1997) Heavy prenatal alcohol exposure with or without physical features of fetal alcohol syndrome leads to IQ deficits. *J Pediatr* **131**: 718–721.

Mattson SN, Riley EP, Gramling LJ, et al. (1998) Neuropsychological comparison of alcohol-exposed children with or without physical features of fetal alcohol syndrome. *Neuropsychology* **12**: 146–153.

Mattson SN, Goodman AM, Caine C, et al. (1999) Executive functioning in children with heavy prenatal alcohol exposure. *Alcohol Clin Exp Res* **23**: 1808–1815.

Mattson SN, Calarco KE, Lang AR (2006) Focused and shifting attention in children with heavy prenatal alcohol exposure. *Neuropsychology* **20**: 361–369.

McGee CL, Fryer SL, Bjorkquist O, et al. (2008a) Social problem solving deficits in adolescents with prenatal exposure to alcohol. *Am J Drug Alcohol Abuse* **34**: 423–431.

McGee CL, Schonfeld AM, Roebuck-Spencer TM, et al. (2008b) Children with heavy prenatal alcohol exposure demonstrate deficits on multiple measures of concept formation. *Alcohol Clin Exp Res* **32**: 1388–1397.

McGee CL, Bjorkquist OA, Riley EP, Mattson SN (2009) Impaired language performance in young children with heavy prenatal alcohol exposure. *Neurotoxicol Teratol* **31**: 71–75.

Nanson JL, Hiscock M (1990) Attention deficits in children exposed to alcohol prenatally. *Alcohol Clin Exp Res* **14**: 656–661.

O'Connor MJ, Kogan N, Findlay R (2002a) Prenatal alcohol exposure and attachment behavior in children. *Alcohol Clin Exp Res* **26**: 1592–1602.

O'Connor MJ, Shah B, Whaley S, et al. (2002b) Psychiatric illness in a clinical sample of children with prenatal alcohol exposure. *Am J Drug Alcohol Abuse* **28**: 743–754.

O'Connor MJ, Frankel F, Paley B, et al. (2006) A controlled social skills training for children with fetal alcohol spectrum disorders. *J Consult Clin Psychol* **74**: 639–648.

O'Hare ED, Kan E, Yoshii J, et al. (2005) Mapping cerebellar vermal morphology and cognitive correlates in prenatal alcohol exposure. *NeuroReport* **16**: 1285–1290.

O'Malley K, Huggins J (2005) Suicidality in adolescents and adults with fetal alcohol spectrum disorders. *Can J Psychiatry* **50**: 125.

Pennington BF, Ozonoff S (1996) Executive functions and developmental psychopathology. *J Child Psychol Psychiatry* **37**: 51–87.

Pulsifer MB (1996) The neuropsychology of mental retardation. *J Int Neuropsychol Soc* **2**: 159–176.

Rasmussen C (2005) Executive functioning and working memory in fetal alcohol spectrum disorder. *Alcohol Clin Exp Res* **29**: 1359–1367.

Riikonen R, Salonen I, Partanen K, Verho S (1999) Brain perfusion SPECT and MRI in foetal alcohol syndrome. *Dev Med Child Neurol* **41**: 652–659.

Riikonen RS, Nokelainen P, Valkonen K, et al. (2005) Deep serotonergic and dopaminergic structures in fetal alcoholic syndrome: a study with nor-ß-CIT-single-photon emission computed tomography and magnetic resonance imaging volumetry. *Biol Psychiatry* 57: 1565–1572.

Riley EP, Mattson SN, Sowell ER, et al. (1995) Abnormalities of the corpus callosum in children prenatally exposed to alcohol. *Alcohol Clin Exp Res* **19**: 1198–1202.

Roebuck TM, Simmons RW, Mattson SN, Riley EP (1998a) Prenatal exposure to alcohol affects the ability to maintain postural balance. *Alcohol Clin Exp Res* **22**: 252–258.

Roebuck TM, Simmons RW, Richardson C, et al. (1998b) Neuromuscular responses to disturbance of balance in children with prenatal exposure to alcohol. *Alcohol Clin Exp Res* **22**: 1992–1997.

Roebuck TM, Mattson SN, Riley EP (1999) Behavioral and psychosocial profiles of alcohol-exposed children. *Alcohol Clin Exp Res* **23**: 1070–1076.

Roebuck TM, Mattson SN, Riley EP (2002) Interhemispheric transfer in children with heavy prenatal alcohol exposure. *Alcohol Clin Exp Res* **26**: 1863–1871.

Roebuck-Spencer TM, Mattson SN (2004) Implicit strategy affects learning in children with heavy prenatal alcohol exposure. *Alcohol Clin Exp Res* **28**: 1424–1431.

Roebuck-Spencer TM, Mattson SN, Marion SD, et al. (2004) Bimanual coordination in alcohol-exposed children: role of the corpus callosum. *J Int Neuropsychol Soc* **10**: 536–548.

Sampson PD, Kerr B, Olson HC, et al. (1997) The effects of prenatal alcohol exposure on adolescent cognitive processing: a speed–accuracy tradeoff. *Intelligence* **24**: 329–353.

Schonfeld AM, Mattson SN, Lang AR, et al. (2001) Verbal and nonverbal fluency in children with heavy prenatal alcohol exposure. *J Stud Alcohol* **62**: 239–246.

Schonfeld AM, Mattson SN, Riley EP (2005) Moral maturity and deliquency after prenatal alcohol exposure. *J Stud Alcohol* **66**: 545–555.

Schonfeld AM, Paley B, Frankel F, O'Connor MJ (2006) Executive functioning predicts social skills following prenatal alcohol exposure. *Child Neuropsychol* **12**: 439–452.

Simmons RW, Wass T, Thomas JD, Riley EP (2002) Fractionated simple and choice reaction time in children with prenatal exposure to alcohol. *Alcohol Clin Exp Res* **26**: 1412–1419.

Sood B, Delaney-Black V, Covington C, et al. (2001) Prenatal alcohol exposure and childhood behavior at age 6 to 7 years: I. Dose–response effect. *Pediatrics* **108**: 34–42.

Sowell ER, Jernigan TL, Mattson SN, et al. (1996) Abnormal development of the cerebellar vermis in children prenatally exposed to alcohol: size reduction in lobules I–V. *Alcohol Clin Exp Res* **20**: 31–34.

Sowell ER, Mattson SN, Thompson PM, et al. (2001a) Mapping callosal morphology and cognitive correlates: effects of heavy prenatal alcohol exposure. *Neurology* 57: 235–244.

Sowell ER, Thompson PM, Mattson SN, et al. (2001b) Voxel-based morphometric analyses of the brain in children and adolescents prenatally exposed to alcohol. *NeuroReport* **12**: 515–523.

Sowell ER, Thompson PM, Mattson SN, et al. (2002a) Regional brain shape abnormalities persist into adolescence after heavy prenatal alcohol exposure. *Cerebral Cortex* **12**: 856–865.

Sowell ER, Thompson PM, Peterson BS, et al. (2002b) Mapping cortical gray matter asymmetry patterns in adolescents with heavy prenatal alcohol exposure. *Neuroimage* **17**: 1807–1819.

Sowell ER, Lu LH, O'Hare ED, et al. (2007) Functional magnetic resonance imaging of verbal learning in children with heavy prenatal alcohol exposure. *NeuroReport* **18**: 635–639.

Sowell ER, Johnson A, Kan E, et al. (2008a) Mapping white matter integrity and neurobehavioral correlates in children with fetal alcohol spectrum disorders. *Journal Neurosci* **28**: 1313–1319.

Sowell ER, Mattson SN, Kan E, et al. (2008b) Abnormal cortical thickness and brain–behavior correlation patterns in individuals with heavy prenatal alcohol exposure. *Cerebral Cortex* **18**: 136–144.

Spohr H-L, Willms J, Steinhausen H-C (2007) Fetal alcohol spectrum disorders in young adulthood. *J Pediatr* **150**: 175–179.

Steinhausen H-C, Spohr H-L (1998) Long-term outcome of children with fetal alcohol syndrome: psychopathology, behavior and intelligence. *Alcohol Clin Exp Res* 22: 334–338.

Steinhausen H-C, Willms J, Metzke CW, Spohr H-L (2003) Behavioural phenotype in foetal alcohol syndrome and foetal alcohol effects. *Dev Med Child Neurol* **45**: 179–182.

Streissguth A (2007) Offspring effects of prenatal alcohol exposure from birth to 25 years: the Seattle prospective longitudinal study. *J Clin Psychol Med Settings* **14**: 81–101.

Streissguth AP, Barr HM, Sampson PD, et al. (1989) IQ at age 4 in relation to maternal alcohol use and smoking during pregnancy. *Dev Psychol* **25**: 3–11.

Streissguth AP, Barr HM, Sampson PD (1990) Moderate prenatal alcohol exposure: effects on child IQ and learning problems at age 7½ years. *Alcohol Clin Exp Res* 14: 662–669.

Streissguth AP, Aase JM, Clarren SK, et al. (1991) Fetal alcohol syndrome in adolescents and adults. *JAMA* **265**: 1961–1967.

Streissguth AP, Barr HM, Olson HC, et al. (1994a) Drinking during pregnancy decreases word attack and arithmetic scores on standardized tests: adolescent data from a population-based prospective study. *Alcohol Clin Exp Res* **18**: 248–254.

Streissguth AP, Barr HM, Sampson PD, Bookstein FL (1994b) Prenatal alcohol and offspring development: the first fourteen years. *Drug Alcohol Depend* **36**: 89–99.

Streissguth AP, Sampson PD, Olson HC, et al. (1994c) Maternal drinking during pregnancy: attention and short-term memory in 14-year-old offspring—a longitudinal prospective study. *Alcohol Clin Exp Res* **18**: 202–218.

Streissguth AP, Bookstein FL, Sampson PD, Barr HM (1995) Attention: prenatal alcohol and continuities of vigilance and attentional problems from 4 through 14 years. *Dev Psychopathol* **7**: 419–446.

Streissguth AP, Barr HM, Kogan J, Bookstein FL (1996) *Final Report: Understanding the Occurrence of Secondary Disabilities in Clients with Fetal Alcohol Syndrome (FAS) and Fetal Alcohol Effects (FAE).* Seattle, WA: University of Washington Publication Services.

Streissguth AP, Bookstein FL, Barr HM, et al. (2004) Risk factors for adverse life outcomes in fetal alcohol syndrome and fetal alcohol effects. *J Dev Behav Pediatr* **25**: 228–238.

Swayze VW, Johnson VP, Hanson JW, et al. (1997) Magnetic resonance imaging of brain anomalies in fetal alcohol syndrome. *Pediatrics* **99**: 232–240.

Thomas SE, Kelly SJ, Mattson SN, Riley EP (1998) Comparison of social abilities of children with fetal alcohol syndrome to those of children with similar IQ scores and normal controls. *Alcohol Clin Exp Res* **22**: 528–533.

Uecker A, Nadel L (1996) Spatial locations gone awry: object and spatial memory deficits in children with fetal alcohol syndrome. *Neuropsychologia* **34**: 209–223.

Uecker A, Nadel L (1998) Spatial but not object memory impairments in children with fetal alcohol syndrome. *Am J Ment Retard* **103**: 12–18.

Victor A, Wozniak JR, Chang P (2008) Environmental correlates of cognition and behavior in children with fetal alcohol spectrum disorders. *J Hum Behav Social Environment* **18**: 288–300.

Wass TS, Persutte WH, Hobbins JC (2001) The impact of prenatal alcohol exposure on frontal cortex development in utero. *Am J Obstet Gynecol* **185**: 737–742.

Wass TS, Simmons RW, Thomas JD, Riley EP (2002) Timing accuracy and variability in children with prenatal exposure to alcohol. *Alcohol Clin Exp Res* **26**: 1887–1896.

Welsh MC, Pennington BF (1988) Assessing frontal lobe functioning in children: views from developmental psychology. *Dev Neuropsychol* **4**: 199–230.

Whaley SE, O'Connor MJ, Gunderson B (2001) Comparison of the adaptive functioning of children prenatally exposed to alcohol to a nonexposed clinical sample. *Alcohol Clin Exp Res* **25**: 1018–1024.

Willford JA, Richardson GA, Leech SL, Day NL (2004) Verbal and visuospatial learning and memory function in children with moderate prenatal alcohol exposure. *Alcohol Clin Exp Res* **28**: 497–507.

Willoughby KA, Sheard ED, Nash K, Rovet J (2008) Effects of prenatal alcohol exposure on hippocampal volume, verbal learning, and verbal and spatial recall in late childhood. *J Int Neuropsychol Soc* **14**: 1022–1033.

Wozniak JR, Mueller BA, Chang P-N, et al. (2006) Diffusion tensor imaging in children with fetal alcohol spectrum disorders. *Alcohol Clin Exp Res* **30**: 1799–1806.

8

EFFECTS OF DRUGS OF ABUSE ON THE FETUS: COCAINE AND OPIATES INCLUDING HEROIN

Lynn T Singer and Sonia Minnes

This chapter will address the current state of knowledge on the developmental effects of two very different drugs of abuse – cocaine and opiates.

Cocaine

HISTORICAL CONTEXT

Cocaine is a potent stimulant drug first popularized in the USA and Europe in the late 1800s. Its refreshing and energizing properties were easily attainable in beverages such as Coca-Cola and through Birney's Catarrhal Powder for stuffy noses. By 1912, its harmful properties had become well recognized and cocaine was made a restricted and illegal substance in the USA under the Federal Drug Administration Act enacted that year. The 1970s and '80s witnessed resurgence in interest in cocaine but its expense restricted its use to the most affluent of the population. Its potential harmful impact was minimized, and even President Carter's 'drug czar' characterized cocaine as a "benign" substance (Bourne 1974). In the late 1980s and early '90s, however, a number of factors converged to create an epidemic of cocaine use among pregnant women, localized largely to poor urban areas of the USA. South American cartels had devised a method to create a cheap, smokable alkaloid form of cocaine ('crack') that was highly addictive and appealing to women. The social and cultural milieu in the USA had become more accepting of drug use since the 1960s, and large numbers of women had become accustomed to smoking cigarettes and marijuana (cannabis).

Epidemiological studies in the USA estimated that hundreds of thousands of infants were born after prenatal exposure to cocaine, primarily in its crack form, during the 1980s and '90s (SAMHSA 1999). Although rates of crack cocaine use by women who are pregnant or of childbearing age have declined substantially in the USA, there has been increasing use in Europe. The European Monitoring Centre for Drugs and Addiction in 2007 found an overall increase in cocaine use among the 15–34 year age group. Average prevalence was 2.6% across Europe, but Spain, the United Kingdom, Italy and Ireland had the highest use, with rates ranging from 3.1% to 5.4%, while Greece, Poland, the Czech Republic and Latvia had the lowest rates. Increasing use was found in the 15–24 year age groups in the Netherlands and Denmark. During the US epidemic a number of small, clinical, uncontrolled studies elicited alarmist media attention to the 'crack baby', construed as hopelessly damaged and unable to learn or make emotional connections (Zuckerman et al. 2002). Several states began punitive efforts to jail pregnant cocaine-using women, and the foster care system was overwhelmed as many infants were removed from their homes in the wake of discovery of maternal cocaine use. While such removal was understandably necessary in many cases, given the violent, dangerous and unstable caregiving environment experienced by some children of drug-using women, developmental scientists expressed concerns about the biases inherent in media reports and the punitive responses of judicial bodies and social services to pregnant cocaine-using women (Chavkin 2001).

To address the scientific questions about fetal harm, a number of National Institute on Drug Abuse longitudinal cohort studies were designed and funded to assess the developmental consequences of prenatal cocaine exposure. Because they were designed to address many of the methodological problems in studies of drug-exposed children, including the impact of confounding factors (low social class, preterm birth, foster care placement, maternal psychological distress, educational disadvantage, experience of violence, and polydrug use, especially tobacco, alcohol and cannabis), these studies, to date, provide the most reliable data on the developmental sequelae of prenatal cocaine exposure. The present review will summarize current findings of many of these ongoing studies, focusing on those that have attained robust retention rates in follow-up.

It should be noted that the studies reviewed in this chapter and the available literature on prenatal cocaine exposure are generalizable largely to the underrepresented minority, low socio-economic status population of the urban US cities where the cocaine epidemic initially flourished. There is little to no information on middle-class users in the USA or on developmental sequelae of prenatal cocaine exposure outside the USA. Since the majority of cocaine users in the studies reviewed here were polydrug users, primarily with alcohol, cannabis and tobacco, the review addresses only those studies that have attempted to control, through research design or statistically, for the effects of other substances before attribution of cocaine effects (Jacobson and Jacobson 2005). Because maternal self-report of alcohol and drug use during pregnancy is so unreliable, this review has also focused on those studies that have used biological markers in conjunction with maternal interview in identification of samples. Urine screens can identify women who have recently used cocaine, and the use of meconium screens for metabolites of cocaine and other drugs can identify infants exposed during the last two trimesters of pregnancy. The use of meconium screens significantly enhances ability to assess the amount of drug exposed to the fetus (Arendt et al. 1999).

MECHANISMS OF ACTION

Cocaine acts on the central nervous system (CNS) primarily through inhibition of dopaminergic reuptake, but also through activation of noradrenergic and serotonergic sites in the basal forebrain and cerebral cortex (Malanga and Kosofsky 1999). A number of mechanisms have been proposed for possible negative effects of cocaine exposure on the developing fetal brain and subsequent developmental sequelae. These mechanisms include fetal hypoxia initiated by maternal arterial vasoconstriction, which may produce generalized effects (Volpe 1992). Direct effects on the monoaminergic neurotransmitter system in areas of the brain involved in attention and arousal (Stanwood et al. 2001) and subsequent evidence for

TABLE 8.1
Effects of prenatal cocaine exposure on infants and school-age children

Deficit	Features
Birth outcomes	Poorer fetal growth outcomes, including lower birthweight, reduced length and head circumference, preterm birth and intrauterine growth retardation
Physical development	Significant catch-up growth, but several studies find shorter stature and symmetrical growth retardation at school age
Infant behaviour	Neurobehavioural abnormalities in the neonatal period include jitteriness, attentional problems, and movement and tone abnormalities
Health	Early cardiac abnormalities, including diastolic alterations and blunted vagal tone in heavily exposed infants. Increased incidence of iron deficiency anaemia
Language	Expressive and receptive language delays
Attention	Impaired visual information processing in infancy. Selective and sustained attentional deficits
Behaviour	Aggressive behaviour, oppositional defiant disorder and hyperactivity appear to be increased but outcomes are dependent on observer
Cognition	Impairments in visuospatial information processing and arithmetic; deficits in perceptual reasoning and abstract categorical processing
Neuroimaging	Volumetric reductions in corpus callosum and parietal areas; reduced maturational white matter pathways in the frontal lobes

alterations in fetal cerebral architecture (Lidow 2003) have been observed primarily in dopamine-rich cortical areas involved in components of executive functioning. Primate studies of prenatal cocaine exposure corresponding to the second trimester in humans have found an attenuation of the number of neurons in the cerebral cortex (Lidow 2003).

BIRTH OUTCOMES AND GROWTH (Table 8.1)

Neurotoxic effects of fetal cocaine exposure can be manifest in fetal and long-term growth outcomes, as well as structural abnormalities, reflecting altered CNS development. Although some early case reports suggested an increase in major and minor congenital anomalies among cocaine-exposed infants, two large prospective well-controlled studies have not found an increased number of major or minor anomalies or a consistent phenotype of abnormalities for cocaine-exposed infants or children (Behnke et al. 2001, Minnes et al. 2005).

Virtually all studies of birth outcomes of cocaine-exposed neonates have identified poorer fetal growth outcomes, including lower birthweight, and decreased length and head circumference, often with inversely linear relationships to the amount of drug exposure (Singer et al. 2000, Frank et al. 2001, Zuckerman et al. 2002). In one large study (Bada et al. 2005) prenatal cocaine exposure predicted an increased likelihood of low birthweight (odds ratio, 3.59), preterm birth (odds ratio, 1.25) and intrauterine growth retardation (odds ratio, 2.24). Synergistic effects of cocaine with alcohol and tobacco have been found to predict reduced head and chest circumference and birth length (Coles et al. 1992, Singer et al. 1994a, Eyler et al. 1998). In the first study to examine cocaine–polydrug effects on birth outcomes while considering possible effects of psychological distress symptoms, Singer et al. (2002b) found higher rates of psychopathological symptoms of depression, anxiety, psychosis and paranoia in cocaine-using women, and these elevated symptoms contributed to prediction of their infants' reduced head circumference and birthweight.

While considerable consistency exists in the reports of reduced fetal growth and preterm birth in cocaine-exposed cohorts, follow-up at later ages suggests significant catch-up growth, although the literature is more limited and findings are more variable. The longest follow-up studies of growth have extended to 6, 7, 8 and 10 years of age, with somewhat disparate findings. Minnes et al. (2005) found a dose–response relationship of prenatal cocaine exposure to lower height and weight-for-height z-scores at 6 years, based on the amount of the cocaine metabolite metahydroxybenzoylecgonine in infant meconium. Covington et al. (2002) also reported a negative effect on height at 7 years, restricted to offspring of cocaine-using women over 30 years of age. In contrast, Lumeng et al. (2007) found catch-up in all growth parameters by 6 months of age and no effects of cocaine at 8 years of age. However, Richardson et al. (2002), using longitudinal growth analysis at four time-points to 10 years, found a late emergence of significant cocaine effects of exposure in the first trimester with increasing age, indicating symmetrical growth retardation. At 10 years, there was a statistically significant 10 pounds (≈4.5 kg) difference in weight, although both exposed and non-exposed children were in the normal growth range. Thus, overall, findings indicate some residual effects of cocaine on growth, as well as catch-up at early ages after fetal growth attenuation.

INFANT BEHAVIOURAL OUTCOMES

Numerous studies have examined the behavioural characteristics of cocaine-exposed neonates. These studies present interpretive difficulties for a number of reasons, including the relatively poor reliability and validity of neonatal assessment instruments, and the dependence on the gestational age of the infant, which is hard to calculate exactly (Singer 2001). It is also not possible to decouple acute drug or alcohol withdrawal effects from more permanent sequelae in the first several weeks after birth.

With these caveats in mind, several large controlled studies comparing cocaine-exposed with non-cocaine-exposed infants have found abnormalities in the early neonatal period, including alterations in alert responsiveness (Eyler et al. 1998), diminished state variability (Richardson et al. 1996) and poorer orientation (Brown et al. 1998). Similar but longer-term studies to 2–4 weeks have identified motor activity and reflex abnormalities (Coles et al. 1992), as well as jitteriness, attentional problems, and movement and tone abnormalities (Singer et al. 2000). Heavily cocaine-exposed infants, who were exposed on average to approximately six 'rocks' of crack cocaine* a day for about two days a week over the prenatal period, were four times as likely to be jittery and twice as likely to have any neurobehavioural abnormality as non-exposed infants. Of particular interest, this study examined the role of maternal distress symptoms, such as depression, anxiety and hostility, in relation to cocaine effects on neurobehavioural outcomes, and found that maternal distress

*Cocaine is usually purchased in 'rocks' of off-white nuggets formed from the cocaine alkaloid. Rocks vary in size making standardized measurement of consumption quantity difficult.

mediated cocaine's negative effects on the infant's early attentional system (Singer et al. 2000). In another large study, heavy cocaine exposure also predicted poorer regulation, higher excitability and more non-optimal reflexes at 1 month of age, replicating earlier findings (Lester et al. 2002).

MATERNAL–CHILD INTERACTION

Because birth outcome and neurobehavioural studies of the cocaine-exposed infant suggest a vulnerable and more difficult to care for infant, with a caregiver whose own psychological state and parenting capacities may be impaired by drug addiction and concomitant social stressors, some researchers have also assessed maternal–infant interactions in cocaine-exposed dyads. At infant age of 1 month, cocaine-using mothers were rated as less flexible and engaged, and had shorter feeding sessions with their infants than controls (Lagasse et al. 2003). In a controlled longitudinal study with time-points at birth, 6.5 and 12 months, cocaine-exposed infants demonstrated poorer clarity of cues during a feeding session with their birth mothers, who were rated as less sensitive to their infants. Heavier cocaine users were also less responsive to their infants than mothers who had not used cocaine during pregnancy (Minnes et al. 2005). In another large study, women who reported continued cocaine use were perceived to be more intrusive and hostile, and less confident in their instructions to their 3-year-old children, and their children were less persistent in task completion than comparison children (Johnson et al. 2002).

HEALTH OUTCOMES

Surprisingly, apart from obstetric outcomes and growth, there are few studies addressing the health of cocaine-exposed children. Early concerns about increased incidence of sudden infant death syndrome have not been substantiated (Klonoff-Cohen and Lam-Kruglick 2001). Similarly, initial reports of elevated incidence of cerebral haemorrhages and other neurological problems (Frank et al. 2001) were not replicated (Behnke et al. 2001), except in cohorts of very-low-birthweight infants (Singer et al. 1994a).

In a series of controlled, prospective studies assessing cardiac function, abnormal decreased heart rate variability was noted in 10% of cocaine-exposed newborn infants vs 2% of controls (p=0.003) (Mehta et al. 2002d) as well as abnormal diastolic cardiac function within the first four days of life (Mehta et al. 2002c). Follow-up at 2–6 months of age indicated a significant recovery of vagal tone in lighter cocaine-exposed infants, but a blunted response (Mehta et al. 2002a) and persistent diastolic alterations in heavily exposed infants (Mehta et al. 2002b). Although no further follow-up of this cohort has occurred, a National Institute of Child Health and Human Development Neonatal Research Network Study of 1388 infants, 600 of whom were cocaine-exposed, found no association of prenatal exposure with hypertension at 6 years. Twenty per cent of exposed children had hypertension compared with 16% of non-exposed children (Shankaran et al. 2006).

Haematological assessments of cocaine-exposed and non-exposed children at 2 and 4 years identified a significantly higher rate of iron-deficiency anaemia in the 4-year-old exposed group, although the overall incidence was quite low. Lead exposure was also measured across the same groups but was not associated with cocaine exposure. However, elevated lead levels were at high rates for all children, with about 28% of exposed and non-exposed children having levels ≥10μg/dL at 2 years (Nelson et al. 2004). Since all children came from disadvantaged environments, the source of lead exposure appears to be from the lead paint characteristic of old housing in the Cleveland, Ohio area.

While thus far no pattern of significant physical health effects of prenatal cocaine exposure has been found, very few studies have addressed health outcomes. Because prenatal stress associated with drug exposure may have long-term effects on the neuroendocrine system, and based on the findings of fetal growth deficits, a number of the major cohort studies plan to investigate whether or not obesity and/or delayed pubertal development may be late sequelae of fetal exposure.

LANGUAGE

Several large longitudinal prospective cohort studies have found stable negative effects on language skills in cocaine-exposed infants and children up to 7 years of age, beyond the effect of the home environment or other confounding factors. In consecutive studies, from 4 months to 3 years (Morrow et al. 2003), and at 3, 4 and 7 years (Bandstra et al. 2004), severity of prenatal cocaine exposure was associated with corresponding deficits in language performance. Singer et al. (2001) noted increased levels of receptive language delays related to attentional deficits as early as 12 months of age in cocaine-exposed infants compared with non-exposed infants of similar age, sex, race and social class. This cohort from the Cleveland, Ohio study was then followed prospectively to 2, 4 and 6 years of age (Lewis et al. 2007), and a constant effect of cocaine exposure was found for both expressive and receptive language, accounting for 0.18 standard deviations (standard error = 0.09) difference in total language score, while all children in this low socio-economic status group declined in skills from 1 to 4 years. Continued follow-up of these cohorts to later ages can determine the specific linguistic deficits and brain functions that underlie these language delays in prenatally cocaine-exposed children, as well as identify modifying environmental factors (Beeghly et al. 2006).

ATTENTION AND COGNITIVE DEVELOPMENT

Data from animal models of prenatal cocaine exposure suggest that alterations in the fetal development of the monoaminergic system can affect later attention, information processing and emotional regulation (Dow-Edwards et al. 1999, Stanwood et al. 2001, Mayes 2002), raising concerns about later learning and school achievement.

In an early critical review of the research, Frank et al. (2002) found no convincing evidence of any consistent specific effect of prenatal cocaine exposure on standard developmental test scores to 6 years of age, possibly reflecting the poor reliability and predictive validity of infant tests prior to 2 years of age (Singer 2001) as well as the lack of prospective controlled studies of prenatally exposed cohorts at the time of the review.

Subsequently, however, impairments in attention, one component of executive neuro-psychological function, have been found across a range of ages, cohorts and assessment instruments in cocaine-exposed populations. Measures of visual information processing in the neonatal period (Singer et al. 1999) and during early infancy (Mayes et al. 1995, Coles

135

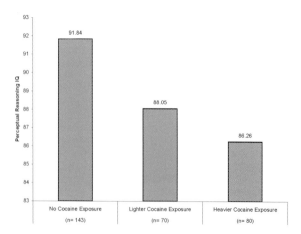

Fig. 8.1. Perceptual reasoning IQ by level of cocaine exposure (F=3.97, df=9, 264, p=0.02) with significant post-hoc mean difference between No Cocaine group and Heavier Cocaine Exposed group (p=0.02). The heavier cocaine group was determined by benzoylecgonine meconium screen (≥216 ng/g) or maternal self-report (≥17.5 units/week) indicating use >70th centile for the cocaine users. The provided mean scores were adjusted for scores on the Home Observation of Maternal Environment (a measure of caregiving quality), parity, maternal number of prenatal visits, biological maternal Peabody Picture Vocabulary–Revised scores, psychological distress at birth, current caregiver's scores on the Block Design subscale of the Wechsler Adult Intelligence Scale–Revised and lead level. (Adapted by permission from Singer et al. 2008.)

et al. 1999) suggest that impairments in these processes can be identified early in life in cocaine-exposed cohorts. Using a measure of visual processing related to cognitive functioning (Fagan and Singer 1983), several researchers noted poorer visual recognition memory at 6.5 months (Jacobson et al. 1996) and 12 months (Singer et al. 2005) in cocaine-exposed cohorts. In the latter study, significant differences in at-risk classification for later developmental delay across exposure groups were found for heavily cocaine-exposed infants at 6.5 months (35% vs 22% non-exposed, p<0.05) and for any cocaine-exposed infant at 12 months (27% vs 17%, p<0.025).

Well-controlled follow-up studies of IQ and cognitive function in cocaine-exposed cohorts have also begun to suggest a convergent finding of specific cognitive deficits in visuospatial information processing rather than generalized IQ differences, although not all studies support this finding (Arendt et al. 2004, Hurt et al. 2005). Although many preschool developmental assessments do not differentiate specific cognitive functions, several cohort studies at 2 and 3 years of age have linked prenatal cocaine exposure to poorer developmental outcome in general (Singer et al. 2002a, Behnke et al. 2006, Richardson et al. 2008). Moreover, among very-low-birthweight (<1500 g) infants, cocaine exposure is related to significant overall developmental delay in the first three years of life (Singer et al. 1994b).

Cocaine-exposed children had deficient performance compared with controls on the Wechsler IQ tests, the WIPPSI-R (Wechsler 1989) at 4 years and the WISC-IV (Williams et al. 2003) at 9 years, reflecting poorer visuospatial information processing (Singer et al.

136

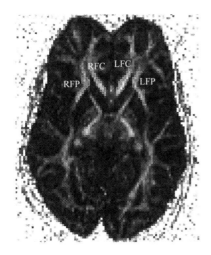

Fig. 8.2. Axial image showing white matter regions of interest. RFP = right frontal projection fibres; RFC = right frontal callosal fibres; LFC = left frontal callosal fibres; LFP = left frontal projection fibres. Cocaine-exposed children showed significantly higher average diffusion in LFC and RFC fibres. (Reprinted by permission from Warner and Behnke 2006.) For colour version of this figure, see plate section at end of book.

2004, 2008). At 4 years, on the WIPPSI-R, Object Assembly performance was negatively affected, as was, for boys, Arithmetic performance. At 9 years, Perceptual Reasoning IQ, a subscale of the WISC-IV Performance IQ that includes Block Design, Picture Concepts and Matrix Reasoning subtests, showed impairments in fluid reasoning and abstract categorical processing. A dose–response relationship, illustrated in Figure 8.1, between the amount and duration of prenatal cocaine exposure and attenuation of Perceptual Reasoning IQ was found in this study at 9 years, replicating a dose–response effect found in the Object Assembly task of the preschool assessment at 4 years (Singer et al. 2004).

Similar findings in a smaller sample followed longitudinally using the Stanford–Binet IQ scales at 4, 6 and 9 years were observed for cocaine-exposed boys on the Abstract/Visual reasoning scale (Bennett et al. 2008) and for cocaine-exposed 8- to 10-year-old children on an experimental measure of visuospatial working memory (Mayes et al. 2007).

The older ages of the children tested, the use of prospective longitudinal models, and the similar findings across four different assessment instruments suggest a stable finding of visuospatial information processing deficits in cocaine-exposed children. This finding is further strengthened by its conceptual relationship to the earlier data on impaired visual attention in infancy, to the preclinical literature that has found prenatal cocaine-induced deficits in behavioural studies of spatial navigation and memory abilities (Trksak et al. 2007), and to neuroimaging studies of cocaine-exposed children that have shown volumetric reductions in the corpus callosum and parietal areas of the brain (Dow-Edwards et al. 2006) and reduced maturational white matter pathways in the frontal lobes (Warner et al. 2006) (Fig. 8.2).

When tests of selective and sustained attention are given, findings from preschool to school-age studies indicate long-term disruptions to the attentional system congruent with the earlier findings of deficits in visual attention and memory in infancy. At 3, 5 and 7 years, Bandstra et al. (2001) found a stable negative influence of cocaine on tests of sustained attention, and, in the same cohort, increases in omission errors and response times (Accornero et al. 2007), confirming findings in a small group of cocaine-exposed children at 6 and 10 years of age (Leech et al. 1999, Richardson et al. 2002). Selective attention deficits were also found in 4-year-old cocaine-exposed children who demonstrated increases in commission errors on a continuous performance task (Noland et al. 2005). Both verbal (Rose-Jacobs et al. 2009) and motor (Bendersky et al. 2003) inhibitory control also appear to be compromised in cocaine-exposed children at school age.

ACADEMIC ACHIEVEMENT

To date, findings on academic achievement tests in cocaine-exposed cohorts have been mixed. Two large studies (Hurt et al. 2005, Singer et al. 2008) did not find achievement differences based on standardized tests. However, cocaine-exposed cohorts have been referred more often for intervention services (Frank et al. 2002, Singer et al. 2008), are more likely to be categorized as discrepant in achievement based on their IQ scores at 7 years, suggesting risk for learning disability (Morrow et al. 2006), and are referred more often for special education (Levine et al. 2008). However, in general, lags in educational achievement are often not detected until the later school years, and currently available outcome studies on cocaine-exposed children have been restricted to earlier school ages.

BEHAVIOUR

Deficits in self-regulatory behaviour, combined with negative environmental conditions, have been hypothesized to increase the rate of externalizing behaviour problems in cocaine-exposed children. While outcomes are still somewhat mixed, there is growing evidence that prenatal cocaine exposure is related to increased rates of conduct disorder, delinquency, inattention and possibly aggression. When evaluating existing data, several factors must be considered including sex, the individual rating the child's behaviour [self, caregiver (birth mother or relative vs foster or adoptive caregiver), teacher or examiner], other pre-natal drug exposures, and other caregiver factors such as psychological symptoms and relationship of the caregiver. In one study, a compilation of behaviour ratings completed by the experimenter, caregiver and teacher indicated that cocaine-exposed boys living in a high-risk environment demonstrated more aggressive behaviour than non-exposed boys (Bendersky et al. 2006). In another study, teacher-rated evaluations at age 6 indicated that cocaine-exposed boys had more behavioural problems, particularly hyperactivity, than non-exposed boys, while cocaine-exposed girls did not show this difference (Delaney-Black et al. 2004). Highlighting the importance of maternal factors in evaluating behavioural outcomes, other studies have found that recent caregiver drug use and psychological symp-toms, but not prenatal cocaine exposure, were predictors of behavioural problems in children from 4 months to 11 years of age (Accornero et al. 2002, 2006; Sheinkopf et al. 2006; Warner et al. 2006). In two studies using self-report, 6-year-old children who were prenatally cocaine exposed demonstrated clinically elevated levels of oppositional defiant disorder and inattention (Linares et al. 2006) and 10-year-old boys demonstrated more aggressive behaviour than non-exposed children (Bennett et al. 2008).

In the limited number of longitudinal studies, caregiver reports indicate more internalizing and externalizing behavioural problems up to age 7 (Bada et al. 2007) and a greater likelihood of delinquent behaviour (Minnes et al. 2010). Among cocaine-exposed children, those living in foster or adoptive care were rated as having more negative behavioural symptoms, including social, thought and attention problems, delinquency, aggression, internalizing and externalizing, than cocaine-exposed children living in birth mother or relative care (Minnes et al. 2010). However, it is unclear whether the cocaine-exposed children in foster/adoptive care were rated as having more problematic behaviours due to higher levels of prenatal cocaine exposure or because foster/adoptive parents are more adept at identifying behavioural problems. Ongoing longitudinal studies will determine whether these findings are precursors to higher rates of substance use disorders and risk-taking behaviours during adolescence and young adulthood.

Environmental Factors

While the above review delineates many of the specific findings indicating biological effects of prenatal cocaine exposure on child developmental outcomes, it is important to recognize the complex environmental contexts exerting additional influences that may add, moderate or minimize initial drug effects. All studies of cocaine-using women in the USA have found the majority to be polydrug users, exposing the fetus to heavier doses of alcohol, cannabis and tobacco, as well as other drugs, than non-cocaine-using women (Coles et al. 1992, Eyler et al. 1998, Frank et al. 2001, Singer et al. 2002b). In addition to cocaine, most of the studies in this review have found additional effects of these other substances on the growth, behavioural, cognitive and other functional domains studied in cocaine-exposed cohorts (see Chapters 7, 9). Studies to date suggest that cocaine is a mild teratogen compared with alcohol and lead (Singer et al. 2008). However, cocaine-exposed children are often exposed to high levels of alcohol and lead as well as cocaine, with additive effects (Singer et al. 2008, Min et al. 2009). Because of the high coexposure to alcohol and other drugs, the cocaine-exposed neonate needs to be monitored for withdrawal symptoms and the possibility of coexistent fetal alcohol syndrome and/or alcohol-related neurodevelopmental deficits evaluated in follow-up.

Cocaine-using pregnant women have high rates of comorbid psychopathology (Singer et al. 2002b, Minnes et al. 2005) that has independent physiological effects on the fetus and can also negatively affect the quality of their parenting (Hans et al. 1999). Many also have histories of child abuse and neglect that place their own children at risk (Min et al. 2007), and poorer intellectual functioning than women who did not use cocaine during pregnancy (Singer et al. 2002b). The identification of significant psychopathology, violent behaviour, and additional drug and alcohol problems in cocaine-using women frequently leads to a need for intervention of social services and foster care placement in the most severe cases (Minnes et al. 2008).

Because many cocaine-exposed children in the US cohorts were placed in foster or adoptive care at birth, they received an unforeseen environmental intervention in homes with more stimulating caregivers, lower lead exposure and less caregiver psychopathology than non-exposed infants or cocaine-exposed infants in their birth families (Frank et al. 2001; Brown et al. 2004; Singer et al. 2004, 2008). These children benefited from alternative and better quality caregiving, with better language scores (Lewis et al. 2004, 2007) and improved developmental outcomes (Frank et al. 2002), and a lower incidence of learning disability (Singer et al. 2004) than cocaine-exposed children in birth mother or kinship care. Interestingly, however, while foster or adoptive care into a more stimulating environment appeared to attenuate the risk of learning disability, cocaine-exposed children were less likely to achieve IQ scores at or above the average IQ of 100, despite their enriched environments (Singer et al. 2004, 2008).

These findings, on balance, suggest that the cocaine-exposed child can benefit substantially from intervention, and that interventions need to address the addiction and mental health needs of the parents while providing appropriate developmental services for the cocaine/polydrug-exposed infant and child. As no specific phenotype of the cocaine-exposed infant or child exists, individual assessments and interventions should be based on outcome domains affected at each developmental stage as needed. The current literature suggests that specific interventions related to feeding and growth, attention, language, visuospatial processing and regulatory behaviour are warranted.

Nevertheless, findings to date suggest that cocaine is a relatively mild behavioural teratogen with sequelae of significant but discrete deficits in growth, visuospatial information processing, selective and sustained attention, and behavioural regulation, after control for polydrug exposure and a wide range of environmental factors. Because these outcomes are preventable, medical and societal efforts should focus on alcohol, drug and mental health intervention efforts for women of childbearing age and pregnant women. Paediatric surveillance efforts should be augmented for children of drug- and alcohol-using women, and environmental lead exposure should be monitored.

Opiates
DRUG CLASSIFICATION AND HISTORY

An opiate is a chemical substance that has an analgesic action in the body. It works by binding to opioid receptors found primarily in the central nervous and digestive systems. Opiates, because of their strong pain-relieving properties, have been widely sought for recreational use and are associated with physiological dependence and tolerance. With heroin, a potent recreational opiate, dependence develops extremely rapidly due to the quick onset of action, profound relaxation and the intense euphoria it creates. Abrupt withdrawal can result in very uncomfortable, but usually not life-threatening, symptoms including restlessness, depression, dilated pupils, perspiration, insomnia, nausea, cramps, diarrhoea, and long-bone and muscle pain. While these symptoms resolve in a week or so, depression and insomnia can be quite protracted (up to six months) (National Institute on Drug Abuse 2005). Exogenous opiates are categorized into three major classes: natural (contained in the resin of the opium poppy, including morphine and codeine), semisynthetic (created from natural opiates, including heroin, hydracodone, oxycodone and buprenorphine), and fully synthetic (fentanyl, methadone and levomethadyl acetate) (Karch 2008).

Opiates have been used for pain relief and cultural ritual since the Neolithic age. Recreational use and dependence was first documented in China during the 17th century. At the end of World War Two the USA and Europe saw great increases in opiate dependence, prompting the development of treatment and rehabilitation programmes. The problem of opiate dependence continues today. The European Monitoring Centre for Drugs and Addiction indicated that in 2007 global opium and heroin production reached record levels, at 8870 and 733 tons respectively. Because of the illicit nature of opiate use, accurate figures regarding consumption are difficult to obtain. Among the estimated 19.9 million (8%) illicit drug users in the USA, 2.5 million of those aged 12 and older reported using pain relievers recreationally for the first time in the year of measurement (2007) and 106 000 reported using heroin; 554 000 reported using the potent time-release opiate oxycontin, typically prescribed for chronic pain. While men use opiates at higher rates than women, there have been, and continue to be, children born to opiate-dependent women or women maintained on opiate maintenance therapy.

OPIATE USE AMONG PREGNANT WOMEN

Reporting of opiate use among pregnant women is especially unreliable due to the illicit nature of the drug and fear of prosecution for child endangerment. Women who abuse opiates are likely to abuse other recreational drugs such as cocaine, cannabis, alcohol and tobacco, largely to manage opiate withdrawal symptoms. The combination of polydrug use and the covert nature of opiate drug use makes epidemiological research of prenatal opiate exposure difficult. Despite the difficulties of gathering accurate information, recent surveys from the USA, UK and Australia indicate that a significant number of women of childbearing years abuse opiates. A survey of pregnant women in the UK obtaining drug treatment indicated that 1.3% were found to be positive for opiates using urine toxicology screening (Sanaullah et al. 2006). In a retrospective chart review of 89 080 births in Australia, among the 0.8% (n=707) women who reported substance use, 29.9% reported methadone use and 12.5% reported heroin use (Kennare et al. 2005). In a multicentre study in the USA, meconium screening was completed for 8527 newborn infants. Results indicated that 10.7% of their mothers used cocaine and opiates prenatally, with 1.2% having used opiates alone (Lester et al. 2001). In a universal screening of women delivering at Louisiana State University Hospital in the USA, 2.1% were positive for opiates. Dependence on opiates among pregnant women continues to be a public health issue worldwide.

Pregnancy in opiate-dependent women is rarely planned and can result in differing behavioural responses (Bell and Harvey-Dodds 2008). According to the Australian Institute on Health and Welfare (2004), most women who use substances and subsequently discover they are pregnant make efforts to reduce or quit their drug use. Researchers report that illicit drug use declined from 17% in non-pregnant women to 6% in pregnant women, but that pregnant women were less likely to reduce tobacco or opiate use than that of other drugs of abuse. Dependent opiate and tobacco users have a very difficult time maintaining abstinence despite efforts to stop. Paradoxically, some drug-dependent women may increase drug use because of the stress of pregnancy and impending parenthood, and ambivalence toward the pregnancy.

PREGNANCY OUTCOME

Opiate use, accompanying polydrug use (primarily tobacco, cocaine and alcohol), and a chaotic and impoverished lifestyle during pregnancy can have negative effects on pregnancy

TABLE 8.2
Effects of prenatal opiate exposure on infants and school-age children

Deficit	Features
Pregnancy and birth outcomes	Neonatal abstinence syndrome (pre- and postnatally) can result in negative pregnancy outcomes including increased rates of stillbirth, premature rupture of membranes, preterm delivery and sudden infant death syndrome, and decreased birthweight, length and head circumference
Central nervous system	Seizures in 2–11% of neonates, high muscle tone, high-pitched cry, difficulty being consoled, irritability, excessive and poor sucking. There is evidence that combined cocaine and opiate exposure results in greater negative effects
Cognition	Suggestion of poor cognitive function at 3 years, lower verbal and performance ability, and impaired reading and arithmetic achievement. Outcome studies suffer from lack of control groups, control for covariates and small sample size
Behaviour	Prenatal opiate exposure is associated with behavioural problems in children, particularly attention-deficit–hyperactivity disorder and disruptive behaviours at 10 years of age
Neuroimaging	9- to 11-year-old opiate-exposed children had smaller brain volumes, thinner cortex, and reduced pallidum and putamen size

outcome. One of the primary risks to fetuses in opiate-dependent women is daily fluctuation of opiate levels causing varying degrees of fetal abstinence syndrome (Bell and Harvey-Dodds 2008). Daily opiate dose fluctuation and fetal abstinence syndrome can result in increased rates of stillbirth, preterm delivery, low birthweight and sudden infant death syndrome (Joseph et al. 2000) (Table 8.2). Adding to the physiological burden of fluctuating opiate levels, opiate-exposed children, as with cocaine-exposed children, are likely to be exposed to other recreational drugs that can also increase the risk of spontaneous abortion, premature rupture of membranes, intrauterine growth retardation, preterm labour, toxaemia, breech presentation and other birth complications (Kennare et al. 2005). Studies have documented the increased risk of the combination of opiate exposure, other drug exposure and health factors common among opiate-using women. Low-birthweight infants exposed to both cocaine and opiates had significantly higher mortality rates than those exposed to either drug alone (Ostrea et al. 1997), and human-immunodeficiency-virus-infected women who also used opiates had children with higher rates of sudden infant death syndrome compared with the general population (Kahlert et al. 2007).

DEVELOPMENTAL OUTCOME (Table 8.2)
Studies of animals exposed to opiate drugs during gestation indicate CNS changes and provide a basis for examining cognitive and behavioural effects of fetal opiate exposure in humans. For example, prenatal morphine exposure in rats has been found to be related to neural tube defects (Nasiraei-Moghadam et al. 2005). Villarreal et al. (2008) found that rats exposed to morphine during gestation had sustained alterations in late long-term potentiation, the cellular mechanisms that underlie the formation of long-term memories. Prenatal exposure to morphine in male and female rats is also related to changes in the norepinephrine and opiate neurotransmitter systems in several brain regions involved in stress responsivity

and maintenance of homeostatic balance (Vathy 2002). Cross-generational effects have also been observed in the behaviour of second-generation morphine-exposed rat pups, with decreased CNS integrity, lower birthweight and morphometric differences (Slamberová et al. 2006).

Evidence of CNS damage in humans exposed prenatally to opiates is mounting, although the effects appear to be specific rather than a more global or overall deficit as seen with some teratogens. Using magnetic resonance imaging in a small number of 9- to 11-year-old opiate-exposed children and controls, smaller brain volumes, thinner cortex, and reduced pallidum and putamen were found in the opiate-exposed children (Walhovd et al. 2007). Associations were found between lower volumes of specific brain regions and cognitive ability and behaviour problems. Opiate-exposed infants had less rhythmic swallowing, were not efficient feeders (Gewolb et al. 2004) and had higher rates of strabismus (Gill et al. 2003) than controls, also indicating CNS insult. Feeding and swallowing differences disappeared by 1 month (Ornoy et al. 2001). No evidence of increased risk for hearing loss was found in prenatally opiate-exposed infants (Grimmer et al. 1999).

Early studies of cognitive and behavioural outcomes found impairments among opiate-exposed children. However, these studies had very small sample sizes and did not adequately control for other drug exposure or environmental conditions and therefore must be evaluated with caution. Three- to 6-year-old children exposed to heroin prenatally were rated by their caregivers as less well adjusted and they performed more poorly on perceptual measures than non-heroin-exposed children (Wilson et al. 1979). Five- to 12-year-old children who were heroin exposed and resided at home or were of low socio-economic status had lower verbal and performance intellectual ability and impaired reading and arithmetic skills (Ornoy et al. 2001). Children who were heroin exposed were more likely to be diagnosed with attention-deficit–hyperactivity disorder, including those reared in higher-quality homes of adoptive caregivers (Ornoy et al. 2001).

Later studies, with larger samples and adequate control for environmental conditions and other drug exposures, also indicate adverse effects of prenatal opiate exposure on developmental outcome. The Maternal Lifestyles Study recruited a large sample (n=1388) of women who used cocaine only, cocaine plus opiate, or opiate only, and their prenatally drug-exposed children, and followed them longitudinally, making it possible to evaluate the effects of cocaine/polysubstance exposure and multiple environmental conditions on birth outcomes and cognitive development. The combination of prenatal cocaine and opiate exposure created the highest odds of CNS/autonomic nervous system symptoms in infancy (Bada et al. 2002). The cocaine–opiate combination of prenatal exposure also had a negative effect on acoustic cry characteristics that reflect compromised reactivity, respiratory and neuronal control (Lester et al. 2002) and neuronal transmission (Lester et al. 2003), supporting results found in early animal studies. It should be noted that these CNS symptoms were also negatively affected by alcohol and cannabis exposure and lower birthweight (Lester et al. 2002). Early feeding behaviour in cocaine- and cocaine/opiate-exposed infants was examined by Lagasse et al. (2003). Opiate-exposed infants had prolonged sucking bursts, fewer pauses, more feeding problems and increased arousal, while opiate-using mothers showed increased activity. Children exposed only to cocaine did not show differences in feeding behaviour.

Investigation of this cohort at ages 1–3 years indicated that there were no cocaine or opiate effects on mental and motor development after controlling for covariates, although opiate-exposed children scored 3.8 points below children not exposed to opiates on psycho-motor function (Messinger et al. 2004). Study of the same cohort at a later age (Bada et al. 2008) demonstrated that children's living arrangements and living stability were related to behavioural problems and adaptive functioning, but there were no opiate-specific outcomes.

Older prenatally opiate-exposed children (aged 7–12 years) who were assessed for attention and autonomic regulation and compared with two control groups (boys whose mothers began opiate use after birth and boys whose mothers did not use opiates) showed a decreased ability to suppress vagal tone, an indicator of sustained attention, compared with both control groups (Hickey et al. 1995, Suess et al. 1997). In another study, opiate-exposed boys also showed a decreased ability to suppress vagal tone compared with control groups when distracters were added to a vigilance task, suggesting that the normal physiological response to increased attention demand may be impaired in boys exposed to opiates (Hickey et al. 1995).

MAINTENANCE THERAPY DURING PREGNANCY

Complete maternal abstinence from opiates after dependence has a high failure rate. In addition, complete abstinence poses danger to the fetus due to abstinence stress. Therefore it has become widely recognized that maintenance therapy with drugs (methadone, buprenorphine, etc.) is beneficial. Maintenance drugs reduce the intense intoxication and withdrawal from recreational drugs such as heroin and reduce drug-seeking behaviour and accompanying social and legal consequences. Their efficacy for use during pregnancy and effects on pregnancy and developmental outcomes has also been investigated.

Methadone

Methadone was originally synthesized for use as an analgesic before World War Two in Germany for fear of opium shortages. At the time, it was generally deemed unfit for regular pain relief use. However, a series of research studies has shown that methadone is useful in the treatment of opiate withdrawal, in reduction of drug-seeking behaviours (craving) and in pain management in some cases. Methadone acts on the opiate receptors but stabilizes withdrawal symptoms through its long duration of action and blockage of the 'rush' experienced during intravenous heroin or morphine use.

Methadone's usefulness as a treatment for withdrawal from heroin was first documented by Isbell and Vogal (1949; see Joseph et al. 2000). Decreasing doses were given over a period of 10 weeks and, although patients were technically withdrawn from heroin, over 90% relapsed after treatment. In the mid-1960s research on methadone maintenance therapy began, in which patients were maintained on stable doses of methadone over an indefinite period of time. Research by Dole et al. (1966), Kreek and Reisinger (1997), Joseph et al. (2000) and others found that patients maintained on methadone over a period of time were not sedated or preoccupied with getting their next dose. Their behaviour became stabilized and their affect was normalized. With the addition of counselling for addiction, personal and social problems, an outpatient model was successfully developed and became the predominant mode of treatment. Methadone maintenance therapy became sanctioned in the USA in the mid-1990s by the Institute of Medicine (Rettig and Yarmolinsky 1995) and the National Institutes of Health (National Consensus Development Panel on Effective Medical Treatment of Opiate Addiction 1998).

Methadone maintenance is recommended for opiate-dependent women who become pregnant (Kaltenbach et al. 1998). The effect of methadone on pregnancy outcome and fetal development has been studied since the 1960s. Methadone maintenance reduces the likelihood of pregnant women using injectable opiates such as heroin as well as other legal and illegal substances, and reduces fetal risk due to abstinence syndrome. However, it cannot be used in isolation without adequate social support, counselling, nutrition and prenatal care. Methadone maintenance is associated with better pregnancy outcomes than no maintenance therapy intervention. These positive effects are due to reduced heroin use, increased social and economic level (Brulet et al. 2007), the possibility of social stabilization and increased rates of prenatal care (Vavrinkova and Binder 2007b).

Pregnancy and developmental outcomes of prenatally methadone-exposed infants have been compared with those of infants exposed to uncontrolled heroin use during pregnancy and to racially and socially matched control groups. Compared with uncontrolled heroin exposure, prenatally methadone-exposed infants had higher birthweights and lower rates of intrauterine growth retardation (Vavrinkova and Binder 2007). Despite attenuating effects of methadone on neonatal abstinence syndrome, 60–87% of infants required treatment. In another small study, hearing, speech and intellectual performance were lower in uncontrolled opiate-exposed children than in children exposed to methadone (Bunikowski et al. 1998). A cohort of African-American prenatally methadone- and other opiate-exposed infants and a control group have been studied longitudinally since 1979 by Hans and colleagues (see Hans 1996). Their cohort was studied during infancy (n=100) and later at 10 (n=77) and 14 (n=74) years of age. Neurodevelopmental assessments completed in infancy (1 day and 4 months) using the Brazelton Neonatal Assessment Scale with the Kansas supplement (Horowitz et al. 1978) indicate that methadone-exposed infants had poorer motor coordination, greater tenseness and higher activity levels than the control group (Marcus et al. 1982). Using the Bayley Scales of Infant Development at 4 months, prenatally methadone-exposed infants performed more poorly than controls in motor function, but not in social or cognitive behaviours (Bernstein et al. 1984). At 12 months, methadone-exposed children had poorer attention (Marcus et al. 1984), higher scores on disorganized and avoidant behaviour, and lower scores on contact-maintaining behaviour (Goodman et al. 1999). The importance of rearing conditions was highlighted in this cohort, with findings that motor delay persisted after 4 months only in methadone-exposed children in poorer families (Hans 1989). Earlier findings of an effect of prenatal methadone exposure on attention were also no longer present at 24 months after control for maternal IQ (Schneider and Hans 1996). Hans (1989) concluded that prenatal methadone exposure may make children more susceptible to the negative effects of an impoverished environment.

Few studies of prenatal methadone exposure extend beyond the infancy period, nor do they have adequate sample size and control for covariates. Studies that have extended through the early childhood years indicate evidence of cognitive delay and increased behavioural problems in opiate-exposed children. For example, lower Bayley Scales of Mental Development (Mental and Motor) scores at 18 months (Rosen and Johnson 1982) were found for methadone-exposed children, but there were no differences in overall cognitive outcomes at age 4 (Kaltenbach and Finnegan 1984). At school age, methadone-exposed children were found by de Cubas and Field (1993) to have lower IQs and more maternal-rated behavioural disturbances including anxiety, aggression, rejection and overall poorer behaviour than non-exposed children. Hans (1996) also reported that methadone-exposed children at age 10 received higher ratings of behavioural problems in the area of attention-deficit–hyperactivity disorder and disruptive behaviour.

To understand more fully the effects of prenatal methadone and opiate exposure on pregnancy and developmental outcome, they have been studied in context with other drug exposures. The combination of tobacco and opiate exposure in utero has been shown to have differential effects on the severity of neonatal abstinence syndrome. Infants of methadone-maintained mothers, who were also exposed to more than 20 cigarettes per day, had higher neonatal abstinence syndrome scores and took longer to reach the highest level of symptoms of neonatal abstinence syndrome than infants exposed to fewer than 10 cigarettes per day (Choo et al. 2004). For additional reviews of literature related to outcomes of children exposed to methadone prenatally, see Kaltenbach and Finnegan (1989), Hans (1996) and Kaltenbach (1996).

Buprenorphine
Buprenorphine is another, more recently developed, synthetic opiate drug that is also prescribed as a maintenance drug for the treatment of heroin addiction. Buprenorphine is approved for the treatment of opiate addiction during pregnancy in the USA, Europe and Australia (Australian Institute of Health and Welfare 2004). The pregnancy outcome effects of buprenorphine compared with methadone and heroin use during pregnancy have been investigated, but long-term studies of developmental outcome have not been completed.

Magnetic resonance imaging studies to evaluate the effects of prenatal buprenorphine exposure on brain development have not found any major structural abnormalities attributable to this maintenance therapy. It is thought that buprenorphine therapy may prevent hypoxic–ischaemic brain changes that can result from uncontrolled heroin use during pregnancy (Kahila et al. 2007). Buprenorphine has protective factors similar to methadone regarding birth size compared with uncontrolled heroin exposure. Heroin-addicted women had children with the lowest birthweights and the greatest number of infants with intrauterine growth retardation (Vavrinkova and Binder 2007a) when compared with prenatally methadone- or buprenorphine-exposed children (Jones et al. 2005). A growing number of studies comparing buprenorphine with methadone maintenance therapy have found better outcomes of higher infant birthweight and gestational age, and lower incidence of neonatal abstinence syndrome and length of hospital stay for buprenorphine-exposed infants (Johnson et al. 2003, Kayemba-Kay's and Laclyde 2003, Schindler et al. 2003, Jones et al. 2005, Fischer et al. 2006, Lejeune et al. 2006, Kakko et al. 2008).

Lack of blinded designs, adequate numbers of participants and control for other drug exposures limit the interpretation of these findings. A National Institute on Drug Abuse agency-funded study called MOTHER is a double-blind, double-dummy, randomized, stratified, parallel-group study comparing the efficacy of methadone and buprenorphine. Evaluation of buprenorphine and methadone is ongoing and holds promise for clarifying the best course of treatment for opiate-addicted women and their children.

SUMMARY

There are very few long-term outcome studies of the developmental effects of either heroin or other illicit opiate exposures during gestation. The abuse of prescription opiates such as vicodin, hydrocodone and oxycontin among pregnant women has not yet been investigated. Evidence suggests that uncontrolled heroin use during pregnancy can have negative effects on pregnancy outcome and has consistently been associated with lower birthweight and intrauterine growth retardation. Evidence from relatively small neonatal studies of prenatally heroin-exposed samples indicates decreased cognitive performance in younger children and increased rates of behaviour problems in 8- to 17-year-olds. Studies that have investigated the effects of opiate maintenance therapy on pregnancy and developmental outcome have found fewer pregnancy complications, greater birthweight, and better developmental and behavioural outcomes than uncontrolled heroin exposure (Kaltenbach et al. 1998). However, compared with control groups with no opiate exposure, rates of early motor delay, attentional problems and compromised regulatory behaviour have been reported. Since long-term outcome studies of prenatally opiate-exposed children are sparse, later propensity for drug use and dependence, reactivity to stressful environmental conditions and mental health outcomes are unknown. The importance of high-quality rearing conditions after prenatal opiate exposure has been highlighted in many studies.

For opiate-addicted pregnant women, early engagement in maintenance therapy is essential for optimal pregnancy and infant developmental outcome. Continued supportive and occupational counselling can help to improve negative environmental conditions, which have been shown to compound the negative developmental effects of gestational opiate exposure. Proper treatment for neonatal abstinence syndrome at birth, early assessment for developmental delay, and ongoing monitoring for attentional problems and environmental and caregiving quality are essential for optimal developmental outcome.

ACKNOWLEDGEMENTS

Research by Lynn Singer and Sonia Minnes was supported by the National Institute on Drug Abuse (grant RO1-DA07957). We would like to thank Terri Lotz-Ganley for manuscript preparation.

REFERENCES

Accornero VH, Morrow CE, Bandstra ES, et al. (2002) Behavioral outcome of preschoolers exposed prenatally to cocaine: role of maternal behavioral health. *J Pediatr Psychol* **27**: 259–269.

Accornero VH, Anthony JC, Morrow CE, et al. (2006) Prenatal cocaine exposure: an examination of childhood externalizing and internalizing behavior problems at age 7 years. *Epidemiol Psichiatr Soc* **15**: 20–29.

Accornero VH, Amado AJ, Morrow CE, et al. (2007) Impact of prenatal cocaine exposure on attention and response inhibition as assessed by continuous performance tests. *J Dev Behav Pediatr* **28**: 195–205.

Arendt RA, Singer LT, Minnes S, Salvator A (1999) Accuracy in detecting prenatal drug exposure. *J Drug Issues* **29**: 203–214.

Arndt R, Short E, Singer LT, et al. (2004) Children prenatally exposed to cocaine: developmental outcomes and environmental risks at seven years of age. *J Dev Behav Pediatr* **25**: 83–90.

Australian Institute of Health and Welfare (2004) *Australia's Health.* Canberra: AIHW.

Bada HS, Bauer CR, Shankaran S, et al. (2002) Central and autonomic system signs with in utero drug exposure. *Arch Dis Child Fetal Neonatal Ed* **87**: F106–F112.

Bada HS, Das A, Bauer CR, et al. (2005) Low birth weight and preterm births: etiologic fraction attributable to prenatal drug exposure. *J Perinatol* **25**: 631–637.

Bada HS, Das A, Bauer CR, et al. (2007) Impact of prenatal cocaine exposure on child behavior problems through school age. *Pediatrics* **119**: e348–e359.

Bada HS, Langer J, Twomey J, et al. (2008) Importance of stability of early living arrangements on behavior outcomes of children with and without prenatal drug exposure. *J Dev Behav Pediatr* **29**: 173–182.

Bandstra ES, Morrow CE, Anthony JC, et al. (2001) Longitudinal investigation of task persistence and sustained attention in children with prenatal cocaine exposure. *Neurotoxicol Teratol* **23**: 545–559.

Bandstra ES, Vogel AL, Morrow CE, et al. (2004) Severity of prenatal cocaine exposure and child language functioning through age seven years: a longitudinal latent growth curve analysis. *Substance Use Misuse* **39**: 25–59.

Beeghly M, Martin B, Rose-Jacobs R, et al. (2006) Prenatal cocaine exposure and children's language functioning at 6 and 9.5 years: moderating effects of child age, birthweight, and gender. *J Pediatr Psychol* **31**: 98–115.

Behnke M, Eyler FD, Garvan CW, Wobie K (2001) The search for congenital malformations in newborns with fetal cocaine exposure. *Pediatrics* **107**: e74.

Behnke M, Eyler FD, Warner TD, et al. (2006) Outcome from a prospective, longitudinal study of prenatal cocaine use: preschool development at 3 years of age. *J Pediatr Psychol* **31**: 41–49.

Bell J, Harvey-Dodds L (2008) Pregnancy and injecting drug use. *BMJ* **336**: 1303–1305.

Bendersky M, Gambini G, Lastella A, et al. (2003) Inhibitory motor control at five years as a function of prenatal cocaine exposure. *J Dev Behav Pediatr* **24**: 345–351.

Bendersky M, Bennett D, Lewis M (2006) Aggression at age 5 as a function of prenatal exposure to cocaine, gender, and environmental risk. *J Pediatr Psychol* **31**: 71–84.

Bennett DS, Bendersky M, Lewis M (2008) Children's cognitive ability from 4 to 9 years old as a function of prenatal cocaine exposure, environmental risk, and maternal verbal intelligence. *Dev Psychol* **44**: 919–928.

Bernstein VJ, Jeremy RJ, Hans SL, Marcus J (1984) A longitudinal study of offspring born to methadone-maintained women. II. Dyadic interaction and infant behavior at 4 months. *Am J Drug Alcohol Abuse* **10**: 161–193.

Bourne P (1974) The great cocaine myth. *Drugs and Drug Abuse Education Newsletter* **5**: 5–7.

Brown JV, Bakeman R, Coles CD, et al. (1998) Maternal drug use during pregnancy: are preterm and full-term infants affected differently? *Dev Psychol* **34**: 540–554.

Brown JV, Bakeman R, Coles CD, et al. (2004) Prenatal cocaine exposure: a comparison of 2-year-old children in parental and nonparental care. *Child Dev* **75**: 1282–1295.

Brulet C, Chanal C, Ravel P, et al. (2007) [Multidisciplinary monitoring and psychosocial support reduce complications of opiate dependence in pregnant women: 114 pregnancies.] *Presse Med* **36**: 1571–1580 (French).

Bunikowski R, Grimmer I, Heiser A, et al. (1998) Neurodevelopmental outcome after prenatal exposure to opiates. *Eur J Pediatr* **157**: 724–730.

Chavkin W (2001) Cocaine and pregnancy—time to look at the evidence. *JAMA* **285**: 1613–1625.

Choo RE, Huestis MA, Schroeder JR, et al. (2004) Neonatal abstinence syndrome in methadone-exposed infants is altered by level of prenatal tobacco exposure. *Drug Alcohol Depend* **75**: 253–260.

Coles CD, Platzman KA, Smith I, et al. (1992) Effects of cocaine and alcohol use in pregnancy on neonatal growth and neurobehavioral status. *Neurotoxicol Teratol* **14**: 23–33.

Coles CD, Bard KA, Platzman KA, Lynch ME (1999) Attentional response at eight weeks in prenatally drug-exposed and preterm infants. *Neurotoxicol Teratol* **21**: 527–537.

Covington CY, Nordstrom-Klee B, Ager J, et al. (2002) Birth to age 7 growth of children exposed to drugs: a prospective cohort study. *Neurotoxical Teratol* **24**: 489–496.

de Cubas MM, Field T (1993) Children of methadone-dependent women: developmental outcomes. *Am J Orthopsychiatry* **63**: 266–276.

Delaney-Black V, Covington C, Nordstrom B, et al. (2004) Prenatal cocaine: quantity of exposure and gender moderation. *J Dev Behav Pediatr* **25**: 254–263.

Dole VP, Nyswander M, Kreek MJ (1966) Narcotic blockade. *Arch Intern Med* **118**: 304–309.

Dow-Edwards D, Mayes L, Spear L, Hurd Y (1999) Cocaine and development: clinical, behavioral, and

148

neurobiological perspectives—a symposium report. *Neurotoxicol Teratol* **21**: 481–490.

Dow-Edwards DL, Benveniste H, Behnke M, et al. (2006) Neuroimaging of prenatal drug exposure. *Neuro-toxicol Teratol* **28**: 386–402.

Eyler FD, Behnke M, Conlon M, et al. (1998) Birth outcome from a prospective, matched study of prenatal crack/cocaine use: II. Interactive and dose effects on neurobehavioral assessment. *Pediatrics* **101**: 237–41.

Fagan JF, Singer LT (1983) Infant recognition memory as a measure of intelligence. In: Lipsitt LP, ed. *Advances in Infancy Research, vol. 2*. Norwood, NJ: Ablex, pp 31–78.

Fischer G, Ortner R, Rohrmeister K, et al. (2006) Methadone versus buprenorphine in pregnant addicts: a double-blind, double-dummy comparison study. *Addiction* **101**: 275–281.

Frank DA, Augustyn M, Knight WG, et al. (2001) Growth, development, and behavior in early childhood following prenatal cocaine exposure: a systematic review. *JAMA* **285**: 1613–1625.

Frank DA, Jacobs RR, Beeghly M, et al. (2002) Level of prenatal cocaine exposure and scores on the Bayley Scales of Infant Development: modifying effects of caregiver, early intervention, and birth weight. *Pediatrics* **110**: 1143–1152.

Gewolb IH, Fishman D, Qureshi MA, Vice FL (2004) Coordination of suck–swallow–respiration in infants born to mothers with drug-abuse problems. *Dev Med Child Neurol* **46**: 700–705.

Gill AC, Oei J, Younan N, et al. (2003) Strabismus in infants of opiate-dependent mothers. *Acta Paediatr* **92**: 379–385.

Goodman G, Hans SL, Cox SM (1999) Attachment behavior and its antecedents in offspring born to methadone-maintained women. *J Clin Child Psychol* **28**: 58–69.

Grimmer I, Bührer C, Aust G, Obladen M (1999) Hearing in newborn infants of opiate-addicted mothers. *Eur J Pediatr* **158**: 653–657.

Hans SL (1989) Developmental consequences of prenatal exposure to methadone. *Ann N Y Acad Sci* **562**: 195–207.

Hans SL (1996) Prenatal drug exposure: behavioral functioning in late childhood and adolescence. *NIDA Res Monogr* **164**: 261–276.

Hans SL, Bernstein VJ, Henson LG (1999) The role of psychopathology in the parenting of drug-dependent women. *Dev Psychopathol* **11**: 957–977.

Hickey JE, Suess PE, Newlin DB, et al. (1995) Vagal tone regulation during sustained attention in boys exposed to opiates in utero. *Addict Behav* **20**: 43–59.

Horowitz FD, Sullivan JW, Linn P (1978) Stability and instability in the newborn infant: the quest for elusive threads. *Monogr Soc Res Child Dev* **43**: 29–45.

Hurt H, Brodsky NL, Roth H, et al. (2005) School performance of children with gestational cocaine exposure. *Neurotoxicol Teratol* **27**: 203–211.

Isbell H, Vogel VH (1949) The addiction liability of methadon (amidone, dolophine, 10820) and its use in the treatment of the morphine abstinence syndrome. *Am J Psychiatry* **105**: 909–914.

Jacobson JL, Jacobson SW (2005) Methodological issues in research on developmental exposure to neuro-toxic agents. *Neurotoxicol Teratol* **27**: 395–406.

Jacobson SW, Jacobson JL, Sokol RJ, et al. (1996) New evidence for neurobehavioral effects of in utero cocaine exposure. *J Pediatr* **129**: 581–590.

Johnson AL, Morrow CE, Accornero VH, et al. (2002) Maternal cocaine use: estimated effects on mother–child play interactions in the preschool period. *J Dev Behav Pediatr* **23**: 191–202.

Johnson RE, Jones HE, Fischer G (2003) Use of buprenorphine in pregnancy: patient management and effects on the neonate. *Drug Alcohol Depend* **70**: S87–S101.

Jones HE, Johnson RE, Jasinski DR, et al. (2005) Buprenorphine versus methadone in the treatment of pregnant opioid-dependent patients: effects on the neonatal abstinence syndrome. *Drug Alcohol Depend* **79**: 1–10.

Joseph H, Stancliff S, Langrod J (2000) Methadone maintenance treatment (MMT): a review of historical and clinical issues. *Mt Sinai J Med* **67**: 347–364.

Kahila H, Kivitie-Kallio S, Halmesmäki E, et al. (2007) Brain magnetic resonance imaging of infants exposed prenatally to buprenorphine. *Acta Radiol* **48**: 228–231.

Kahlert C, Rudin C, Kind C, et al. (2007) Sudden infant death syndrome in infants born to HIV-infected and opiate-using mothers. *Arch Dis Child* **92**: 1005–1008.

Kakko J, Heilig M, Sarman I (2008) Buprenorphine and methadone treatment of opiate dependence during pregnancy: comparison of fetal growth and neonatal outcomes in two consecutive case series. *Drug Alcohol Depend* **96**: 69–78.

Kaltenbach K, Berghella V, Finnegan L (1998) Opioid dependence during pregnancy. Effects and management. *Obstet Gynecol Clin N Am* **25**: 139–151.

Kilenbach KA (1996) Exposure to opiates: behavioral outcomes in preschool and school-age children. *NIDA Res Monogr* **164**: 230–241.

Kilenbach K, Finnegan LP (1984) Developmental outcome of children born to methadone maintained women: a review of longitudinal studies. *Neurobehav Toxicol Teratol* **6**: 271–275.

Kilenbach KA, Finnegan LP (1989) Prenatal narcotic exposure: perinatal and developmental effects. *Neurotoxicology* **40**: 597–604.

Kath SB (2008) *Karch's Pathology of Drug Abuse*. Boca Raton, FL: CRC Press.

Kajemba-Kay's S, Laclyde JP (2003) Buprenorphine withdrawal syndrome in newborns: a report of 13 cases. *Addiction* **98**: 1599–1604.

Kemare R, Heard A, Chan A (2005) Substance use during pregnancy: risk factors and obstetric and perinatal outcomes in South Australia. *Aust N Z J Obstet Gynaecol* **45**: 220–225.

Klonoff-Cohen H, Lam-Kruglick P (2001) Maternal and paternal recreational drug use and sudden infant death syndrome. *Arch Pediatr Adolesc Med* **155**: 765–770.

Krek MJ, Reisinger M (1997) The addict as patient. In: Lowinson JH, Ruiz P, Millman RB, Langrod JG, eds. *Substance Abuse: a Comprehensive Textbook, 3rd edn*. Baltimore: Williams & Wilkins, pp 822–823.

Lagasse L, Messinger D, Lester BM, et al. (2003) Prenatal drug exposure and maternal and infant feeding behavior. *Arch Dis Child Fetal Neonatal Ed* **88**: F391–F399.

Leech SL, Richardson GA, Goldschmidt L, Day NL (1999) Prenatal substance exposure: effects on attention and impulsivity of 6-year-olds. *Neurotoxicol Teratol* **21**: 109–118.

Lejeune C, Simmat-Durand L, Gourarier L, et al. (2006) Prospective multicenter observational study of 260 infants born to 259 opiate-dependent mothers on methadone or high-dose buprenophine substitution. *Drug Alcohol Depend* **82**: 250–257.

Lester BM, ElSohly M, Wright LL, et al. (2001) The Maternal Lifestyle Study: drug use by meconium toxicology and maternal self-report. *Pediatrics* **107**: 309–317.

Lester BM, Tronick EZ, LaGasse L, et al. (2002) The Maternal Lifestyle Study: effects of substance exposure during pregnancy on neurodevelopmental outcome in 1-month-old infants. *Pediatrics* **110**: 1182–1192.

Lester BM, Lagasse L, Seifer R, et al. (2003) The Maternal Lifestyle Study (MLS): effects of prenatal cocaine and/or opiate exposure on auditory brain response at one month. *J Pediatr* **142**: 279–285.

Levine TP, Liu J, Das A, et al. (2008) Effects of prenatal cocaine exposure on special education in school-aged children. *Pediatrics* **122**: e83–e91.

Lewis BA, Singer LT, Short EJ, et al. (2004) Four-year language outcomes of children exposed to cocaine in utero. *Neurotoxicol Teratol* **26**: 617–627.

Lewis BA, Kirchner HL, Short EJ, et al. (2007) Prenatal cocaine and tobacco effects on children's language trajectories. *Pediatrics* **120**: e78–e85.

Lidow MS (2003) Consequences of prenatal cocaine exposure in nonhuman primates. Dev Brain Res 147: 23–36.

Linares TJ, Singer LT, Kirchner HL, et al. (2006) Mental health of cocaine exposed children at 6 years of age. *J Pediatr Psychol* **61**: 85–97.

Lumeng JC, Cabral HJ, Gannon K, et al. (2007) Pre-natal exposures to cocaine and alcohol and physical growth patterns to age 8 years. *Neurotoxicol Teratol* **29**: 446–457.

Malanga CJ, Kosofsky BE (1999) Mechanisms of action of drugs of abuse on the developing fetal brain. *Clin Perinatol* **26**: 17–37.

Marcus J, Hans SL, Jeremy RJ (1982) Patterns of 1-day and 4-month motor functioning in infants of women on methadone. *Neurotoxicol Teratol* **4**: 473–476.

Marcus J, Hans SL, Jeremy RJ (1984) A longitudinal study of offspring born to methadone-maintained women. III. Effects of multiple risk factors on development at 4, 8, and 12 months. *Am J Drug Alcohol Abuse* **10**: 195–207.

Mayes LC (2002) A behavioral teratogenic model of the impact of prenatal cocaine exposure on arousal regulatory systems. *Neurotoxicol Teratol* **24**: 385–395.

Mayes LC, Bornstein MH, Chawarska K, Granger RH (1995) Information processing and developmental assessments in 3-month-old infants exposed prenatally to cocaine. *Pediatrics* **95**: 539–545.

Mayes L, Snyder PJ, Langlois E, Hunter N (2007) Visuospatial working memory in school-aged children exposed in utero to cocaine. *Child Neuropsychol* **13**: 205–218.

Mehta SK, Super DM, Connuck D, et al. (2002a) Autonomic alterations in cocaine-exposed infants. *Am Heart J* **114**: 1109–1115.

Mehta SK, Super DM, Connuck D, et al. (2002b) Diastolic alterations in infants exposed to intrauterine cocaine: a follow-up study by color kinesis. *J Am Soc Echocardiogr* **158**: 1361–4366.

150

Mehta SK, Super DM, Salvator A, et al. (2002c) Diastolic filling abnormalities by color kinesis in newborns exposed to intrauterine cocaine. *J Am Soc Echocardiogr* **15**: 447–453.

Mehta SK, Super DM, Salvator A, et al. (2002d) Heart rate variability by triangular index in infants exposed prenatally to cocaine. *Ann Noninvasive Electrocardiol* **7**: 374–378.

Messinger DS, Bauer CR, Das A, et al. (2004) The maternal lifestyle study: cognitive, motor, and behavioral outcomes of cocaine-exposed and opiate-exposed infants through three years of age. *Pediatrics* **113**: 1677–1685.

Min MO, Farkas K, Minnes S, Singer LT (2007) Impact of childhood abuse and neglect on substance use and psychological distress in adulthood. *J Trauma Stress* **20**: 833–844.

Min MO, Singer LT, Kirchner HL, et al. (2009) Cognitive development and low-level lead exposure in poly-drug exposed children. *Neurotoxicol Teratol* **31**: 225–231.

Minnes M, Singer LT, Kirchner HL, et al. (2010) The effects of prenatal cocaine exposure on problem behavior in children 4–10 years. *Neurotoxicol Teratol* **32**: 443–451.

Minnes S, Singer LT, Arendt R, Satayathum S (2005) Effects of prenatal cocaine/polydrug use on maternal–infant feeding interactions during the first year of life. *Dev Behav Pediatr* **26**: 194–200.

Minnes S, Singer LT, Humphrey-Wall R, Satayathum S (2008) Psychosocial and behavioral factors related to the post-partum placements of infants born to cocaine-using women. *Child Abuse Negl* **32**: 353–366.

Morrow CE, Bandstra ES, Anthony JC, et al. (2003) Influence of prenatal cocaine exposure on early language development: longitudinal findings from four months to three years of age. *J Dev Behav Pediatr* **24**: 39–50.

Morrow CE, Culbertson JL, Accornero VH, et al. (2006) Learning disabilities and intellectual functioning in school-aged children with prenatal cocaine exposure. *Dev Neuropsychol* **30**: 905–931.

Nasiraei-Moghadam S, Sahraei H, Bahadoran H, et al. (2005) Effects of maternal oral morphine consumption on neural tube development in Wistar rats. *Brain Res Dev Brain Res* **159**: 12–17.

National Consensus Development Panel on Effective Medical Treatment of Opiate Addiction (1998) Effective medical treatment of opiate addiction. *JAMA* **280**: 1936–1943.

National Institute on Drug Abuse (2005) *Heroin abuse and addiction. Research Report. US Department of Health and Human Services.* Bethesda, MD: National Institutes of Health.

Nelson S, Lerner E, Needlman R, et al. (2004) Cocaine, anemia, and neurodevelopmental outcomes in children: a longitudinal study. *J Dev Behav Pediatr* **25**: 1–9.

Noland JS, Singer LT, Short EJ, et al. (2005) Prenatal drug exposure and selective attention in preschoolers. *Neurotoxicol Teratol* **27**: 429–438.

Ornoy A, Segal J, Bar-Hamburger R, Greenbaum C (2001) Developmental outcome of school-age children born to mothers with heroin dependency: importance of environmental factors. *Dev Med Child Neurol* **43**: 668–675.

Ostrea EM, Ostrea AR, Simpson PM (1997) Mortality within the first 2 years in infants exposed to cocaine, opiate, or cannabinoid during gestation. *Pediatrics* **100**: 79–83.

Rettig RA, Yarmolinsky A, eds (1995) *Federal Regulation of Methadone Treatment.* Washington, DC: National Academy Press.

Richardson GA, Hamel SC, Goldschmidt L, Day NL (1996) The effects of prenatal cocaine use on neonatal neurobehavioral status. *Neurotoxicol Teratol* **18**: 519–528.

Richardson GA, Ryan C, Willford J, et al. (2002) Prenatal alcohol and marijuana exposure: effects on neuro-psychological outcomes at 10 years. *Neurotoxicol Teratol* **24**: 309–320.

Richardson GA, Goldschmidt L, Willford J (2008) The effects of prenatal cocaine use on infant development. *Neurotoxicol Teratol* **30**: 96–106.

Rose-Jacobs R, Waber D, Beeghly M, et al. (2009) Intrauterine cocaine exposure and executive functioning in middle childhood. *Neurotoxicol Teratol* **31**: 159–168.

Rosen TS, Johnson HL (1982) Children of methadone-maintained mothers: follow-up to 18 months of age. *J Pediatr* **101**: 192–196.

SAMHSA (1999) *National Household Survey on Drug Abuse Population Estimates, 1998.* Rockville, MD: US Department of Health and Human Services, Substance Abuse Mental Health Services Administration.

Sanaullah F, Gillian M, Lavin T (2006) Screening of substance misuse during early pregnancy in Blyth: an anonymous unlinked study. *J Obstet Gynaecol* **26**: 187–190.

Schindler SD, Eder H, Ortner R, et al. (2003) Neonatal outcome following buprenorphine maintenance during conception and throughout pregnancy. *Addiction* **98**: 103–110.

Schneider JW, Hans SL (1996) Effects of prenatal exposure to opioids on focused attention in toddlers during free play. *J Dev Behav Pediatr* **17**: 240–247.

Shankaran S, Das A, Bauer CR, et al. (2006) Fetal origin of childhood disease: intrauterine growth restriction in term infants and risk for hypertension at 6 years of age. *Arch Pediatr Adolesc Med* **160**: 977–981.

Sheinkopf SJ, Lester BM, LaGasse LL, et al. (2006) Interactions between maternal characteristics and neonatal behavior in the prediction of parenting stress and perception of infant temperament. *J Pediatr Psychol* **31**: 27–40.

Singer LT (2001) Randomized clinical trials in infancy: methodologic issues. *Semin Neonatol* **6**: 393–401.

Singer LT, Arendt R, Song LY, et al. (1994a) Direct and indirect interactions of cocaine with childbirth outcomes. *Arch Pediatr Adolesc Med* **148**: 959–964.

Singer L, Yamashita TS, Hawkins S, et al. (1994b) Increased incidence of intraventricular hemorrhage and developmental delay in cocaine-exposed, very low birth weight infants. *J Pediatr* **124**: 765–771.

Singer LT, Arendt RA, Fagan J, et al. (1999) Neonatal visual information processing in cocaine-exposed and non-exposed infants. *Infant Behav Dev* **22**: 1–15.

Singer LT, Arendt R, Minnes S, et al. (2000) Neurobehavioral outcomes of cocaine-exposed infants. *Neurotoxicol Teratol* **22**: 653–666.

Singer LT, Arendt RA, Minnes S, et al. (2001) Developing language skills of cocaine-exposed infants. *Pediatrics* **107**: 1057–1064.

Singer LT, Arendt R, Minnes S, et al. (2002a) Cognitive and motor outcomes of cocaine-exposed infants. *JAMA* **287**: 1952–1960.

Singer LT, Salvator A, Arendt R, et al. (2002b) Effects of cocaine/polydrug exposure and maternal psychological distress on infant birth outcomes. *Neurotoxicol Teratol* **24**: 127–135.

Singer LT, Minnes S, Short E, et al. (2004) Cognitive outcomes of preschool children with prenatal cocaine exposure. *JAMA* **291**: 2448–2456.

Singer LT, Eisengart LJ, Minnes S, et al. (2005) Prenatal cocaine exposure and infant cognition. *Infant Behav Dev* **28**: 431–444.

Singer LT, Nelson S, Short E, et al. (2008) Prenatal cocaine exposure: drug and environmental effects at 9 years. *J Pediatr* **153**: 105–111.

Slamberová R, Pometlová M, Charusová P (2006) Postnatal development of rat pups is altered by prenatal methamphetamine exposure. *Prog Neuropsychopharmacol Biol Psychiatry* **30**: 82–88.

Stanwood GD, Washington RS, Shumsky JS, Levitt P (2001) Prenatal cocaine exposure produces consistent developmental alterations in dopamine-rich regions of the cerebral cortex. *Neuroscience* **106**: 5–14.

Suess PE, Newlin DB, Porges SW (1997) Motivation, sustained attention, and autonomic regulation in school-age boys exposed in utero to opiates and alcohol. *Exp Clin Psychopharmacol* **5**: 375–387.

Trksak GS, Glatt SJ, Mortazavi F, Jackson D (2007) A meta-analysis of animal studies on disruption of spatial navigation by prenatal cocaine exposure. *Neurotoxicol Teratol* **29**: 570–577.

Vathy I (2002) Prenatal opiate exposure: long-term CNS consequences in the stress system of the offspring. *Psychoneuroendocrinology* **27**: 1–2.

Vavrinková B, Binder T (2007a) [The effect of substitution therapy on the birth weight of the newborn, its postpartum adaptation, trophic and course of the neonatal abstinence syndrome.] *Ceska Gynekol* **72**: 247–253 (Czech).

Vavrinková B, Binder T (2007b) [Socioeconomic data, the course of pregnancy and delivery in opioid-addicted women and women under substitution therapy.] *Ceska Gynekol* **72**: 330–335 (Czech).

Villarreal DM, Derrick B, Vathy I (2008) Prenatal morphine exposure attenuates the maintenance of late LTP in lateral perforant path projections to the dentate gyrus and the CA3 region in vivo. *J Neurophysiol* **99**: 1235–1242.

Volpe J (1992) Effect of cocaine use on the fetus. *N Engl J Med* **327**: 399–407.

Walhovd KB, Moe V, Slinning K, et al. (2007) Volumetric cerebral characteristics of children exposed to opiates and other substances in utero. *Neuroimage* **36**: 1331–1344.

Warner TD, Behnke M, Eyler FD, et al. (2006) Diffusion tensor imaging of frontal white matter and executive functioning in cocaine-exposed children. *Pediatrics* **118**: 2014–2024.

Wechsler D (1989) *Weschler Adult Intelligence Scale—Revised.* San Antonio: Psychological Corporation.

Williams PE, Weiss LG, et al. (2003). *WISC-IV. Technical Report 1: Theoretical Model and Test Blueprint.* San Antonio: Psychological Corporation.

Wilson GS, McCreary R, Kean J, Baxter JC (1979) The development of preschool children of heroin-addicted mothers: a controlled study. *Pediatrics* **63**: 135.

Zuckerman B, Frank DA, Mayes L (2002) Cocaine-exposed infants and developmental outcomes: "crack kids" revisited. *JAMA* **287**: 1990–1991.

9
CANNABIS USE DURING PREGNANCY: ITS EFFECTS ON OFFSPRING FROM BIRTH TO YOUNG ADULTHOOD

Peter A Fried

In spite of a surge in interest in cannabis (marijuana/hashish) in both the public media and the scientific community there is a relative dearth of information dealing with how cannabis use during pregnancy may impact upon the cognitive development of the offspring. That this is much more than an academic exercise is evidenced by the fact that women have been, and are presently, the subject of legal actions both within the criminal justice system and in the civil child welfare system based on their use of this drug during pregnancy.

Rate of use

Cannabis is the most commonly used illicit drug among women of childbearing age. In recent years a relatively consistent 15% of women between the ages of 18 and 25 report using cannabis in the past month (SAMHSA 2006).

The most recent US government figure for cannabis smoking during pregnancy (SAMHSA 2005) was 3.6% use during the past month. These pregnancy usage figures reported by surveys may well be conservative in their estimates. In a number of longitudinal, prospective cohort studies investigating cannabis use and pregnancy, rates ranging from 10% to 16% in predominantly middle-class samples (Fried et al. 1980, Greenland et al. 1982, Gibson et al. 1983, Bailey et al. 2008) to 23–30% in inner-city populations (Tennes et al. 1985, Richardson et al. 1989, Day et al. 1994a) have been reported.

Longitudinal studies

The potential consequences of cannabis use during pregnancy can be examined from a number of perspectives, including the drug's effect upon the course of pregnancy and, postnatally, the morphology, growth and cognitive behaviour from the newborn period onward. Almost all of the available data to be described in this chapter, particularly in offspring older than 3 years (some of which I have reviewed elsewhere: Fried 2002, 2004), arise from two longitudinal studies with very different sample characteristics. (For a comparison and summary of outcome in these studies, see Table 9.1.)

Since 1978, the Ottawa Prenatal Prospective Study (OPPS) has been investigating the effects of cannabis and tobacco inhaled during pregnancy. The sample consisted of low-

TABLE 9.1
The impact of prenatal cannabis use as assessed in the Ottawa Prenatal Prospective Study (OPPS)
and the Maternal Health Practices and Child Development Study (MHPCD)*

Variable	Age	OPPS	MHPCD
Sample characteristics		Low-risk, white, predominantly middle class (Fried 1982)	High-risk, approximately 50% African-American, low socio-economic status (Goldschmidt et al. 2000)
Morphological abnormalities	Birth	None (Fried et al. 1983)	None (Day et al. 1991)
Fetal growth	Birth	No relationship (Fried et al. 1999)	Birth length reduced (Day et al. 1991)
Postnatal growth	1–6 years	No relationship (Fried et al. 1999)	No relationship (Day et al. 1994a)
Neonatal behaviour	1 month	Some CNS effects (Fried et al. 1987)	No relationship (Richardson et al. 1995)
Infant cognitive development	9–12 months	No relationship (Fried and Watkinson 1988)	Lower mental scores on Bayley Scales (Richardson et al. 1995)
Toddler cognitive tests	18–24 months	No relationship (Fried and Watkinson 1988)	No relationship (Richardson et al. 1995)
Short-term memory	3–4 years	Negative relationship (Fried and Watkinson 1990)	Negative relationship (Day et al. 1994b)
Verbal outcomes	3–4 years	Negative relationship (Fried and Watkinson 1990)	Negative relationship (Day et al. 1994b)
Overall IQ	3–4 years	No relationship (Fried and Watkinson 1990)	No relationship (Day et al. 1994b)
Aspects of attention	6 years	Negative relationship (Fried et al. 1992)	Negative relationship (Day et al. 1991)
Rating by mothers	6–12 years	Increased inattention and impulsivity (Fried et al. 1992)	Increased inattention and impulsivity (Day et al. 1991)
Abstract visual skills	9–12 years	Negative relationship (Fried and Watkinson 2001)	Negative relationship (Richardson et al. 2002)

*Only those outcomes evaluated in both longitudinal studies and carried out when the offspring were approximately the same age are included in this summary table. Further descriptions of the variables and outcomes are given in text.

risk, white, predominantly middle-class families, and was representative of the English-speaking Ottawa population (Fried 1982). Upon volunteering, each participant was interviewed once during each of the trimesters remaining in her pregnancy. Birth data were collected from 682 women in the Ottawa area (Fried 1982). For pragmatic reasons, approximately 180 offspring were chosen to be followed from the neonatal period to young adulthood. Details describing the assessment procedures at various ages are presented throughout this chapter.

The second longitudinal study that has reported on a number of outcomes of prenatal exposure to cannabis in children ranging in ages from infancy to early adolescence is the Maternal Health Practices and Child Development Study (MHPCD) based in Pittsburgh

(Goldschmidt et al. 2000). This study was initiated in 1982 and has focused upon the consequences of prenatal use of cannabis, alcohol and cocaine. In contrast to the OPPS sample, the participants in this cohort are considered to be of high-risk, low socio-economic status, with just over half being African-American.

In the discussion of the OPPS and MHPCD findings, as well as other studies, unless otherwise stated, the results described have been reported in the original articles as being statistically significant after controlling for potential confounding, mediating or moderating variables.

COURSE OF PREGNANCY

Cross-placental transfer of delta-9-tetrahydrocannabinol, the main psychoactive component of cannabis, is approximately one-third of maternal plasma levels (Behnke and Eyler 1993). In the OPPS sample (Fried et al. 1984), statistically significant reduction of approximately one week in the gestational age of infants born to mothers who used cannabis six or more times per week was noted. In a California-based sample (Greenland et al. 1982), precipitate labour was significantly more frequent among women who reported using cannabis, an observation that is consistent with folk medicine (Abel 1980) and may be related to the shortened gestation noted in the OPPS sample. In and of itself, the approximate one-week reduction in gestation length observed is of questionable clinical significance. However, as the shortened gestation length was dose related, it may take on clinical significance if large amounts of the drug are consumed, if the delta-9-tetrahydrocannabinol concentration levels are now higher than those of the cannabis used in the early 1980s (Hardwick and King 2008), and/or if lifestyle habits include other risk factors such as alcohol. Some (Gibson et al. 1983, Hatch and Bracken 1986) but not all researchers (Tennes et al. 1985, Day et al. 1991) have reported an association between cannabis use during pregnancy and preterm delivery.

Maternal use of cannabis was not associated with miscarriage rates, types of presentation at birth, Apgar status, or the frequency of neonatal complications or major physical abnormalities in the OPPS sample (Fried 1982, Fried et al. 1983). No patterns of minor physical anomalies were noted among the offspring of cannabis users, although two anomalies, true ocular hypertelorism and severe epicanthus, were observed, but only among children of heavy users of cannabis (O'Connell and Fried 1984). The majority of researchers have not reported an association between prenatal cannabis use and morphological abnormalities in offspring (e.g. Day et al. 1991), and, as reviewed elsewhere (O'Connell and Fried 1984, Dalterio and Fried 1992), the few reports of increased physical abnormalities may reflect a lack of control for confounding factors (e.g. prenatal exposure to alcohol) and/or the relative risk status of the women in the study.

That lifestyle and concomitant risk status appears to be an important interactive component in determining prenatal cannabis outcomes is evident from both the human and animal literature. For example, in the low-risk sample of the OPPS, no evidence of increased meconium staining was noted among the newborn infants of the heavy cannabis users (Fried et al. 1983). This observation contrasts with the first but not the second of two reports by Greenland and associates (1982, 1983). A primary difference between these two reports was the generally higher standard of living and health among the sample in the later (Greenland et al. 1983) report, with these families being quite similar, demographically, to the OPPS sample. A study, utilizing animal models, that manipulated non-cannabis factors (Charlebois and Fried 1980) provides support for the critical role that lifestyle factors may have in interacting with the teratogenic effects of the drug. Briefly, different groups of pregnant rats were exposed to cannabis smoke while receiving diets varying in protein content. The combination of cannabis smoke with a low-protein diet markedly potentiated compromised pregnancies, but, conversely, cannabis smoke coupled with a high-protein diet attenuated some risks associated with the cannabis exposure.

GROWTH

The role of lifestyle, interacting with the prenatal effect of cannabis, is also to be observed in investigations examining fetal growth (Fried et al. 1999). Most studies have not found cannabis to have a negative impact upon fetal growth. However, in some samples drawn from high-risk environments, a small but significant negative relationship between first trimester cannabis use and birth length (Tennes et al. 1985, Day et al. 1991) or birthweight and length (Zuckerman et al. 1989) has been reported. In the limited number of studies that have examined offspring beyond the newborn stage, cannabis exposure was not significantly related to weight and height at 8 months (Day et al. 1992), 1 year (Tennes et al. 1985, Fried et al. 1999), 4 years (Fried et al. 1999), 6 years (Day et al. 1994, Fried et al. 1999) or adolescence (Fried et al. 2001). One growth parameter in the OPPS sample, a smaller head circumference, observed as a trend at all ages (birth, 1, 2, 3, 4 and 6 years) reached statistical significance among early adolescents (Fried et al. 1999) born to daily cannabis users but was not significant during mid-adolescence (Fried et al. 2001). In the OPPS sample, maternal cannabis use was not associated with the timing of pubertal milestones in either adolescent males or females (Fried et al. 2001).

NEONATAL AND INFANT BEHAVIOUR

In the OPPS sample, using the Brazelton Neonatal Assessment Scale (Brazelton 1973), cannabis use was associated, at less than 1 week of age, with increased fine tremors typically accompanied by exaggerated and prolonged startles, both spontaneous and in response to mild stimuli (Fried et al. 1980, Fried 1982, Fried and Makin 1987). In the same sample, maternal cannabis use was associated with relatively similar observations in 9- and 30-day-old infants (Fried et al. 1987). At 9 days, hand-to-mouth behaviour was also associated with cannabis use during pregnancy. Many of the behaviours seen both in the newborn infant and at 9 and 30 days are consistent with, but milder in degree than, those found among infants undergoing opioid withdrawal.

Although these particular indicants of impairments in the regulation of the nervous system were not detected by some researchers (Tennes et al. 1985, Richardson et al. 1995), altered autonomic arousal has been reported in other outcome measures. Newborn infants of maternal cannabis users have been identified as having an increased likelihood of exhibiting a high-pitched cry (Lester and Dreher 1989) and to spend less time in quiet sleep (Scher et al. 1988).

A widely used indicant of nervous system integrity in infants is habituation to stimuli. This measure has been shown in a number of studies to be affected by prenatal exposure to cannabis. In the OPPS sample, 4-day-old infants born to cannabis users had poorer habituation to visual, but not auditory, stimuli (Fried 1982, Fried and Makin 1987). This finding is consistent with a primate study in which the behaviour distinguishing offspring of mothers who were administered cannabis from controls was a failure to habituate to novel visual stimuli (Golub et al. 1981).

The vulnerability of facets of visual functioning in the neonate is a finding that recurs in the longer-term assessment of the offspring in both the OPPS and MHCPD cohorts, as well as in a polydrug study (Griffith et al. 1994), and will be elaborated in later parts of this chapter.

NEUROCOGNITIVE OUTCOMES IN LATE INFANCY AND PRESCHOOL CHILDREN

The literature describing the teratogenic effects of prenatal cannabis exposure on offspring beyond infancy is intriguingly consistent among different cohorts. Most researchers (including the OPPS), all using the Bayley Scales of Infant Development (Bayley 1969), have reported no effect of cannabis use during pregnancy on infant cognitive or motor development (Tennes et al. 1985, Fried and Watkinson 1988, Astley and Little 1990). In contrast, in the high-risk MHPCD cohort, the use of one or more 'joints' (cannabis cigarettes) per day during the third trimester was associated with lower mental scores on the Bayley Scales at 9 months of age but no longer at 18 months (Richardson et al. 1995). The findings at 9 months may reflect, once again, the possible role of other non-cannabis risk factors potentiating the impact of prenatal cannabis exposure.

In children involved in the OPPS, this lack of effect of prenatal cannabis exposure persisted until 3 years of age (Fried and Watkinson 1988, 1990). However, at 4 years (Fried and Watkinson 1990), an association with prenatal cannabis exposure that remained significant, after controlling for confounding factors, was observed with the children born to women who had smoked an average of five or more joints per week, scoring significantly lower than the remainder of the sample on a number of memory and verbal outcome measures using the McCarthy Scales of Children's Abilities (McCarthy 1972). These observations are strikingly similar to those reported by Day et al. (1994b) in their high-risk sample in which the 3-year-old offspring of daily cannabis users were impaired on the short-term memory, verbal and abstract/visual reasoning subscales of the Stanford–Binet Intelligence Test (Thorndike et al. 1986). Griffith et al. (1994), investigating the interaction between the prenatal use of cocaine and a number of drugs including cannabis, also noted, in 3-year-old offspring, that maternal cannabis use (the amount was not specified) was predictive of poorer performance on abstract/visual reasoning.

In these three studies with preschool children, maternal use during pregnancy was not associated with an overall lowered IQ. As will be emphasized below, this has major interpretative and theoretical implications in evaluating the findings in older children who had been prenatally exposed to cannabis. Reports focusing on the cognitive effects of prenatal cannabis exposure in offspring older than 3 years are limited to observations derived from the very different OPPS and MHCPD cohorts.

157

Executive function

A domain of functioning that may be negatively impacted in school-age offspring by in utero exposure to cannabis is the behavioural/cognitive construct of executive function (e.g. Fried 1998, 2002; Fried and Smith 2001). Executive function is a term that connotes overarching, 'top-down' mental control processes (Denckla 1993) manifested in future-oriented behaviours that include cognitive flexibility in problem solving, focused attention, inhibiting prepotent responses, and monitoring, evaluating and adjusting self-directed responses and working memory (the temporary storage of information while processing incoming data). Executive function can thus be thought of as a shorthand describing a multiple, nonunitary set of behavioural/cognitive abilities critical in effortful, nonroutine, goal-oriented situations (Fried 1998).

Clinical and empirical evidence has revealed that executive function is primarily subserved by various subregions of the prefrontal area of the brain with its many reciprocal connections to other cortical and subcortical (e.g. hippocampus, cerebellum) regions. These anatomical pathways subserve the integrative nature of executive function and its involvement with subordinate cognitive processes (e.g. Denckla 1993, Lezak 1995). Critical to the findings discussed in this chapter, the morphological development of the prefrontal lobes continues well after birth, full maturation being achieved in late adolescence with different regions within the prefrontal area functionally maturing at different times. It is quite feasible that certain facets or factors of executive function may be vulnerable to prenatal cannabis exposure, whereas other aspects of executive function may not show any impact of the drug.

A further characteristic of executive function that has high relevance for the present chapter is that this construct is not associated with typical measures of overall intelligence. This observation is based both on clinical reports in which injury to the frontal lobes has occurred and on studies that examine the normative developmental course of executive function in children (Welsh et al. 1991, Denckla 1993, Lezak 1995). As elaborated elsewhere (Fried 1998, 2002), executive function distinguishes between the types of intelligence required to carry out adaptive, goal-directed behaviour and the sort of intelligence captured by global performance on standardized psychometric intelligence tests. Because of the structure of these latter evaluations, the assessment of such key components of executive function as integration of domains, goal setting, planning and self-monitoring is problematic. Global IQ tests evaluate established cognitive sets and well-learned information ('crystallized intelligence') – those that may not tap into executive function. However, this does not preclude the fact that general IQ and executive function share some variance, particularly when the subtests involve the ability to reason logically and abstractly ('fluid intelligence') in problem-solving tasks that are timed and/or do not involve familiar, well-learned information.

The finding, described in earlier sections of this chapter, that maternal cannabis use appeared to have no effect in offspring beyond the neonatal period until the age of 3 years (Fried and Watkinson 1988, Day et al. 1994b, Griffith et al. 1994) or 4 years (Fried and Watkinson 1990) is consistent with the prolonged developmental course of the prefrontal lobes and, concomitantly, executive function. Furthermore, the behavioural/cognitive functioning in these studies of preschoolers exposed prenatally to cannabis – the combination of an absence of an impact upon global IQ but a negative association with subtests that assess memory and abstract/visual reasoning – is congruent with the interpretation that in utero cannabis exposure impacts negatively on particular facets of executive function.

Adding to the hypothesis of a link between prenatal cannabis exposure and executive function in offspring are studies examining the distribution and concentration of cannabinoid receptors in fetal, neonatal and adult human brain. Binding sites are widely distributed throughout the brain, with the highest density being in the middle gyrus of the frontal lobe, the hippocampus, cingulate gyrus and cerebellum. Glass et al. (1997) concluded that one of the major cannabinoid receptor sites in the human brain is in that portion of the forebrain associated with higher cognitive functions.

NEUROCOGNITIVE OUTCOMES IN YOUNG SCHOOL-AGED CHILDREN
Employing global tests of cognition and language, maternal use of cannabis was not found to be associated with lowered IQ in 5- and 6-year-old offspring (Fried et al. 1992a). As mentioned in the section above concerning executive function and intelligence, it is possible that the instruments used in this work evaluated broad and general cognitive abilities and may have been inappropriate for the identification of nuances associated with prenatal cannabis exposure. Studies were undertaken in order to investigate this possibility.

In the OPPS sample, participants between the ages of 9 and 12 were examined, taking two different approaches. In the first (Fried and Watkinson 2001), a battery was used that included a combination of tests evaluating various aspects of executive function as well as global intelligence. The second study was a direct investigation of the putative role that prenatal cannabis exposure may have on 'top-down' visuoperceptual function (Fried and Watkinson 2000).

Consistent with the results found in the OPPS participants at younger ages, prenatal cannabis exposure was not associated in the 9- to 12-year-olds with a lowered Full Scale IQ as assessed by the Wechsler Intelligence Scale for Children–III (WISC-III) with its 13 subtests (Wechsler 1991). Indeed, among the subtests only two, Block Design and Picture Completion, significantly differentiated children who were exposed to different levels of cannabis prenatally, suggesting that in utero exposure to cannabis affects particular rather than global aspects of intelligence. From an interpretative cause-and-effect perspective it may be noteworthy to recall that, as described in the Neonatal and Infant Behaviour section of this chapter, when the children in the OPPS sample were less than 1 week old, prenatal cannabis exposure was associated with visual cognitive functioning as manifested by poorer visual habituation (Fried 1982, Fried and Makin 1987).

The Block Design subtest requires children to assemble blocks to form a design identical to one presented in a picture. This nonverbal, concept formation task places demands on perceptual organization, spatial visualization and abstract conceptualization. The Picture Completion subtest requires the child to identify a missing aspect of an incompletely drawn picture. This task requires the participant to differentiate essential from non-essential visual details.

A detailed statistical analysis (Fried and Watkinson 2000) revealed that the impact of prenatal cannabis exposure persisted after controlling for basic spatial and motor abilities, supporting the interpretation that prenatal cannabis exposure has its impact on these visual subtests in a 'top-down' rather than a 'bottom-up' fashion. The basic abilities are not impaired; rather the utilization of these abilities in an integrated, higher-order cognitive manner is impaired in these offspring. Also consistent with this purported linkage to executive function is the clinical literature, describing patients with damage to the prefrontal area. Individuals with such an injury are not impaired on basic visuo-perceptual tasks but are markedly impacted on tasks that require visuo-perceptual planning and integration (Luria 1973, Stuss 1992).

These negative relationships between the two subtests and maternal cannabis use are strikingly consistent with the other cohort undertakings, focusing upon prenatal cannabis exposure (Day et al. 1994b, Griffith et al. 1994). In these other studies, when the offspring were assessed at 3 years of age, a statistically significant impact of the drug was noted in the sphere of abstract/visual reasoning skills as assessed using form boards and block designs. This consistency among different cohorts continued to be observed at 10 years of age. In the MHCPD study (Richardson et al. 2002), using block design, a progressive matrices task and a copying of geometric shapes task, in utero cannabis exposure continued to be negatively associated with abstract/visual reasoning.

As mentioned earlier, the 9- to 12-year-olds in the OPPS cohort, as well as being assessed via the WISC-III, were also tested using six non-WISC outcomes that examined aspects of executive function (Fried et al. 1998). The results were consistent with and extend the observations for the cannabis groups gleaned from the WISC tasks. Of the two non-WISC tests that maximally discriminated among the cannabis groups, one required the application of visual deduction to a problem-solving task while the other was an assessment of impulsivity. Thus, of the six tests thought to assess aspects of executive function, the two that were found to be associated with cannabis involve impulse control, visual analysis and hypothesis testing. This is consistent with the WISC-III results, as the two subtests in that battery associated with prenatal cannabis use – Block Design and Picture Completion – require visual analysis and hypothesis testing.

The dual vulnerability of visual analysis and impulsivity, but not other facets of executive function, to in utero cannabis exposure supports the conceptualization, as discussed earlier in this chapter, of executive function as a non-unitary process. Developmental research utilizing a factor analytic approach to examine executive function in children at different ages (Welsh et al. 1991) provides an important additional avenue of support for the cannabis findings from two perspectives. Welsh et al. (1991), using an extensive battery of tests with a sample of normal children, identified three independent factors in the developmental course of executive function reflecting planning, verbal fluency and hypothesis testing, while controlling prepotent responding. This last was derived from a convergence of cognitive processes based on visual hypothesis testing and impulse control. These components contributing to this factor, labelled 'Hypothesis Testing and Impulse Control', are strikingly similar to those neurobehavioural outcomes negatively associated with prenatal cannabis exposure in the 9- to 12-year-old OPPS participants (Fried et al. 1998). In terms of the developmental time course of the Hypothesis Testing and Impulse Control factor, competence is normally achieved at around 10 years of age (Welsh et al. 1991). This is consistent with the observation that the negative effect of cannabis in this dimension of executive function manifested itself in the 9- to 12-year-olds.

A possible mechanism for the impact of prenatal cannabis exposure upon higher-order visual functioning may be found in a study using animal models in which pregnant rats were administered a cannabis receptor agonist and the offspring were examined behaviourally, electrophysiologically and neurochemically (Mereu et al. 2003). At electrophysiological and neurochemical levels, prenatal exposure was linked to alterations in hippocampal long-term potentiation and glutamate release in juvenile and young adult offspring. The hippocampus is known to play a vital role in visuospatial cognitive mapping (O'Keefe and Nadel 1978) and, as mentioned earlier, along with the frontal and cerebellar region, has the highest density of cannabinoid receptors in the brain (Glass et al. 1997, Biegon and Kerman 2001).

Attention control
An additional body of findings suggesting an association between cannabis use during pregnancy and facets of executive function comes from research investigating various as-pects of attention. This domain of functioning is considered to be a complex, multidimensional behaviour (Barkley 1996) encompassing processes that overlap with many aspects of executive function (Barkley 1997), including the ability to withhold prepotent but inappropriate response tendencies, the ability to screen out distracting or irrelevant stimuli while con-centrating on the task at hand, and the faculty of both flexibility and sustainability of focus when appropriate.

The OPPS and MHCPD cohorts have been assessed at various ages to investigate this complex behaviour, with negative effects noted in both cohorts. In both samples, inattention and impulsivity were assessed using the Continuous Performance Task (CPT). Essentially, the CPT involves a serial presentation of stimuli over a designated period of time. The participant's task is to press a response button or computer key when a particular stimulus (or sequence of stimuli) is presented and to withhold response when non-target stimuli occur. Dependent variables that can be measured in this sort of assessment include correct identification (hits), errors of omission (misses) and errors of commission (false alarms) (Greenberg and Kindschi 1996).

In both the OPPS (Fried et al. 1992b) and MHCPD (Leech et al. 1999) samples, children at age 6 were assessed using the CPT. In the OPPS offspring, prenatal cannabis exposure was significantly predictive, in a dose–response fashion, of decreased attentiveness as mani-fested by increased omission errors and a decreased number of hits. Furthermore, as the CPT progressed, children born to regular users (more than five joints per week) increased their omission errors, suggestive of a particular vulnerability of sustained attention. Among the 6-year-olds in the MHCPD cohort, prenatal cannabis exposure was found to impact upon attentional processes in terms of an increase in errors of commission, possibly reflecting impulsivity. The authors speculated that in utero exposure to cannabis may slow processing speed and that this deficit would manifest itself to a greater degree over a longer task, particularly if there were time pressure demands upon the child. Further, the MHCPD investigators, consistent with the earlier interpretation by the OPPS researchers, argued that

161

prenatal cannabis exposure impacts upon attention and impulsivity and thereby decreases the ability to plan and execute tasks (Leech et al. 1999), critical aspects of executive function.

In the OPPS work (Fried et al. 1992b), in addition to the CPT assessment, the mothers were asked to rate their offspring using a behavioural checklist (Conners 1989). Paralleling and extending the observations on the laboratory CPT task, the children exposed prenatally to cannabis were rated as more impulsive and hyperactive. A very similar observation was reported in the MHPCD sample when the children, at 10 years of age, were rated by their mothers (Day et al. 1991). Increased reports of hyperactivity, inattention and impulsivity were associated with cannabis use during the first and third trimester.

In this MHPCD study (Day et al. 1991), an additional finding was that, based on both maternal ratings and teacher reports, in utero cannabis exposure was related to increased levels of delinquency and externalizing behaviour. Using a path analysis statistical procedure, it appeared that poor attentional skills mediated these observations. The association between prenatal cannabis exposure and negative behavioural outcomes in the offspring is similar to the finding of an earlier preliminary report in the OPPS sample when the cohort was between 9 and 12 years of age (O'Connell and Fried 1991). At this age, mothers who had used cannabis regularly during pregnancy rated their children as having a higher rate of conduct disorders. However, this difference did not retain significance after extraneous variables were controlled. Possibly the trend in the low-risk OPPS sample versus the statistical difference in the high-risk MHPCD sample may reflect, once again, the importance of non-cannabis lifestyle and concomitant risk factors (many of which cannot be controlled statistically) that may potentiate the impact of prenatal cannabis exposure.

NEUROCOGNITIVE OUTCOMES IN ADOLESCENTS AND YOUNG ADULTS
Facets of attention have also been studied in older children participating in the OPPS (Fried and Watkinson 2001). At the ages of 13–16 years an assessment battery was used that permitted the investigation of a number of components of attention, similar to those described in a multifactorial model of attention developed by Mirsky (1996). Among adolescents heavily exposed to cannabis in utero, CPT reaction times became less consistent as the test proceeded, coupled with increased CPT omissions. This stability factor is interpreted as relating to the reliability or consistency of attention effort over time (Conners 1989, Halperin 1996, Mirsky 1996). Response variability, particularly in combination with the more ubiquitously reported outcome variables such as omission errors (false alarms), is viewed as a critically sensitive indicant of performance on sustained attention tasks (Barkley 1996, Sergeant 1996).

The negative association of prenatal cannabis exposure and increased errors of omission noted in these OPPS adolescents (Fried and Watkinson 2001) is similar to the findings when the children were assessed at 6 years using a CPT (Fried et al. 1992b). The wide range of ages over which this impact has been found in this domain is consistent with the developmental course of sustained attention, which, unlike some other elements of attention, continues to develop throughout childhood and adolescence (McKay et al. 1994).

Two recent studies, utilizing the OPPS participants between the ages of 18 and 22 years, examined aspects of attention employing functional magnetic resonance imaging (fMRI) (Smith et al. 2004, 2006). Briefly, fMRI relies on the changes in blood oxygenation that occur with changes in neuronal activity. As neuronal activity increases, so too does the oxygenation of the blood. With the increase in oxygenated blood, there is an increase in magnetic signal, quantifiable with fMRI. This noninvasive technique can map neural activity during many cognitive processes (Ogawa et al. 1993), including executive functioning.

The neurophysiological effects of prenatal cannabis exposure on response inhibition/ impulsivity – a facet of executive function and attention – were assessed in young adults in the OPPS using a Go/No-Go task while neural activity was monitored with fMRI (Smith et al. 2004). In this paradigm, the participant was required to press a button to a particular stimulus (Go) and to withhold responding to a different stimulus (No-Go). The frequency of presentation of the Go and No-Go stimuli varied across the course of the task, resulting in the manipulation of the participant's expectancy of the target stimulus.

At a behavioural level, consistent with the findings at earlier ages that prenatal exposure to cannabis impacts aspects of attention (Fried et al. 1992b, Leech et al. 1999, Fried and Watkinson 2001), exposed young adults had significantly more commission errors (impulsivity) than non-exposed participants, but all the participants were able to perform the task with more than 85% accuracy. The major finding from the fMRI portion of the study was that prenatal exposure to cannabis significantly increased bilateral neural activity in the prefrontal cortex – the region widely accepted as critical for mediating inhibitory functions (reviewed by Smith et al. 2004). The increased activity was interpreted as representing an increased effort in the performance of the task.

The other region of the brain that was found, in this OPPS fMRI study, to show a significant positive relationship between the level of prenatal cannabis exposure and neural activity was the right premotor cortex – an area involved in response inhibition and the preparatory process leading to correct initiation or suppression of movement. Together, the neurophysiological and behavioural findings suggest that prenatal cannabis exposure is related to changes in neural activity during response inhibition tasks (a facet of executive function) that last, at least, into young adulthood.

A second investigation with the OPPS young adults using fMRI procedures looked at the effect of prenatal cannabis exposure on visuospatial working memory (Smith et al. 2006). Visuospatial working memory encompasses several aspects of executive functioning, including the capacity to mentally hold visual information while utilizing or manipulating it. This ability, recognized as a facet of attention (Mirskey 1996), has been shown to be adversely affected at a behavioural level, at younger ages, by prenatal cannabis exposure (Day et al. 1994b; Griffith et al. 1994; Fried and Watkinson 2000, 2001). Previous neuroimaging studies have shown that the prefrontal cortex (critical in executive function) is involved in visuospatial working memory, along with the posterior parietal cortex, visual cortex and cerebellum (reviewed in Smith et al. 2006). The role of the hippocampus has also been implicated in the utilization of spatial information and memory (O'Keefe and Nadel 1978). The identification of these neurological sites, functioning in visuospatial working memory, is of particular interest in cannabis research as the cerebellum and the hippocampus, in addition to the frontal lobe, contain the highest density of cannabinoid receptors in the adult brain (Glass et al. 1997).

The visuospatial task used in the study with the young OPPS adults (Smith et al. 2006) involved presenting a particular letter in one of nine different positions on a screen. Participants were required to press a button every time the letter was projected in the same position that it was two presentations before. Several aspects of executive function were required in this 2-back task, including manipulation, maintenance and active processing of stored information, spatial attention and selection of a response based on active processing.

Prenatal cannabis exposure had a significant robust impact on the neural activity in a number of areas in the prefrontal cortex, the parahippocampal gyrus and the cerebellum. These sites, with the highest density of cannabinoid receptors, play a critical role in the carrying out of a visuospatial working memory task. The roles of the prefrontal area of the brain in executive function and the hippocampus in spatial localization and memory have been described earlier in this chapter. The impact on the cerebellar region may be linked to the observation, noted in previous imaging studies (Belger et al. 1998), that when a cognitive task requires increased concentration because of difficulty, there is an increase in activity in this region.

Overall conclusions and summary

Although predicated upon a limited body of literature, the consequences of prenatal cannabis exposure are subtle but suggest a relatively consistent, albeit nascent, theoretical picture. However, examining the findings and applying them in practice requires the critical recognition of the limitations of the observations. The longitudinal research that forms the basis of the bulk of the observations reported in this chapter is quasi-experimental in nature (i.e. many variables were not under the control of the investigators) and, as such, raises issues of interpretation that the reader must recognize. Perhaps the most critical is the inability to manipulate the host of factors ranging from non-cannabis drug use to caregiver variables that potentially influence outcomes of interest.

However, both of the major cohort studies (OPPS and MHPCD) upon which the vast majority of findings are drawn have made considerable efforts to statistically compensate for these limitations. The fact that the two cohorts, although differing enormously in terms of socio-economic, racial and educational backgrounds, have demonstrated such similar consequences of prenatal exposure to cannabis confirms the robustness of the findings and the interpretation of the observations.

Evidence from a number of cohorts suggests mild effects upon fetal growth and central nervous system functioning, with the impact during the course of pregnancy and upon the neonate appearing to be considerably moderated by other risk factors. During the toddler stage, there is little evidence for a prenatal cannabis effect upon either growth or behaviour. However, beyond the age of 3, suggestive findings indicate an association between prenatal cannabis exposure and the aspects of cognitive behaviour associated with executive function. The facets of this construct that show the greatest impact are in the domains of attention/impulsivity and problem-solving situations requiring integration and manipulation of basic visuoperceptual skills. Both behavioural and fMRI data lead to these conclusions. Supporting this proposed association is the developmental literature that, via factor analysis, has identified that these two cognitive processes follow a single maturational course (Welsh et al. 1991, McKay et al. 1994). These domains continue to be the ones that appear vulnerable in the offspring of maternal cannabis users, up to and including adolescence and young adulthood, noted in the long-term longitudinal studies over a 20-year study period.

As described at the outset of this chapter, use of cannabis during pregnancy in the previous month occurred in 3.5% of mothers (SAMHSA 2005). Breaking down this figure by age revealed some important trends. Among pregnant 26- to 44-year-olds the rate of using cannabis in the past month was approximately 2%; among 18- to 25-year-old pregnant women the rate increased to just over 6%, while among the pregnant 15- to 17-year-olds the rate of use in the past month was a striking 12%. The dramatic inverse relationship between the age of the mother-to-be and the likelihood of using cannabis on a regular basis during pregnancy strongly suggests that female adolescents may be the most important target for dissemination of information regarding the possible impact cannabis use may have upon the developing fetus.

Finally, the strength of cannabis has increased over the past decade and it is therefore likely that the findings of the long-term studies described above will be strengthened as the observed effects were clearly dose related (Hardwick and King 2008).

ACKNOWLEDGEMENT

Research utilizing subjects from the OPPS was supported by grants from the National Institute on Drug Abuse.

REFERENCES

Abel EL (1980) *Marijuana: The First Twelve Thousand Years.* New York: Plenum Press.

Astley S, Little R (1990) Maternal marijuana use during lactation and infant development at one year. *Neurotoxicol Teratol* **12**: 161–168.

Bailey JA, Hill KG, Hawkins, JD, et al. (2008) Men's and women's patterns of substance use around pregnancy. *Birth* **35**: 50–59.

Barkley RA (1996) Critical issues in research on attention. In: Lyon GR, Krasnegor NA, eds. *Attention, Memory, and Executive Function.* Baltimore: Brookes, pp. 45–56.

Barkley RA (1997) Behavioral inhibition, sustained attention, and executive functions: constructing a unifying theory of ADHD. *Psychol Bull* **121**: 65–94.

Bayley N (1989) *Bayley Scales of Infant Development.* New York: Psychological Corporation.

Behnke M, Eyler FD (1993) The consequences of prenatal substance use for the developing fetus, newborn and young child. *Int J Addict* **28**: 1341–1391.

Belger A, Puce A, Krystal JH, et al. (1998) Dissociation of mnemonic and perceptual processes during spatial and nonspatial working memory using fMRI. *Hum Brain Mapp* **6**: 14–32.

Biegon A, Kerman IA (2001) Autoradiographic study of pre- and postnatal distribution of cannabinoid receptors in human brain. *NeuroImage* **14**: 1463–1468.

Brazelton TB (1973) *Neonatal Behavioral Assessment Scale. Clinics in Developmental Medicine No. 50.* London: Spastics International Medical Publications.

Charlebois AT, Fried PA (1980) The interactive effects of nutrition and cannabis upon rat perinatal development. *Dev Psychobiol* **13**: 591–605.

Conners CK (1989) *Manual for Conners' Rating Scales.* Toronto: Multi-Health Systems.

Dalterio SL, Fried PA (1992) The effects of marijuana use on offspring. In: Sonderegger TB, ed. *Perinatal Substance Abuse.* Baltimore, MD: Johns Hopkins University Press, pp. 161–183.

Day N, Sambamoorthi U, Taylor P, et al. (1991) Prenatal marijuana use and neonatal outcome. *Neurotoxicol Teratol* **13**: 329–334.

Day N, Cornelius M, Goldschmidt L, et al. (1992) The effects of prenatal tobacco and marijuana use on offspring growth from birth through 3 years of age. *Neurotoxicol Teratol* **14**: 407–414.

Day NL, Richardson GA, Geva D, Robles N (1994a) Alcohol, marijuana, and tobacco: effects of prenatal exposure on offspring growth and morphology at age six. *Alcohol Clin Exp Res* **18**: 786–794.

Day N, Richardson G, Goldschmidt L, et al. (1994b) The effect of prenatal marijuana exposure on the cognitive development of offspring at age three. *Neurotoxicol Teratol* **16**: 169–175.

Denckla MB (1993) Measurement of executive function. In: Lyon GR, ed. *Frames of Reference for the Assessment of Learning Disabilities: New Views on Measurement Issues.* Baltimore, MD: Paul H Brookes, pp. 117–142.

Fried PA (1982) Marihuana use by pregnant women and effects on offspring: an update. *Neurotoxicol Teratol* **4**: 451–454.

Fried PA (1998) Behavioral evaluation of the older infant and child. In: Slikker W, Chang LW, eds. *Handbook of Developmental Neurotoxicology.* San Diego, CA: Academic Press, pp. 469–486.

Fried PA (2002) Conceptual issues in behavioral teratology and their application in determining long-term sequelae of prenatal marihuana exposure. *J Child Psychol Psychiatry* **43**: 81–102.

Fried PA (2004) Pregnancy and effects on offspring from birth through adolescence. In: Grotenhermen F, ed. *Cannabis und Cannabinoide. Pharmakologie, Toxikologie und therapeutisches Potenzial. 2nd edn.* Bern: Verlag Hans Huber, pp. 329–338.

Fried PA, Makin JE (1987) Neonatal behavioural correlates of prenatal exposure to marihuana, cigarettes and alcohol in a low risk population. *Neurotoxicol Teratol* **9**: 1–7.

Fried PA, Smith A (2001) A literature review of the consequences of prenatal marihuana exposure: an emerging theme of a deficiency in aspects of executive function. *Neurotoxicol Teratol* **23**: 1–11.

Fried PA, Watkinson B (1988) 12- and 24-month neurobehavioural follow-up of children prenatally exposed to marihuana, cigarettes and alcohol. *Neurotoxicol Teratol* **10**: 305–313.

Fried PA, Watkinson B (1990) 36- and 48-month neurobehavioral follow-up of children prenatally exposed to marijuana, cigarettes and alcohol. *J Dev Behav Pediatr* **11**: 49–58.

Fried PA, Watkinson B (2000) Visuoperceptual functioning differs in 9- to 12-year olds prenatally exposed to cigarettes and marihuana. *Neurotoxicol Teratol* **22**: 11–20.

Fried PA, Watkinson B (2001) Differential effects on facets of attention in adolescents prenatally exposed to cigarettes and marihuana. *Neurotoxicol Teratol* **23**: 421–430.

Fried PA, Watkinson B, Grant A, Knights RK (1980) Changing patterns of soft drug use prior to and during pregnancy: a prospective study. *Drug Alcohol Depend* **6**: 323–343.

Fried PA, Buckingham M, Von Kulmiz P (1983) Marijuana use during pregnancy and perinatal risk factors. *Am J Obstet Gynecol* **144**: 922–924.

Fried PA, Watkinson B, Willan A (1984) Marijuana use during pregnancy and decreased length of gestation. *Am J Obstet Gynecol* **150**: 23–27.

Fried PA, Watkinson B, Dulberg CS, Dillon R (1987) Neonatal neurological status in a low risk population following prenatal exposure to cigarettes, marihuana and alcohol. *J Dev Behav Pediatr* **8**: 318–326.

Fried PA, O'Connell CM, Watkinson B (1992a) 60- and 72-month follow-up of children prenatally exposed to marijuana, cigarettes and alcohol: cognitive and language assessment. *J Dev Behav Pediatr* **13**: 383–391.

Fried PA, Watkinson B, Gray R (1992b) A follow-up study of attentional behavior in 6-year-old children exposed prenatally to marihuana, cigarettes and alcohol. *Neurotoxicol Teratol* **14**: 299–311.

Fried PA, Watkinson B, Gray R (1998) Differential effects on cognitive functioning in 9- to 12-year-olds prenatally exposed to cigarettes and marihuana. *Neurotoxicol Teratol* **20**: 293–306.

Fried PA, Watkinson B, Gray R (1999) Growth from birth to early adolescence in offspring prenatally exposed to cigarettes and marihuana. *Neurotoxicol Teratol* **21**: 513–525.

Fried PA, James DS, Watkinson B (2001) Growth and pubertal milestones during adolescence in offspring prenatally exposed to cigarettes and marihuana. *Neurotoxicol Teratol* **23**: 431–436.

Gibson GT, Bayhurst PA, Colley DP (1983) Maternal alcohol, tobacco and cannabis consumption and the outcome of pregnancy. *Aust N Z J Obstet Gynaecol* **23**: 15–19.

Glass M, Dragunow M, Faull RL (1997) Cannabinoid receptors in the human brain: a detailed anatomical and quantitative autoradiographic study in the fetal, neonatal and adult human brain. *Neuroscience* **77**: 299–318.

Goldschmidt L, Day NL, Richardson GA (2000) Effects of prenatal marijuana exposure on child behavior problems at age 10. *Neurotoxicol Teratol* **22**: 325–336.

Golub MS, Sassenrath EN, Chapman CF (1981) Regulation of visual attention in offspring of female monkeys treated chronically with delta-9-tetrahydrocannabinol. *Dev Psychobiol* **14**: 507–512.

Greenberg LM, Kindschi CL (1996) *T.O.V.A. Test of Variables of Attention. Clinical Guide.* Los Alamitos, CA: Universal Attention Disorders.

Greenland S, Staisch KJ, Brown N, Gross SJ (1982) The effects of marijuana use during pregnancy. I. A preliminary epidemiologic study. *Am J Obstet Gynecol* **143**: 408–413.

Greenland S, Richwald GA, Honda GD (1983) The effects of marijuana use during pregnancy. II. A study in a low risk home-delivery population. *Drug Alcohol Depend* **11**: 359–366.

Griffith DR, Azuma SD, Chasnoff IJ (1994) Three-year outcome of children exposed prenatally to drugs. *J Am Acad Child Adolesc Psychiatry* **33**: 20–27.

Halperin JM (1996) Conceptualizing, describing and measuring components of attention. A summary. In: Lyon GR, Krasnegor NA, eds. *Attention, Memory, and Executive Function.* Baltimore, MD: Brookes, pp. 119–136.

Hardwick S, King L (2008) *Home Office Cannabis Potency Study 2008.* St Albans, Hertfordshire: Home Office Scientific Development Branch.

Hatch EE, Bracken MR (1986) Effects of marijuana use in pregnancy on fetal growth. *Am J Epidemiol* **124**: 986–993.

Leech SL, Richardson G, Goldschmidt L, Day NL (1999) Prenatal substance exposure: effects on attention and impulsivity of 6-year-olds. *Neurotoxicol Teratol* **21**: 109–118.

Lester B, Dreher BM (1989) Effects of marijuana use during pregnancy on newborn cry. *Child Dev* **60**: 765–771.

Lezak MD (1995) *Neuropsychological Assessment, 3rd edn.* New York: Oxford University Press.

Luria AR (1973) *The Working Brain. An Introduction to Neuropsychology.* London: Penguin.

McCarthy P (1972) *McCarthy Scales of Children's Abilitites.* New York: Psychological Corporation.

McKay KE, Halperin JM, Schwartz ST, Sharma V (1994) Developmental analysis of three aspects of information processing: sustained attention, selective attention and response organization. *Dev Neuropsychol* **10**: 121–132.

Mereu G, Fà M, Ferraro L, et al. (2003) Prenatal exposure to a cannabinoid agonist produces memory deficits linked to dysfunction in hippocampal long-term potentiation and glutamate release. *Proc Natl Acad Sci USA* **100**: 4915–4920.

Mirsky AF (1996) Disorders of attention. A neuropsychological perspective. In: Lyon GR, Krasnegor NA, eds. *Attention, Memory, and Executive Function.* Baltimore, MD: Brookes, pp. 71–96.

O'Connell CM, Fried PA (1984) An investigation of prenatal cannabis exposure and minor physical anomalies in a low risk population. *Neurotoxicol Teratol* **6**: 345–350.

O'Connell CM, Fried PA (1991) Prenatal exposure to cannabis: a preliminary report of postnatal consequences in school-age children. *Neurotoxicol Teratol* **13**: 631–639.

Ogawa S, Menon RS, Tank DW, et al. (1993) Functional brain mapping by blood oxygenation level-dependent contrast magnetic imaging. A comparison of signal characteristics with a biophysical model. *Biophys J* **64**: 803–812.

O'Keefe J, Nadel L (1978) *The Hippocampus as a Cognitive Map.* Oxford: Oxford University Press.

Richardson G, Day N, Taylor P (1989) The effect of prenatal alcohol, marijuana, and tobacco exposure on neonatal behavior. *Infant Behav Dev* **12**: 199–209.

Richardson GA, Day NL, Goldschmidt L (1995) Prenatal alcohol, marijuana, and tobacco exposure on neonatal behavior. *Neurotoxicol Teratol* **17**: 479–487.

Richardson GA, Ryan C, Willford J, et al. (2002) Prenatal alcohol and marijuana exposure: effects on neuropsychological outcomes at 10 years. *Neurotoxicol Teratol* **24**: 309–320.

SAMHSA (2005) *Results from the 2004 National Survey on Drug Use and Health: National Findings.* Rockville, MD: Office of Applied Studies, US Department of Health and Human Services (NSDUH Series H-28, DHHS Publication No. SMA 05-4062).

SAMHSA (2006) *Results from the 2005 National Survey on Drug Use and Health: National Findings.* Rockville, MD: Office of Applied Studies, US Department of Health and Human Services (NSDUH Series H-30, DHHS Publication No. SMA 06-4194).

Scher MG, Richardson G, Coble P, et al. (1988) The effects of prenatal alcohol and marijuana exposure: disturbances in neonatal sleep cycling and arousal. *Pediatr Res* **24**: 101–105.

Sergeant J (1996) A theory of attention. An information perspective. In: Lyon GR, Krasnegor NA, eds. *Attention, Memory, and Executive Function.* Baltimore, MD: Brookes, pp. 57–69.

Smith AM, Fried PA, Hogan MJ, Cameron I (2004) Effects of prenatal marijuana on response inhibition: an fMRI study of young adults. *Neurotoxicol Teratol* **26**: 533–542.

Smith AM, Fried PA, Hogan MJ, Cameron I (2006) Effects of prenatal marijuana exposure on visuospatial working memory: an fMRI study in young adults. *Neurotoxicol Teratol* **28**: 286–295.

Stuss DT (1992) Biological and psychological development of executive functions. *Brain Cogn* **20**: 8–23.

Tennes K, Avitable N, Blackard C, et al. (1985) Marijuana: prenatal and postnatal exposure in the human. *NIDA Res Monogr* **59**: 48–60.

167

Thorndike RL, Hagen E, Sattler J (1986) *The Standford–Binet Intelligence Scale, 4th edn.* Chicago: Riverside Publishing.

Welsh MC, Pennington BF, Grossier DB (1991) A normative–developmental study in executive function: a window on prefrontal function in children. *Dev Neuropsychol* **7**: 131–149.

Weschler D (1991) *Weschler Intelligence Scale for Children, 3rd edn.* New York: Psychological Corporation.

Zuckerman B, Frank D, Hingson R, et al. (1989) Effects of maternal marijuana and cocaine use on fetal growth. *N Engl J Med* **320**: 762–768.

10

IN UTERO EXPOSURE TO THE POPULAR 'RECREATIONAL' DRUGS MDMA (ECSTASY) AND METHAMPHETAMINE (ICE, CRYSTAL): PRELIMINARY FINDINGS

Derek G Moore, John J D Turner, Julia E Goodwin, Sarah E Fulton, Lynn T Singer and Andrew C Parrott

Chapters 8 and 9 outlined, in detail, findings on the emerging longitudinal outcomes of two of the most popular so-called recreational drugs, cannabis and cocaine. In contrast, there are far fewer data on the impact on the developing human fetus of other increasingly popular synthetic amphetamine derivatives MDMA (3,4-methylenedioxy-N-methylamphetamine), commonly known as 'ecstasy', and methamphetamine ([2S]-N-methyl-1-phenyl-propan-2-amine), known as 'meth', 'ice' or 'crystal'. MDMA and methamphetamine are increasingly popular recreational drugs worldwide, and the study of their effects on the development of human infants has only recently begun. This chapter reports what we currently know about the likely pattern of MDMA and methamphetamine use and the possible neurocognitive effects that these drugs may have on mothers. We review the animal literature on the effects they may have in utero and report the currently limited data on their effects on human infants.

Neurochemical effects

MDMA is a so-called 'synthetic' amphetamine and is a powerful, indirect, monoaminergic agonist which inhibits the reuptake and promotes the release of serotonin and, to a lesser extent, dopamine (Green et al. 2003). MDMA also causes serotonergic neurotoxicity in laboratory animals (Morton 2005). Neuroimaging literature suggests structural changes in adult recreational MDMA users, and data show some broad parallels with the animal data on serotonergic changes, although it is an area of active discussion and debate (see Buchert et al. 2003).

Amphetamine (racemic-B-phenylisopropylamine) is a powerful stimulant of the central nervous system. In adults it causes increased wakefulness, alertness, mood elevation, elation and euphoria, and its effects are reported to be similar in some respects to those of cocaine. These effects are caused by stimulation of the release and blocking of reuptake of the neurotransmitters dopamine, norepinephrine and serotonin. Methamphetamine is an altered form of amphetamine with the addition of a methyl group. It is more readily absorbed into brain tissue than amphetamine (Barr et al. 2006) and importantly produces differential effects in the prefrontal cortex and nucleus accumbens to the parent compound, which appears to result in a less inhibited net reward effect (Shoblock et al. 2003). Taken together with a less negative peripheral sympathomimetic profile than amphetamine (see Iversen 2006), this means that methamphetamine can be taken and tolerated at higher doses and, overall, is more addictive than amphetamine. While methamphetamine is often compared to cocaine in its effects, it has been suggested that it may be more neurotoxic. The effects result from a cascading release of dopamine and also of other monoamine neurotransmitters including norepinephrine and serotonin (Kokoshka et al. 1998). The release of dopamine occurs by a number of mechanisms, including displacement of vesicles and inhibition of monoamine oxidase, and through enhancing dopamine transport across the plasma membrane, increasing dopamine concentration in synapses (for a review, see Scott et al. 2007). As with MDMA, research suggests that structural changes may occur in adult recreational methamphetamine users in specific neural pathways, specifically in dopamine-rich fronto-striato-thalamo-cortical loops (Cass 1997).

Prevalence in young adults

According to the British Crime Survey, 24.1% of 16- to 24-year-olds in England and Wales reported having used one or more illicit substances in the last year (Nicholas et al. 2007). Whilst men are more likely to use illicit substances than women, recent UK and EU data from the European Monitoring Centre for Drugs and Drug Addiction (www.emcdda. europa.eu) show that this gap between the sexes is narrowing and that the experiences and drug-use patterns of young men and women are increasingly similar, even if the effects of the drugs may differ across the sexes.

There is evidence of widespread use of MDMA by adolescents and young adults in the USA. The 2004 'Monitoring the Future' study indicated that rates of MDMA use had increased at accelerated rates from 1998 until 2001, reaching levels as high as 9.2% for 12th graders and college students alike (Johnston et al. 2005a,b). While rates of MDMA have decreased somewhat over a three-year period based on the 2004 survey, 4% of 12th graders reported using MDMA in the past year and 7.5% reported lifetime use (Johnston et al. 2005a).

In the UK and USA the use of MDMA has been associated with 'raves', all-night dance parties where ecstasy use is common, but it is increasingly used in private social settings as well (Singer et al. 2004). The Community Epidemiology Workgroup of the National Institute on Drug Abuse, reporting on the 2003 data on community substance use (NIDA-CEWG 2004), indicated that MDMA use in the USA has spread beyond raves to a variety of urban, suburban and rural areas, including greater use on college campuses. There has been an increasing effort to document the rave and other MDMA-use cultures in the USA, and to estimate rates of MDMA use both alone and in conjunction with other drugs. According to data collected from emergency room visits in the USA, MDMA is most frequently combined with alcohol, cannabis and cocaine.

Methamphetamine is also becoming one of the most dominant drugs of abuse, with an estimated 30 million users worldwide (United Nations Office on Drugs and Crime 2004). There has, in particular, been a steep rise in production and use in south-east and east Asia (see McKetin et al. 2008). Use worldwide has increased from around 2.5% of adolescents and adults over 12 years of age in 1997 to around 5.5% in 2002 (United Nations Office on Drugs and Crime 2004). Thus, MDMA and methamphetamine present serious public health concerns.

In the UK, the use of so-called recreational drugs is commonplace, and MDMA and methamphetamine are often taken together* and in temporal proximity with alcohol, tobacco, powder cocaine, cannabis and other psychoactive substances (Drug Abuse Warning Network 2000; Johnston et al. 2001; Yacoubian et al. 2003; Parrott 2004, 2006; Scholey et al. 2004; Singer et al. 2004), making it very difficult to establish their specific effects. Users may use one drug to counter the negative effects of another (Miliani et al. 2005), and there are also likely to be interaction effects, with these recreational drugs being differentially potentiated by alcohol and tobacco (Ben Hamida et al. 2008).

Prevalence in pregnant drug-using women

The use of recreational drugs is not limited to low socio-economic status groups, and dependent users are not necessarily the same population of women who would regularly be using cannabis, powder cocaine, MDMA and methamphetamine. Many men and women in the UK who use recreational drugs do not also use 'crack' cocaine, heroin or other opiates, and many continue to hold down jobs and raise a family. These 'non-dependent'/recreational users are less likely to be identified by health professionals unless they voluntarily disclose their use, as they do not present with obvious problems.

However, the profile of use of drugs differs across countries, adding difficulties in interpreting data. For example, Ho et al. (2001) surveyed pregnant women who contacted a drug information and helpline in Canada and found that MDMA users were more likely to be younger, single and white, and to be binge drinkers. They were more likely to have unplanned pregnancies, smoking and polydrug use were common, and over a third of the women reported psychiatric problems. Thus, a range of factors need to be accounted for in these developmental studies, and we need to take account of the differing social profiles across countries and cultures.

The accuracy of reported data on drug use is also an issue. In the UK, while some women may disclose their drug use during pregnancy to their midwife, it is likely that many more do not, for fear they might be negatively judged or receive differential health care. Some may simply believe it to be a private issue and that the drugs they take are harmless. General information on the potential negative effects of drug taking is given to UK mothers but is not detailed except with respect to smoking and drinking, and this may contribute to a perception that the dangers are not great. Cannabis in particular is a drug which young women seem to consider less harmful than other illicit drugs (Pearson and Shiner 2002), and levels

*In some cases tablets are sold as 'ecstasy' but in fact contain methamphetamine, which is cheaper to produce (Kalasinsky et al. 2004).

of use in the UK may be high. In one UK survey around 5% of pregnant women were estimated to have used cannabis in pregnancy (Fergusson et al. 2002).

However, profiles of use of recreational drugs across different trimesters are likely to be uneven, and different recreational drugs may have different profiles of use. Specifically, some drugs may be more prevalent during early pregnancy. As MDMA and methamphetamine are more predominant in party/rave contexts and such parties are less likely to be attractive to women once pregnant, then levels of use of these drugs are likely to decline. However, early in pregnancy, prior to confirmation that they are pregnant, many young women will still be attending parties and may take a range of recreational substances. Thus, the prevalence of MDMA and methamphetamine use in pregnant women in early pregnancy could be high.

Establishing levels of use in pregnancy through standard health networks may also be problematic. Anecdotal reports suggest that at antenatal interviews arranged under the National Health Service (NHS) in the UK, while midwives routinely ask questions on drug use, these are often passed over quickly and there is unlikely to be in-depth questioning. Thus, data on recreational drug use collected through these routes may underreport use, and may provide an unreliable picture of the combinations of drugs mothers are likely to expose their infants to across trimesters.

To address this issue, the Drugs and Infancy Study (DAISY) was initiated. As the study was university based and outside the NHS, mothers who come forward seemed willing to disclose their full patterns of use. We interviewed women about their use of a wide range of legal and illicit drugs in their life up to pregnancy, in the year before pregnancy and over each trimester. We are also following up their infants to age 2 years. This began in 2001 and to date we have recruited a cohort of 96 pregnant recreational drug-using women (Moore et al. 2009). Of these women, 68 had used cannabis, 55 amphetamines and 54 MDMA, with the majority having smoked tobacco and having drunk alcohol in their lifetimes.

Our data have revealed that 35% of mothers who used MDMA at some point in their life before pregnancy also used MDMA in the first trimester, and of those mothers who had used amphetamines in their lifetime 9% used them at some point in the first trimester. However, only 4% of pregnant women used MDMA in the following trimesters and only one used amphetamines. We also found that the vast majority of MDMA users also used cannabis, and that the majority of women who used MDMA in the first trimester also drank, smoked or used cannabis in pregnancy, with around a third of the women continuing to use cannabis throughout all three trimesters.

The data confirm that, in the UK at least, infants of polydrug-using mothers are most at risk of MDMA or methamphetamine exposure in the first trimester, and that it is rare for users to take MDMA or methamphetamine in later pregnancy, but quite common for these women to continue taking cannabis and to drink and smoke at reduced levels (Moore et al. 2009). This highlights the need to consider the effects of drugs in combination, as in the real world women rarely use drugs in isolation.

Possible impact on the health and neuropsychological functioning of mothers
While there are some mixed reports on the impact of taking MDMA on daily living, chronic

MDMA use has increasingly been shown to be associated with poorer general psychological health (Parrott et al. 2001, 2000; Thomasius et al. 2006), specifically with depression (MacInnes et al. 2001, de Win et al. 2004, Lamers et al. 2006) and increased anxiety (Lamers et al. 2006). As already outlined (Chapter 5), maternal depression and anxiety are known to be significant risk factors for infant development.

Chronic MDMA use may also lead to impairments in aspects of everyday memory, prospective memory, frontal executive processing, problem solving, decision taking and social and emotional intelligence (Rodgers 2000; Fox et al. 2001, 2002; Rodgers et al. 2003; Fisk et al. 2005; Reay et al. 2006; Rendell et al. 2007). These cognitive and social difficulties may act as contributory factors to adverse parenting, possibly leading to reduced child-focused attention, poorer verbal and nonverbal communication and reduced sensitivity to the communications of their infants, and a higher risk of confusion or cognitive overload that could have an additional impact on affect and mood. Thus, from simple forgetting of tasks to generally poorer cognitive engagement and control, past and continuing drug use could significantly impact upon mother–child relations and therefore child outcomes.

While the exact nature of the long-term effect of exposure to methamphetamine on the adult brain is debated, there is consensus that methamphetamine has specific effects on episodic memory, executive function, speed of processing, motor skills, language, visuo-constructional abilities and other aspects of fronto-striatal and limbic related functioning; and clinical reports also suggest this population may be more distractible and inattentive (for a review, see Scott et al. 2007). Acute neuropsychiatric effects of amphetamine and methamphetamine in adult users include agitation, tremor, hyperreflexia, irritability, confusion, aggressiveness and panic states, among others. This is usually followed by fatigue and depression. Withdrawal effects can also be severe, and chronic injecting users appear more susceptible to psychosis (McKetin et al. 2006). Again, these effects will have a significant impact on women's capacities for caring for their infants.

In addition to long-term neurocognitive effects, acute physical reactions to MDMA and methamphetamine have been recorded. MDMA specifically appears to contribute to rapid body temperature elevation (hyperthermia) and this may have subsequent effects on the liver, brain and cardiovascular systems, sometimes sadly resulting in the sudden death of users (Green et al. 2003, Freedman et al. 2005). While death is rare, these physiological effects, especially hyperthermia, could have significant negative consequences for fetal and pregnancy outcomes, and be additional mechanisms by which MDMA may alter pregnancy outcomes and infant development. MDMA can also lead to a demonstrated reduction in appetite and food intake during the week after use, and in some cases it may be deliberately used as an appetite suppressant (Curran and Robjant 2006, Kobeissy et al. 2008). Poor nutrition is known to lead to poor outcomes during pregnancy (Georgieff 2007). MDMA and methamphetamine may also have an impact on maternal immunity, which may also have adverse effects on pregnancy outcomes as yet unnoticed (Connor 2004, Talloczy et al. 2008, Martinez et al. 2009).

The use of MDMA and methamphetamine in combination with other drugs is also of particular concern, with many studies concluding that MDMA, amphetamines and cannabis are associated with more pronounced psychobiological problems in adult users (Rodgers

2000, Parrott et al. 2001). These adult neuropsychobiological effects are likely to have important influences upon the behaviour of young women who are pregnant and, if use is continued throughout and beyond pregnancy, may have significant impact on their ability to care for their children once born.

Furthermore, while there is some debate, researchers (Liechti et al. 2001, Allot and Redman 2007) have suggested that females may be more vulnerable and show somewhat different MDMA effects than men, even allowing for bodyweight. Verheyden et al. (2002) found that female MDMA users tended to report midweek feelings of depression, whereas males were more prone to aggression during the post-MDMA period. Milani et al. (2004) and ter Bogt and Engels (2005) have reported sex-specific patterns of psychobiological and psychosocial sequelae as a result of MDMA use, and more recently Dluzen and Liu (2008) have reported a similar effect for methamphetamine, with women using it commonly presenting with depression. Thus, to understand the impact of methamphetamine and MDMA on mothers it is important to consider these specific effects and to consider the developing literature on MDMA effects in adults in this light. Certainly the findings suggest that MDMA- and methamphetamine-using mothers may be more at risk for depression before, during and after pregnancy.

Medical outcomes of exposed infants
Animal studies of the impact of amphetamines have observed increased mortality, retinal eye defects, cleft palate, rib malformations, decreased physical growth and delayed motor development. There are also isolated reports of cardiac defects, cleft lip and biliary atresia after in utero exposure in human infants; reduced growth and increased fetal distress have also been reported (Erikson et al. 1978, 1981; Billing et al. 1980; Dixon and Bejar 1989; Catanzarite and Stein 1995; Plessinger 1998).

To date only a handful of studies have examined the outcomes after maternal MDMA use during pregnancy in human infants. There is some suggestive, but inconclusive, evidence that MDMA use by mothers may have an impact on early cardiac and limb formation. A study by the Teratology Information Service for the National Institute for Public Health and Environment in the Netherlands has followed 43 cases (van Tonnigen-van Driel et al. 1999). Of 40 liveborn infants, one had a cardiac malformation, but it was noted that other substances were used by the mothers that were also potentially harmful in pregnancy.

Similarly, MDMA use in the UK has been tracked through the National Teratology Information Service, which collected prospective follow-up outcomes on 136 pregnancies (McElhatton et al. 1999). Approximately 45% of these pregnant women were reported to have been taking MDMA only, with the remainder taking MDMA with other drugs of abuse during pregnancy, primarily amphetamines, cocaine, cannabis and LSD. The women ranged in age between 16 and 36 years. Although this study is a case series, with associated methodological limitations, reported prenatal MDMA exposure was found to be associated with a significantly increased risk of congenital malformations, particularly cardiovascular anomalies and musculoskeletal anomalies, four to seven times greater than expected. Even after taking into account the higher prevalence of malformations associated with high-risk pregnancies, there was a two-fold increase in malformations associated with

MDMA. However, it should be noted that the accuracy of data on drug use was limited in this study, with the mothers being referred by health professionals after revealing that they had taken MDMA. They were not fully interviewed about their use of other drugs, and so it is not clear that these are genuinely MDMA-only users. Indeed, from our study and other reports it is clear that MDMA is often used alongside other drugs and rarely in isolation. Thus, these effects need to be considered in the context of the drug reporting methods used.

Neurocognitive effects of in utero exposure in animals
While to date only limited data are available on the effects of MDMA on the neurocognitive functioning of human infants, there is a growing literature of its effects in utero and post partum on the functioning of animals (for reviews, see Piper 2007, Skelton et al. 2008). One of the earliest studies was of 1-day-old chicks (Bronson et al. 1994). In this study it was found that prenatal exposure to MDMA produced effects such as distress vocalization, wing extension, tremors, flat body posture, loss of righting reflex and convulsion-like kicking. Similarly, subsequent studies of MDMA exposure in fetal rats revealed subtle behavioural alterations to the pups and significant reductions in maternal (dam) weights (Omer et al. 1991). Meyer et al. (2004) also found that neonatal MDMA exposure in rat pups (equivalent to the third trimester in humans, see also Chapter 3) led to significant reductions in serotonin levels in the hippocampus, the brain region associated with memory.

While some of these early studies of prenatal exposure failed to demonstrate any lasting neurobehavioural effects in rat pups (Colado et al. 1997, Aguirre et al. 1998), Broening et al. (2001) reported evidence that exposure to MDMA in rats during stages analogous to early and late third trimester human fetal brain development induced long-term learning and memory impairments. Further, while MDMA exposure had no effect on survival of neonatal rats, it did affect bodyweight gain during treatment. Dose-related impairments on sequential and spatial learning and memory were noted with exposure on postnatal days 11–20, the developmental period in rats proposed to be equivalent to the third trimester in humans in terms of neuroanatomical development.* Similarly, methamphetamine exposure at postnatal days 11–20 in rats seems to lead to difficulties in water-maze learning and may interfere with neurotrophic factors that are important for neuronal proliferation, survival and differentiation. Skelton et al. (2007) found that methamphetamine exposure in rats leads to increases in brain-derived neurotrophic factors in the hippocampus that may be responsible for water-maze learning and memory problems reported in rats. These studies raise concerns about the impact of methamphetamine and MDMA during stages of brain development analogous to the late human fetal period.

However, recent data from the DAISY study cited above (Moore et al. 2009) suggest that, in the UK at least, the majority of prenatal exposure to MDMA and methamphetamine will occur in the first trimester when young women are still socializing at parties and before they are aware that they are pregnant. Thus, work by Koprich et al. (2003) in neonatal rat pups is perhaps most relevant. In their study, early prenatal exposure, equivalent to the first

---

*See Figure 3.1 (p. 24) for equivalent data on mice development in relation to human gestation.

trimester in humans, was also sufficient to produce significant neurochemical and behavioural alterations. Prenatally MDMA-exposed animals had reduced birthweight, reduced dopamine and serotonin metabolites in several brain areas, and increased locomotor activity, and they showed a lack of habituation in a novel cage environment, suggesting persistent neurochemical and behavioural alterations following prenatal exposure.

The mechanism of MDMA-induced developmental effects has yet to be determined, but serotonin is known to have neurotrophic effects on neuronal development. Mazer et al. (1997) and Broening et al. (2001) have shown that interfering with serotonin synthesis during development can lead to long-term reductions in microtubule-associated protein, a synaptic marker. This suggests that the impact of MDMA is more on the role of serotonin in connectivity rather than in neurotransmission. While the experiment of Mazer et al. (1997) used the tryptophan hydroxylase inhibitor p-chlorophenylalanine, and that by Broening et al. (2001) used the serotonin-releaser MDMA, both studies share the finding of long-term learning and memory impairments in the absence of long-term changes in brain serotonin levels.

Thus both MDMA and methamphetamine exposure in utero may produce lasting changes in dopamine and serotonin systems, and animal work suggests that both first and third trimester exposure may have an impact on the neurobiology of human infants with corresponding consequences for cognition, learning and social development.

Preliminary evidence of the neurocognitive effects of methamphetamine and MDMA on human infants

Predicting what the long-term neurobehavioural outcomes will be for human infants exposed to MDMA and methamphetamine in utero is not straightforward. The animal literature outlined above has largely been restricted to chicks and rats, and although there are some clear effects on motor functioning in animals exposed to large doses of MDMA and methamphetamine in utero, it is not clear to what extent these findings can be generalized to human infants. The frequency or size of dose in animal studies is likely to be larger than that to which the typical human infant has been exposed, and the human neurological system clearly differs markedly from that of a rat or chick.

Furthermore, literature that has explored the effects of MDMA and methamphetamine exposure on the adult human brain, while useful in determining how exposure might affect maternal behaviour, may not allow us to clearly predict what the effects of exposure will be on the developing infant brain. The developing infant brain has a large degree of plasticity, and in the initial stages of neuronal development cognitive functions and corresponding brain structures and pathways are not as localized and specialized as in adulthood (Johnson 2003). Thus the elements of the serotonergic and dopamine systems that may be vulnerable to MDMA and methamphetamine effects in adults may not necessarily be those that are affected in infancy, nor, even if the same pathways are involved, does this necessarily mean that the same insult will lead to the same outcomes.

It is, however, reasonable to postulate that children with a history of fetal MDMA or methamphetamine exposure are more likely to perform poorly on overall measures of cognition, language, emotional functioning and behavioural competence, and may show differences in motor skills reflecting, for example, the problems found by Bronson et al. (1994) in chicks. Further, if it is safe to extrapolate from the adult literature and literature on the additive effects of polydrug use, we might also predict that there may be particular deficits in neuropsychological functions. In particular, polydrug use may impact on developing executive functions, attentional processes, and visuospatial and language skills. Note, however, that in infants of polydrug-using women, these effects may not be distinguishable from those reported for cannabis, although there could be an additive or interaction effect of polydrug use.

While the neurocognitive effects of MDMA and methamphetamine on human infants are only now being researched, there are some limited longitudinal data on the impact of unmodified amphetamine on the neurocognitive development of exposed infants. Billing and colleagues followed infants from birth through to 14 years (Billing et al. 1980, 1985, 1988, 1994; Eriksson et al. 1981, 1989; Cernerud et al. 1996). In the first few months infants showed increased drowsiness, and infants exposed to amphetamines throughout all trimesters of pregnancy showed more social communicative problems at age 1 year (Billing et al. 1980). By age 8, exposure was found to be related to later aggressive behaviour and problems with peers. At age 14, children showed problems with maths, language and physical activities (Cernerud et al. 1996). It must be noted, however, that this study was limited in sample size and lacked a control group, and it was not possible to separate the effects of methamphetamine from those of other drugs. Also, as noted above, the action of amphetamines and methamphetamine differ in the intensity of their effects.

There have been two magnetic resonance imaging studies of children exposed prenatally specifically to methamphetamine, investigating possible structural changes and behavioural functioning (Smith et al. 2001, Chang et al. 2004). They examined a small sample of 7- to 8-year-olds (n=13) exposed prenatally to methamphetamine and other substances (alcohol and tobacco), and a control group of unexposed children. Smith et al. (2001) used proton magnetic resonance spectroscopy to evaluate neurochemical alterations, and found possible alterations in cellular energy metabolism in the basal ganglia of the methamphetamine-exposed group. Chang et al. (2004) performed volumetric analysis and revealed bilateral reductions in the volume of the globus pallidus, putamen and hippocampus. In contrast, no differences were found in the thalamus, midbrain or cerebellum. However, the study did not control for polydrug use, so the specific effect of methamphetamine may not be determined.

More recently, two studies funded by the National Institute on Drug Abuse have begun in the USA and UK to examine the impact of MDMA and methamphetamine. The DAISY study, already referred to, has directly recruited a cohort of over 100 polydrug- and MDMA-using pregnant women and is shortly to publish data on infant outcomes. The other study is the IDEAL (Infant Development, Environment and Lifestyle) study (Smith et al. 2006). This is a multisite, longitudinal study of methamphetamine and has screened an initial cohort of almost 14 000 women. Around a fifth of this sample drank alcohol, around 6% used cannabis, and the incidence of methamphetamine use at some point in pregnancy was around 5% (Aria et al. 2006). From this larger sample they have recruited 74 methamphetamine users and 92 comparison women into a prospective longitudinal study.

Infants born to the mothers recruited who took methamphetamine were 3.5 times more likely to be small and to have lower birthweight for gestational age, even controlling for tobacco and alcohol effects (Smith et al. 2003), and initial findings of the impact of methamphetamine exposure on the neurological and motor functioning of newborn (up to 5 days old) infants indicate some dose-dependent effects on infant arousal (Smith et al. 2008). Infants were assessed using the Neonatal Intensive Care Unit Network Neurobehavioral Scale (NNNS; Lester and Tronick 2004), and methamphetamine exposure in the first trimester was related to lower arousal, more lethargy and elevated stress indicators (those behaviours that are also typically associated with abstinence/withdrawal in opiate-exposed infants). Also, methamphetamine exposure in the third trimester was related to poorer quality of movement.

These neonatal effects were also found alongside a higher prevalence of depressive symptoms in the methamphetamine-using mothers (Paz et al. 2009), which in turn were associated with decreased arousal and increased stress in the infants, although this factor did not add to the overall direct effect of methamphetamine. Thus, high levels of methamphetamine use may be impacting directly on neurological development and also indirectly via the impact of maternal depression. This study is ongoing, and the longer-term effects of methamphetamine on neurological functioning are yet to be determined.

Conclusions

Although studies are limited, there is some emerging evidence for the teratogenic effects of MDMA and methamphetamine from both preclinical and human studies, and the IDEAL study has begun to find some specific effects of methamphetamine in the infant period. In addition, animal studies suggest that MDMA or methamphetamine use by mothers will impact on the fetal seretonergic and dopamine systems. However, extrapolating from animal effects to effects in human infants is not simple.

Data from the DAISY study to date show that, in the UK, MDMA exposure is likely to occur predominantly in the first trimester, and that this exposure is unlikely to occur in isolation but rather alongside other drugs. Animal models need to be further developed to reflect these likely patterns of use, so we can better extrapolate these findings to human development in utero. These drugs may not have a simple additive effect in utero but may interact in their effects in ways yet to be determined.

What is clear is that, to understand the ramifications of fetal exposure to these increasingly popular drugs, there need to be more prospective longitudinal studies of polydrug users, with adequate sample sizes that allow the statistical control of the many confounding variables. However, our experience in the UK is that it is difficult to recruit pregnant recreational drug users via the typical health service routes, and future studies will need to use a variety of recruitment techniques to gain a large enough sample to consider a range of extraneous factors.

Studies also need to use a broad number of outcome measures sensitive to neuropsychological dysfunction, similar to those used in studies on cannabis, as outlined in Chapter 9. These studies need to have extended follow-ups into late childhood to be sure of capturing the potential long-term effects. Investigations of the indirect effects of maternal psychological status and caretaking behaviours are also needed to provide information essential to the development of effective maternal drug treatment and child intervention programmes. The examination of interaction effects of various drugs is key. The DAISY and IDEAL studies are longitudinally documenting outcomes of a prospectively recruited sample of exposed infants whose prenatal exposure has been characterized through maternal biological and self-report measures throughout pregnancy, and whose caregiving environment, including maternal psychological status, has been characterized postnatally. Findings from the IDEAL study are now beginning to be published and we will also be reporting infant outcomes from the DAISY study in the near future.

ACKNOWLEDGEMENTS

We thank the women and their babies for their continuing involvement in the DAISY study. The work was funded by the National Institute on Drug Abuse (NIH, USA), grant DA14910.

REFERENCES

Aguirre N, Barrionuevo M, Lasheras B, Del Rio J (1998) The role of dopaminergic systems in the perinatal sensitivity to 3,4-methylenedioxymethamphetamine-induced neurotoxicity in rats. *J Pharmacol Exp Ther* **286**: 1159–1165.

Allott K, Redman J (2007) Are there sex differences associated with the effects of ecstasy/3,4-methylenedioxymethamphetamine (MDMA)? *Neurosci Biobehav Rev* **31**: 327–347.

Arria AM, Derauf C, LaGasse LL, et al. (2006) Methamphetamine and other substance use during pregnancy: preliminary estimates from the Infant Development, Environment, and Lifestyle (IDEAL) study. *Matern Child Health J* **10**: 293–302.

Barr AM, Panenka WJ, MacEwan W, et al. (2006) The need for speed: an update on methamphetamine addiction. *J Psychiatry Neurosci* **31**: 301–313.

Ben Hamida S, Plute E, Cosquer B, et al. (2008) Interactions between ethanol and cocaine, amphetamine, or MDMA in the rat: thermoregulatory and locomotor effects. *Psychopharmacology* **197**: 67–82.

Billing L, Eriksson M, Larsson G, Zetterström R (1980) Amphetamine addiction and pregnancy. III. One year follow-up of the children. Psychosocial and pediatric aspects. *Acta Paediatr Scand* **69**: 675–680.

Billing L, Eriksson M, Steneroth G, Zetterström R (1985) Preschool children of amphetamine-addicted mothers. I. Somatic and psychomotor development. *Acta Paediatr Scand* **74**: 179–184.

Billing L, Eriksson M, Steneroth G, Zetterström R (1988) Predictive indicators for adjustment in 4-year-old children whose mothers used amphetamine during pregnancy. *Child Abuse Negl* **12**: 503–507.

Billing L, Eriksson M, Jonsson B, et al. (1994) The influence of environmental factors on behavioral problems in 8-year-old children exposed to amphetamine during fetal life. *Child Abuse Negl* **18**: 3–9.

Broening HW, Morford LL, Inman-Wood SL, et al. (2001) 3,4-Methylenedioxymethamphetamine (ecstasy)-induced learning and memory impairments depend on the age of exposure during early development. *J Neurosci* **21**: 3228–3235.

Bronson ME, Jiang W, Clark CR, DeRuiter J (1994) Effects of designer drugs on the chicken embryo and 1-day-old chicken. *Brain Res Bull* **34**: 143–150.

Buchert R, Thomasius R, Nebeling B, et al. (2003) Long-term effects of "ecstasy" use on serotonin transporters of the brain investigated by PET. *J Nucl Med* **44**: 375–384.

Cass WA (1997) Decreases in evoked overflow of dopamine in rat striatum after neurotoxic doses of methamphetamine. J Pharmacol Exp Ther 280: 105–113.

Catanzarite VA, Stein DA (1995) 'Crystal' and pregnancy—methamphetamine-associated maternal deaths. *West J Med* **162**: 454–457.

Cernerud L, Eriksson M, Jonsson B, et al. (1996) Amphetamine addiction during pregnancy: 14-year follow-up of growth and school performance. *Acta Paediatr* **85**: 204–208.

Chang L, Smith LM, LoPresti C, et al. (2004) Smaller subcortical volumes and cognitive deficits in children with prenatal methamphetamine exposure. *Psychiatry Res* 132: 95–106.

Colado MI, O'Shea E, Granados R, et al. (1997) A study of the neurotoxic effect of MDMA ('ecstasy') on 5-HT neurones in the brains of mothers and neonates following administration of the drug during pregnancy. *Br J Pharmacol* **121**: 827–833.

Connor TJ (2004) Methylenedioxymethamphetamine (MDMA, 'ecstasy'): a stressor on the immune system. *Immunology* **111**: 357–367.

Curran HV, Robjant K (2006) Eating attitudes, weight concerns and beliefs about drug effects in women who use ecstasy. *J Psychopharmacol* **20**: 425–431.

De Win MM, Reneman L, Reitsma JB, et al. (2004) Mood disorders and serotonin transporter density in ecstasy users—the influence of long-term abstention, dose and gender. *Psychopharmacology* **173**: 376–382.

Dixon SD, Bejar R (1989) Echoencephalographic findings in neonates associated with maternal cocaine and methamphetamine use: incidence and clinical correlates. *J Pediatr* **115**: 770–778.

Dluzen DE, Liu B (2008) Gender differences in methamphetamine use and responses: a review. *Gend Med* **5**: 24–35.

Drug Abuse Warning Network (DAWN) (2000) *Club Drugs.* Rockville, MD: US Department of Health and Human Services.

Eriksson M, Larsson G, Winbladh B, Zetterström R (1978) The influence of amphetamine addiction on pregnancy and the newborn infant. *Acta Paediatr Scand* **67**: 95–99.

Eriksson M, Larsson G, Zetterström R (1981) Amphetamine addiction and pregnancy. II. Pregnancy, delivery, and the neonatal period. Socio-medical aspects. *Acta Obstet Gynecol Scand* **60**: 253–259.

Eriksson M, Billing L, Steneroth G, Zetterström R (1989) Health and development of 8-year-old children whose mothers abused amphetamine during pregnancy. *Acta Paediatr Scand* **78**: 944–949.

Fergusson DM, Horwood LJ, Northstone K (2002) Maternal use of cannabis and pregnancy outcome. *BJOG* **109**: 21–27.

Fisk JE, Montgomery C, Wareing M, Murphy PN (2005) Reasoning deficits in ecstasy (MDMA) polydrug users. *Psychopharmacology* **181**: 550–559.

Fox H, Parrott AC, Turner JJD (2001) Ecstasy/MDMA related cognitive deficits: a function of dosage rather than awareness of problems. *J Psychopharmacol* **15**: 273–281.

Fox HC, McLean A, Turner JJD, et al. (2002) Neuropsychological evidence of a relatively selective profile of temporal dysfunction in drug-free MDMA ("ecstasy") polydrug users. *Psychopharmacology* **162**: 203–214.

Freedman RR, Johnson CE, Tancer ME (2005) Thermoregulatory effects of 3,4-methylenedioxymethamphetamine (MDMA) in humans. *Psychopharmacology* **183**: 248–256.

Georgieff MK (2007) Nutrition and the developing brain: nutrient priorities and measurement. *Am J Clin Nutr* **85**: 614–620.

Green AR, Mechan AO, Elliott JM, et al. (2003) The pharmacology and clinical pharmacology of 3,4-methylene-dioxy-meth-amphetamine (MDMA, "ecstasy"). *Pharmacol Rev* **55**: 463–508.

Ho E, Karimi-Tabesh L, Koren G (2001) Characteristics of pregnant women who use ecstasy (3,4-methylene-dioxymethamphetamine). *Neurotoxicol Teratol* **23**: 561–567.

Iversen L (2006) *Speed, Ecstasy, Ritalin: The Science of Amphetamines.* Oxford: Oxford University Press.

Johnson MH (2003) The development of human brain function. *Biol Psychiatry* **54**: 1312–1316.

Johnston LD, O'Malley PM, Bachman JG (2001) *Monitoring the Future: National Results on Adolescent Drug Use.* Washington, DC: National Institute on Drug Abuse, US Department of Health and Human Services.

Johnston LD, O'Mally PM, Brachman JG, Schulenberg JF (2005a) *Monitoring the Future: National Results on Adolescent Drug Use: Overview and Key Findings, 2004.* (NIH Publication No. 05-5726.) Bethesda, MD: National Institute on Drug Abuse.

Johnston LD, O'Mally PM, Brachman JG, Schulenberg JF (2005b) *Monitoring the Future: National Survey Results on Drug Use, 1975–2004: Vol. II. College Students and Adults Ages 19–45.* (NIH Publication No. 05-5728.) Bethesda, MD: National Institute on Drug Abuse.

Kalasinsky KS, Hugel J, Kish SJ (2004) Use of MDA (the "love drug") and methamphetamine in Toronto by unsuspecting users of ecstasy (MDMA). *J Forensic Sci* **49**: 1106–1112.

Kobeissy FH, Jeung JA, Warren MW, et al. (2008) Changes in leptin, ghrelin, growth hormone and neuro-peptide-Y after an acute model of MDMA and methamphetamine exposure in rats. *Addict Biol* **13**: 15–25.

Kokoshka JM, Metzger RR, Wilkins DG, et al. (1998) Methamphetamine treatment rapidly inhibits serotonin, but not glutamate, transporters in rat brain. *Brain Res* **799**: 78–83.

Koprich JB, Chen EY, Kanaan NM, et al. (2003) Prenatal 3,4-methylenedioxymethamphetamine (ecstasy) alters exploratory behaviour, reduces monoamine metabolism, and increases forebrain tyrosine hydroxylase fiber density of juvenile rats. *Neurotoxicol Teratol* **25**: 509–517.

Lamers CTJ, Bechara A, Rizzo M, Ramaekers JG (2006) Cognitive function and mood in MDMA/THC users, THC users and non-drug using controls. *J Psychopharmacol* **20**: 302–311.

180

Lester BM, Tronick EZ (2004) The Neonatal Intensive Care Unit Network Neurobehavioral Scale (NNNS) – Procedures. *Pediatrics* **113**: 641–667.

Liechti ME, Gamma A, Vollenweider FX (2001) Gender differences in the subjective effects of MDMA. *Psychopharmacology* **154**: 161–168.

MacInnes N, Handley SL, Harding GFA (2001) Former chronic methylenedioxymethamphetamine (MDMA or ecstasy) users report mild depressive symptoms. *J Psychopharmacol* **15**: 181–186.

Martinez LR, Mihu MR, Gácser A, et al. (2009) Methamphetamine enhances histoplasmosis by immunosuppression of the host. *J Infect Dis* **200**: 131–141.

Mazer C, Muneyyirci J, Taheny K, et al. (1997) Serotonin depletion during synaptogenesis leads to decreased synaptic density and learning deficits in the adult rat: a possible model of neurodevelopmental disorders with cognitive deficits. *Brain Res* **760**: 68–73.

McElhatton PR, Bateman DN, Evans C, et al. (1999) Congenital anomalies after prenatal ecstasy exposure. *Lancet* **354**: 1441–1442.

McKetin R, McLaren J, Lubman DI, Hides L (2006) The prevalence of psychotic symptoms among methamphetamine users. *Addiction* **101**: 1473–1478.

McKetin R, Kozel N, Douglas J, et al. (2008) The rise of methamphetamine in southeast and east Asia. *Drug Alcohol Rev* **27**: 220–228.

Meyer JS, Grande M, Johnson K, Ali SF (2004) Neurotoxic effects of MDMA ("ecstasy") administration to neonatal rats. *Int J Dev Neurosci* **22**: 261–271.

Milani R, Parrott AC, Turner JJD, Fox HC (2004) Gender differences in self-reported anxiety, depression, and somatization among ecstasy/MDMA polydrug users, alcohol/tobacco users, and nondrug users. *Addict Behav* **29**: 965–971.

Milani RM, Parrott AC, Schifano F, Turner JJ (2005) Pattern of cannabis use in ecstasy polydrug users: moderate cannabis use may compensate for self-rated aggression and somatic symptoms. *Hum Psychopharmacol* **20**: 249–261.

Moore DG, Turner JD, Parrott AC, et al. (2009) During pregnancy, recreational drug-using women stop taking ecstasy (3,4-methylenedioxy-N-methylamphetamine) and reduce alcohol consumption but continue to smoke tobacco and cannabis initial findings from the Development and Infancy Study. *J Psychopharmacol* (epub ahead of print) doi: 10.1177/0269881109348165.

Morton J (2005) Ecstasy: pharmacology and neurotoxicity. *Curr Opin Pharmacol* **5**: 79–86.

Nicholas S, Kershaw C, Walker A, eds (2007) *Crime in England and Wales 2006/07. 4th edn.* London: Home Office.

NIDA-CEWG (2004) *National Institute on Drug Abuse. Community Epidemiology Work Group. Epidemiologic Trends in Drug Abuse. Vol 1. Proceedings of the Community Epidemiology Work Group. Highlights and Executive Summary. June 2004.* Bethesda, MD: US Department of Health and Human Services.

Omer VW, Ali SF, Holson RR, et al. (1991) Behavioral and neurochemical effects of prenatal methylenedioxymethamphetamine (MDMA) exposure in rats. *Neurotoxicol Teratol* **13**: 13–20.

Parrott AC (2002) Recreational ecstasy/MDMA, the serotonin syndrome, and serotonergic neurotoxicity. *Pharmacol Biochem Behav* **71**: 837–844.

Parrott AC (2004) MDMA (3,4-methylenedioxymethamphetamine) or ecstasy: the neuropsychobiological implications of taking it at dances and raves. *Neuropsychobiology* **50**: 329–335.

Parrott AC (2006) MDMA in humans: factors which influence the neuropsychobiological profiles of recreational ecstasy users, the integrative role of bio-energetic stress. *J Psychopharmacol* **20**: 147–163.

Parrott AC, Sisk E, Turner J (2000) Psychobiological problems in heavy 'ecstasy' (MDMA) polydrug users. *Drug Alcohol Depend* **60**: 105–110.

Parrott AC, Milani R, Parmar R, Turner JJD (2001) Ecstasy polydrug users and other recreational drug users in Britain and Italy: psychiatric symptoms and psychobiological problems. *Psychopharmacology* **159**: 77–82.

Paz MS, Smith LM, LaGasse LL, et al. (2009) Maternal depression and neurobehavior in newborns prenatally exposed to methamphetamine. *Neurotoxicol Teratol* **31**: 177–182.

Pearson G, Shiner M (2002) Rethinking the generation gap. Attitudes to illicit drug among young people and adults. *Criminol Crim Justice* **2**: 71–86.

Piper BJ (2007) A developmental comparison of the neurobehavioral effects of ecstasy (MDMA). *Neurotoxicol Teratol* **29**: 288–300.

Plessinger MA (1998) Prenatal exposure to amphetamines. Risks and adverse outcomes in pregnancy. *Obstet Gynecol Clin North Am* **25**: 119–138.

Reay JL, Hamilton C, Kennedy DO, Scholey AB (2006) MDMA polydrug users show process-specific central executive impairments coupled with impaired social and emotional judgement processes. *J Psychopharmacol* **20**: 385–388.

Rendell PG, Gray TJ, Henry JD, Tolan A (2007) Prospective memory impairment in "ecstasy" (MDMA) users. *Psychopharmacology* **194**: 497–504.

Rodgers J (2000) Cognitive performance amongst recreational users of "ecstasy". *Psychopharmacology* **151**: 19–24.

Rodgers J, Buchanan T, Scholey AB, et al. (2003) Patterns of drug use and the influence of gender on self reports of memory ability in ecstasy users: a web based study. *J Psychopharmacol* **17**: 379–386.

Scholey AB, Parrott AC, Buchanan T, et al. (2004) Increased intensity of ecstasy and polydrug usage in the more experienced recreational ecstasy/MDMA users: a WWW study. *Addict Behav* **29**: 743–752.

Scott JC, Woods SP, Matt GE, et al. (2007) Neurocognitive effects of methamphetamine: a critical review and meta-analysis. *Neuropsychol Rev* **17**: 275–297.

Shoblock JR, Sullivan EB, Maisonnueve IM, Glick S (2003) Neurochemical and behavioral differences between d-methamphetamine and d-amphetamine in rats. *Psychopharmacology* **165**: 359–369.

Singer LT, Linares TJ, Ntiri S, et al. (2004) Psychosocial profiles of older adolescent ecstasy users in the United States. *Alcohol Drug Depend* **74**: 245–252.

Skelton MR, Williams MT, Vorhees CV (2006) Treatment with MDMA from P11-20 disrupts spatial learning and path integration learning in adolescent rats but only spatial learning in older rats. *Psychopharmacology* **189**: 307–318.

Skelton MR, Williams MT, Vorhees CV (2008) Developmental effects of 3,4-methylenedioxymethamphetamine: a review. *Behav Pharmacol* **19**: 91–111.

Smith LM, Chang L, Yonekura ML, et al. (2001) Brain proton magnetic resonance spectroscopy in children exposed to methamphetamine in utero. *Neurology* **57**: 255–260.

Smith L, Yonekura ML, Wallace T, et al. (2003) Effects of prenatal methamphetamine exposure on fetal growth and drug withdrawal symptoms in infants born at term. *J Dev Behav Pediatr* **24**: 17–23.

Smith LM, LaGasse LL, Derauf C, et al. (2006) The infant development, environment, and lifestyle study: effects of prenatal methamphetamine exposure, polydrug exposure, and poverty on intrauterine growth. *Pediatrics* **118**: 1149–1156.

Smith LM, LaGasse LL, Derauf C, et al. (2008) Prenatal methamphetamine use and neonatal neurobehavioral outcome. *Neurotoxicol Teratol* **30**: 20–28.

Tallóczy Z, Martinez J, Joset D, et al. (2008) Methamphetamine inhibits antigen processing, presentation, and phagocytosis. *PLoS Pathog* **4**: e28.

ter Bogt TF, Engels RC (2005) "Partying" hard: party style, motives for and effects of MDMA use at rave parties. *Subst Use Misuse* **40**: 1479–1502.

Thomasius R, Zapletalova P, Petersen K, et al. (2006) Mood, cognition and serotonin transporter availability in current and former ecstasy (MDMA) users: the longitudinal perspective. *J Psychopharmacol* **20**: 211–225.

Thompson BL, Levitt P, Stanwood GD (2009) Prenatal exposure to drugs: effects on brain development and implications for policy and education. *Nat Rev Neurosci* **10**: 303–312.

United Nations Office on Drugs and Crime (2004) *World Drug Report 2004. Vol 1. Analysis.* New York: UNODC.

van Tonningen-van Driel MM, Garbis-Berkvens JM, Reuvers-Lodwijks WE (1999) [Pregnancy outcome after ecstasy use, 43 cases followed by the Teratology Information Service of the National Institute for Public Health and Environment (RIVM).] *Ned Tijdschr Geneeskd* **143**: 27–31 (Dutch).

Verheyden SL, Hadfield J, Calin T, Curran HV (2002) Sub-acute effects of MDMA (+/-3,4-methylene-dioxymethamphetamine, "ecstasy") on mood: evidence of gender differences. *Psychopharmacology* **161**: 23–31.

Yacoubin GS, Boyle C, Harding CA, Loftus EA (2003) It's a rave new world: estimating the prevalence and perceived harm of ecstasy and other drug use among club rave attendees. *J Drug Educ* **33**: 187–196.

11

THE SHORT-TERM AND LONG-TERM DEVELOPMENTAL CONSEQUENCES OF MATERNAL SMOKING DURING PREGNANCY

Kate E Pickett and Lauren S Wakschlag

Prevalence and patterns of smoking in pregnancy

In the UK in 2005, 32% of women smoked cigarettes in the year before they became pregnant (Office for National Statistics 2006), and although most would like to quit (British Medical Association 2004), only half of these women manage to quit just before or during pregnancy, which means that 17% of women are persistent smokers throughout – exposing around 120 000 infants each year. Elsewhere, in common with the UK, most women who smoke prior to pregnancy fail to quit, and although prevalence rates are slightly lower in other countries – 11% in the USA, 12% in Canada and 11% in Sweden (Salihu and Wilson 2007) – this nevertheless translates into very large numbers of exposed infants.

Establishing whether a fetus has been exposed to maternal smoking during pregnancy is not straightforward. Most women receiving antenatal care will have been asked if they are smoking and the answer will be recorded in their medical record. However, this is an unreliable guide to actual exposure. As well as being an incorrect record if women fail to admit to smoking or care providers fail to enquire, we have found substantial variations in smoking across pregnancy for individual mothers (Pickett et al. 2003, 2005). A mother might quit upon learning that she is pregnant, then relapse and quit again multiple times. She may cut down, but later smoke more heavily during times of stress. So her answer to any question about her smoking status at a given point in time may be entirely truthful, yet an unhelpful guide to the timing, intensity and duration of fetal exposure over the pregnancy as a whole (particularly, as is usually the case, if the query occurs at the outset of pregnancy). This is also true of exposure measured by biological assessment of the by-products of smoking in women's urine, blood or saliva. Whilst such approaches provide a more direct method of assessing actual exposure, they only tell us the woman's smoking pattern over the past couple of days and thus do not provide a measure of pregnancy smoking history. As women may quit smoking before the usual time of entry into antenatal care, it is almost impossible to measure very early exposure in real time, but if women are asked to recall previous smoking in a non-judgemental way, first trimester exposure can be estimated (Pickett et al. 2009a).

Who smokes during pregnancy?

Although most pregnant women want to quit and feel guilty about smoking, many feel powerless to change their behaviour (Copeland 2003). Compared with those who manage to quit, women who smoke throughout pregnancy tend to be younger, less educated and unemployed (Hanna et al. 1994, Graham and Der 1999, Agrawal et al. 2008, Martin et al. 2008). They are more likely to be depressed (Hanna et al. 1994, Pritchard 1994), stressed (Paarlberg et al. 1999), single or cohabiting (Thue et al. 1995, Kiernan and Pickett 2006), and to have a partner who smokes (Wakefield et al. 1993, Appleton and Pharoah 1998) or who abuses them (McFarlane et al. 1996). They have less social support (Dejin-Karlsson et al. 1996), and are more likely to be living in a working-class neighbourhood (Pickett et al. 2002, Sellström et al. 2008).

We have also shown, in studies in both the UK and USA, that women who quit and women who continue to smoke differ in the ways they relate to other people, in how well they cope with day-to-day life, and in their likelihood of engaging in other risky health behaviours (Wakschlag et al. 2003, Kodl and Wakschlag 2004, Weaver et al. 2008, Pickett et al. 2009b). All this adds up to the fact that smoking in pregnancy is embedded in a very complex psychological and social context, and this has important implications for interpreting some of the research on the effects of smoking in pregnancy, particularly long-term outcomes.

Established consequences of maternal smoking during pregnancy

HEALTH PROBLEMS IN INFANCY

Congenital malformations

Although smoking during pregnancy does not seem to be related to an overall increase in the risk of birth defects, babies born to mothers who smoke are more likely to have cleft lip and cleft palate (Beaty et al. 1997), limb reductions (Kallen 1997b) and malformations of the genitourinary tract (Kalle 1997a).

Low birthweight, fetal growth restriction and preterm birth

There is a robust body of evidence showing that smoking in pregnancy can cause low birthweight (<2500 g), a consequence of these infants being 1.5–2 times more likely to be born preterm (<37 weeks gestation) and/or to have experienced fetal growth restriction (US Surgeon General 2001, British Medical Association 2004). The babies of women who smoke are 200–250 g lighter than babies of non-smokers, and this deficit is greater among babies of women who smoked very heavily. There is also increasing evidence that women who do not smoke during pregnancy, but are exposed to tobacco smoke at home or in the workplace, are also more likely to have infants with low birthweight (Peacock et al. 1998, US Surgeon General 2001).

A full review of the consequences of preterm delivery and low birthweight is beyond the scope of this chapter (see Paneth 1995); here we simply note that these infants are at increased risk of mortality during their first year and a range of physical illnesses in infancy, childhood and throughout the life course (Goldenberg 1994, Barker 1999), as well as mental health problems (Breslau and Chilcoat 2000) and educational difficulties (Resnick et al. 1999).

Infant mortality and sudden infant death syndrome

Babies born to mothers who smoke in pregnancy are 40% more likely to die in the first four weeks after birth than those born to non-smokers (Ahlsten et al. 1993). However, the risk of infant death is even higher among the offspring of smokers, in comparison with non-smokers, after the first month of life (Salihu et al. 2003), and this risk is higher among infants born to heavy smokers.

Sudden infant death syndrome (SIDS) is the sudden and unexplained death of an apparently healthy child during the first year of life. Most SIDS deaths occur between 2 and 4 months of age. Maternal smoking during pregnancy is a well-established cause, doubling the risk of SIDS (British Medical Association 2004, Salihu and Wilson 2007). As the risk of SIDS is notably increased if babies are exposed to tobacco smoking after birth, as well as before, it is of vital importance that infants are not exposed to passive smoking in their living or sleeping environments.

HEALTH PROBLEMS IN CHILDHOOD AND BEYOND

Lung function and respiratory illnesses

Lung function is reduced in infants (Stocks and Dezateux 2003) and young children (Cunningham et al. 1994, Wang et al. 1994) who were exposed to maternal smoking during pregnancy, and this reduced function persists into adulthood (Svanes et al. 2004). This appears to be a result of the impaired development of airways, rather than an overall reduction in the volume of lung capacity. In clinical terms, this means that children up to 2 years of age are more likely to suffer from wheezing (estimates range from 30% to 100% more likely), and older children are 80% more likely to suffer from asthma and three times as likely to have persistent wheezing (Milner et al. 2007).

Tobacco-exposed infants and children have more hospital admissions for lower respiratory tract infections, such as pneumonia, and for bronchitis, bronchiolitis and croup (British Medical Association 2004). As with SIDS, these risks are compounded by exposure to environmental tobacco smoke after birth, and it is essential that previously exposed infants and children are provided with a smoke-free domestic environment.

Obesity

Children of mothers who smoked in pregnancy have been shown consistently to have a higher body mass index (BMI) than children of non-smokers, despite the fact that they tend to have lower birthweights (Rogers 2008). This appears to be a dose–response relationship: the more the mother smoked, the higher the risk that her child will be overweight (BMI >90th centile) or obese (BMI >97th centile) (von Kries et al. 2002). The greatest risk appears to result from exposure during the first trimester of pregnancy (Oken et al. 2005). In a very large follow-up study of American children aged from 1 to 8 years it was apparent that the exposed children were born smaller than non-exposed children, but soon caught up and exceeded the weight of non-exposed children, whilst remaining shorter (Chen et al. 2006). Maternal smoking during pregnancy seems to increase the risk of childhood obesity by around 60% (Dubois and Girard 2006).

Diabetes

Children of mothers who smoked during pregnancy have a greater risk of developing type II diabetes (Rogers 2008). This risk is related to how heavily the mother smoked. A follow-up study of a large sample of British children born in 1958 looked at whether or not they developed diabetes between the ages of 16 and 33 years (Montgomery and Ekbom 2002). If the mother had smoked heavily during pregnancy, offspring were 4.5 times more likely to develop diabetes than the children of non-smokers.

These risks are not surprising, as a pattern of low birthweight, followed by overweight and obesity, carries a particularly high risk for the development of diabetes, cardiovascular disease and metabolic disorders. Children and young adults who were exposed to maternal smoking during pregnancy should therefore be encouraged to maintain a healthy body weight, be physically active and avoid becoming smokers themselves, as all these can help to prevent the onset of these chronic diseases.

Cancer

Smoking is a well-established cause of a number of cancers, and tobacco smoke contains many known carcinogens, such as nicotine, cadmium and benzene (Rogers 2008). As many of the substances in tobacco smoke can cross the placental barrier, the impact of maternal smoking in pregnancy on the development of cancer in offspring has been widely researched, but no consistent effects have been observed (Sasco and Vainio 1999). There is, however, some evidence that exposure to maternal smoking may increase the risk of brain tumours, leukaemia and lymphoma (Sasco and Vainio 1999, Brooks et al. 2004). Infants of mothers who smoked during pregnancy have higher rates of chromosomal instability and damage than infants born to non-smoking mothers, and these chromosomal problems are related to a higher risk of developing cancer (de la Chica et al. 2005, Zalacain et al. 2006).

Understanding the impact of maternal smoking during pregnancy on the intellectual development and behaviour of children

METHODOLOGICAL ISSUES

Much controversy surrounds the issue of whether or not exposure to maternal smoking during pregnancy causes (a) deficits in cognitive function and IQ, and (b) behavioural problems. In both cases, it is difficult to know whether observed links of exposure and later problems are *caused* by the mother's smoking, or whether smoking is a *marker* for maternal genetic vulnerability to these problems, and/or are due to the context of psychosocial adversity in which smoking in pregnancy is embedded.

As the methodological issues involved in examining these relationships are the same for cognitive development and behaviour, we will discuss them here and then go on to look at the body of evidence related to each.

It would, of course, be unethical to conduct a randomized controlled trial of smoking in pregnancy, assigning some women to smoke and others not, and then following the offspring to examine their cognitive development and behaviour. An alternative might be to study the children born to women who have been enrolled in randomized trials of smoking cessation interventions. Two problems arise with this approach. First, such trials enrol only women who are smoking while pregnant, and if smoking in early pregnancy is relevant for later intelligence and behaviour, then whether or not women manage to quit later in pregnancy would be irrelevant and both quitters and persistent smokers would confer similar risks on their offspring – comparing these two groups would be pointless. Second, the current standard interventions for stopping smoking in pregnancy are relatively ineffective, and they tend to be least effective with heavier, more addicted smokers. These heavy smokers differ from lighter smokers, who are more susceptible to intervention in ways which are likely to also affect their children's risk of intellectual deficits and behaviour problems. Further, given the high rates of spontaneous quitting and the relatively low success rates of the current interventions, it is unlikely that the experimental group in such a study would differ sufficiently from the comparison group to test causal hypotheses.

For these reasons, researchers are reliant on observational studies, and the major methodological problem they face in such studies is dealing with potential confounding factors. They need to measure, and account for, all the characteristics of the mother, her family and her social context that are related to whether or not she smokes, quits or never smokes in pregnancy and are independently related to children's risks of developing problems.

In a review of the literature on maternal smoking and behaviour outcomes in offspring, we identified six domains of characteristics that researchers need to address in these studies (Wakschlag et al. 2002). They also apply to studies of smoking in pregnancy and cognitive development in offspring. They are

1. Socio-demographic factors, such as maternal age, socio-economic status, ethnicity, marital status, etc.
2. Parental psychiatric and psychological factors, such as a history of antisocial behaviour, depression, poor interpersonal skills, etc. Ideally, researchers would have such information for both parents.
3. Parenting and quality of the home environment.
4. Exposure to other substances during pregnancy, such as alcohol, drugs, medications, etc.
5. Perinatal factors, such as low birthweight, preterm delivery.
6. Exposure to environmental tobacco smoke in infancy and childhood.

Assessing whether or not a particular exposure causes a particular outcome, when only observational studies are available, is an inexact science. No single study can provide a definitive answer. Instead, we need to look at the body of evidence as a whole and assess the likelihood that the association is causal. Researchers look for evidence such as consistency across time, place, population and study design, the strength of the associations, dose–response relationships, biological plausibility, and, most importantly, whether or not the relationships can be explained by any of the kinds of factors we have listed above.

COGNITIVE DEVELOPMENT

The idea that fetal exposure to maternal smoking during pregnancy might have an impact on cognition is certainly plausible, as exposure affects brain development (Jauniaux and Burton 2007). Many studies have shown that smoking during pregnancy is indeed associated with impaired cognitive development, including worse performance on tests of language abilities, and poor overall school performance (British Medical Association 2004). These associations have been examined in follow-up studies of cohorts of children in the UK, Canada, Finland, New Zealand and the USA, and the literature was reviewed in 1998 (Lassen and Oei 1998). At that time, there were 16 such studies and 12 showed significant deficits in cognitive development among exposed children, compared to non-exposed children. Among those that did not show significant reductions, small sample sizes were a problem, and one studied the presence or absence of learning disabilities, rather than differences in intelligence (IQ) test scores. Others found significant associations between exposure and deficits in cognitive development that disappeared after controlling for the quality of the home environment. At the time of that review the body of evidence was inconsistent, and alternative explanations of the associations, particularly aspects of parenting, appeared potentially important. Also, few of these older studies controlled for children's passive exposure to environmental tobacco smoke after birth. However, many studies reported dose–response relationships, with heavier smoking associated with greater deficits in IQ.

Only two early studies, with conflicting findings, adjusted for mother's IQ, which is potentially an important confounder. Low IQ is related to smoking and poor success at quitting smoking, and mother's IQ is also strongly related to offspring IQ. To address this methodological issue, Batty et al. (2006) used the US National Longitudinal Survey of Youth 1979 – a sample of 5578 children born to 3145 mothers. They found that, before adjustment, children who had been exposed to maternal smoking of 20 or more cigarettes per day had IQ scores almost 3 points lower than non-exposed children. When they controlled first for mother's education and second for mother's IQ, this difference was substantially reduced. For a separate test of mathematical ability, there was no effect of exposure after adjustment for mother's IQ.

Another important study of the effect of exposure on cognitive development was conducted by Gilman et al. (2008) in the US Collaborative Perinatal Project. A unique methodological development was that the authors used a genetically informative design – comparing the cognitive outcomes of siblings with different exposure – that allowed them to control for genetic and environmental characteristics shared by the siblings, which had not actually been measured in the study. The effects of smoking on IQ and academic achievement disappeared entirely after this adjustment. In a large Swedish study, Lambe et al. (2006) found that if the mother had smoked in her first pregnancy, but not in a second pregnancy, the younger child was at the same increased risk of poor school performance as the exposed child, leading them to conclude that associations between maternal smoking during pregnancy and poor cognitive performance in offspring are not causal.

Taken together, these recent studies suggest that smoking during pregnancy may be a marker for children having a higher risk of cognitive deficits but not a causal factor. If this is true, then the remaining question is whether exposure is a marker for a genetic risk of cognitive deficit, or an environmental risk. If the increased risk is environmental, then if the child is brought up in a different environment, there may be no increased risk at all. If the risk is genetic, then it may well be modified by bringing up the child in an enriched environment.

BEHAVIOUR PROBLEMS

There is now a substantial body of literature looking at maternal smoking during pregnancy and behavioural issues in offspring, including disruptive behaviour disorders and symptoms,

TABLE 11.1
Behaviours in offspring associated with exposure to maternal smoking during pregnancy

Behavioural issue	Definition	Age at onset
Temperament	A pattern of behavioural regulation and reactivity	Evident at birth and stable across the lifespan
Negativity	Measured as an index of 3 behaviours (impulsivity, risk taking and rebelliousness) thought to predict later unconventionality and poor emotional control	Evident by 2 years of age
Externalizing problems/symptoms	Problems such as disobedience, being aggressive towards other children, being restless and unable to sit still. Usually assessed by either (a) observation, or (b) symptom checklists completed by parents, teachers or, when they are older, the children themselves	Can be measured from around 1 year onwards
Oppositional defiant disorder	A pattern of hostile, argumentative behaviour, including loss of temper, defiance and swearing	Usually appears in childhood or early adolescence
Conduct disorder	A repetitive and persistent pattern of aggressive and/or antisocial behaviour, such as vandalism, substance abuse, and lying	Childhood or adolescence
Antisocial personality disorder	Impulsive, destructive behaviour that disregards the rights and feelings of others; characterized by lack of guilt, intolerance of frustration, problems with relationships and the law	Adults, cannot be diagnosed before age 18 years
Attention-deficit–hyperactivity disorder	A pattern of high level of activity and/or difficulty in attending to tasks. Affected persons are restless, unable to sit still for more than a few minutes, inattentive and impulsive	Onset usually between ages 3 and 7 years
Delinquency	Unlawful behaviour, i.e. antisocial or illegal behaviour or acts, not necessarily resulting in involvement in the justice system	Any age, a child not old enough to be held responsible for a crime may still commit acts of delinquency
Criminal offending	Unlawful behaviour resulting in criminal charge	Jurisdictions vary in the age at which a child is considered to become criminally responsible and can be charged with a crime. In the UK, this is 10 years, in Scotland 8 years, Canada 12 years, Sweden 15 years. In some US states it is as low as 6 years

delinquency and criminal activity, and substance use (Table 11.1 lists and defines the problems that have been associated with smoking in pregnancy). Of note, this association is specific to behaviour problems rather than mental health problems in general.

The biological plausibility of this association is discussed by Slotkin (1998), who examined the effects of nicotine on neural development in animal models. By exposing fetal animals to nicotine alone, Slotkin ensured that it was the nicotine, rather than lack of oxygen or exposure to other constituents of cigarette smoke, that caused the fetal brain damage observed. Nicotine acts directly on the fetal brain and affects growth in the number of cells and the ways in which cells develop, so that the brains of exposed animals have fewer brain cells and reductions in neural activity. Slotkin says that exposure also affects "the eventual programming of synaptic competence. Accordingly, defects may appear after a prolonged period of apparent normality…" Perhaps most surprisingly, this research showed that nicotine is far more toxic to the developing brain than exposure to crack cocaine.

Looking at the research literature as a whole, how strong are the associations between smoking in pregnancy and behavioural problems? For severe antisocial behaviour problems, including diagnosed conduct disorder, oppositional defiant disorder, delinquency and criminal offending, relative risks range from around 1.5 to 4.0, meaning that exposed children are between 50% and 300% more likely to develop these problems than non-exposed children (Wakschlag et al. 2002). Although less consistent than findings linking exposure and antisocial behaviour, across a number of studies reviewed by Linnet et al. (2003) relative risks for attention-deficit–hyperactivity disorder are around 3.0 (200% higher risk) for exposed versus non-exposed offspring. For substance use in offspring, including cigarette smoking, alcohol and illegal drugs, relative risks range from 2.0 to 3.0 (Button et al. 2007). These relative risks are moderately strong, and comparable to the increased risk of low birthweight and SIDS among the offspring of smokers.

As mentioned earlier, it is difficult to measure smoking in pregnancy, and this means that in research studies some women will be classified as non-smokers when in fact they smoked. If this kind of misclassification is substantial in a research study, then the strength of the effect of smoking on adverse outcomes will be underestimated and the true relative risks might be bigger than those we describe above. Whilst pregnant smokers with antisocial problems of their own might report heavier or more persistent smoking than is true, because of lack of social inhibition, and this could possibly mean that relative risks are being overestimated, underestimation seems the more likely scenario of the two.

There is some evidence from epidemiological studies, as well as from animal studies, of a dose–response relationship between exposure and behavioural outcomes. Problems in accurately measuring the timing, intensity and duration of exposure, i.e. the number of cigarettes smoked per day at different time points during pregnancy, are a critical limitation to being able to establish a precise dose–response effect. No studies have been able to precisely establish a threshold beyond which exposure is most damaging, nor do we know much about whether quitting at particular time-point in pregnancy is protective. The first trimester is important for the development and differentiation of neural systems, but the third trimester is important for growth in size of the fetal brain.

Effects of smoking during pregnancy on behavioural outcomes in boys have been found in many different populations, at different times and using different study designs. Whereas early studies were mainly of adolescents, there is also now evidence of a consistent developmental pattern of affected behaviour from infancy onwards. Exposure has been linked to lower scores of easy temperament in 9-month-old infants (Martin et al. 2006, Pickett et al. 2008); to negativity (Brook et al. 2000) and a pattern of escalating behaviour problems

(Wakschlag et al. 2006a) in toddlers; to disruptive behaviour in 3-year-old children (Hutchinson et al. 2010); and to earlier onset of delinquency in school-aged youth (Wakschlag et al. 2006b). Linnet et al. (2003) found a consistent effect of smoking in pregnancy on attention-deficit–hyperactivity disorder in studies conducted over 30 years, although it is possible that this effect only exists because children with attention-deficit–hyperactivity disorder often have comorbid oppositional defiant disorder or conduct disorder (Wakschlag et al. 2006b, Huijbregts et al. 2007).

Findings are less consistent for girls (Wakschlag et al. 2002). Some of this inconsistency is probably due to the fact that behavioural disorders are less common in girls, and so bigger studies are needed to detect significant effects of smoking in pregnancy. Inconsistency may also arise from the ways in which oppositional defiant disorder and conduct disorder are defined as disorders; the ways in which girls exhibit behavioural problems differ from boys. For example, behaviour problems in girls may manifest as promiscuous behaviour, whilst boys may be violent, and current diagnostic criteria are based on problems that are characteristically male. Exposure may also have less effect on girls; animal experiments suggest that the male fetus may be more vulnerable to toxic exposures in the womb. In our study of infant temperament, we found that the effects of smoking were stronger for male babies compared to females (Pickett et al. 2008).

In boys, the effect of exposure to maternal smoking on psychological problems seems to be specific to disruptive behaviour disorders and unrelated to other mental health problems, such as depression and anxiety. Indeed, Monuteaux et al. (2006) found that exposure was not related to 'covert' behaviour problems, such as theft, but was related to 'overt' problems, such as physical aggression, particularly among the most deprived children they studied.

Increasingly, studies of smoking in pregnancy and behavioural problems in offspring have begun to control for maternal (and occasionally, paternal) antisocial behaviour, parenting problems, substance use, etc., and generally these studies have found that the effect of smoking is not explained by these characteristics. However, Maughan et al. (2004) found that women who smoked in pregnancy were more likely to be antisocial, and to have children with antisocial men, and that controlling for this reduced the estimated effect of smoking by half. Recently, in a Dutch study of toddlers, Roza et al. (2009) reported no effect of smoking after controlling for a wide range of factors. In contrast, Huijbregts et al. (2008) demonstrated that the behavioural risks of exposure were heightened when combined with having an antisocial parent.

Apart from the child's sex, do any other factors modify the apparent impact of smoking in pregnancy on behaviour? One study found that smoking was related to behavioural problems in families with low socio-economic status, but not in other families (Monuteaux et al. 2006); another found that exposed boys whose mothers were unresponsive were at increased risk of conduct disorder, whereas exposed boys with more responsive mothers were not (Wakschlag and Hans 2002). Batstra et al. (2003) found that effects of smoking were modified by single motherhood, medication use during pregnancy, and obstetric complications such as instrumental delivery. Postnatal exposure to cigarette smoke modified the impact of prenatal exposure in a large study of the 1970 British Birth Cohort (Maughan et al. 2001). Mothers who started smoking only after pregnancy had children with an increased risk of conduct problems, and mothers who smoked heavily in pregnancy but then quit had children with no greater risk of behavioural problems than non-smokers.

Five studies have used innovative study designs (kinship studies and sophisticated statistical methods) to examine whether or not the effect of smoking in pregnancy on behaviour is either (a) entirely due to genetic confounding (i.e. smoking in pregnancy is a marker for a genotype that is also causative of behavioural problems in children), or (b) a gene–environment interaction, whereby exposure to cigarette smoke in utero affects the expression of genetic vulnerability to behavioural problems. In a study of twins, Silberg et al. (2003) used a technique called latent variable modelling and reported that the link between exposure and conduct problems in boys was due to the intergenerational transmission of an unmeasured genetic risk. Similarly, Maughan et al. (2004) used a special statistical technique to separate out genetic and environmental influences on child behaviour in a twin study; however, they found that genetic factors and prenatal exposure to tobacco smoke independently affected the risk of conduct problems in children aged 5 and 7 years. D'Onofrio et al. (2008) studied sibling pairs. Comparing exposed children with non-exposed siblings, they found no effect of smoking on behaviour, which suggests that the association between maternal smoking during pregnancy and behavioural problems in children might be due to unidentified environmental factors. Sen and Swaminathan (2007) also used sophisticated statistical models in a kinship design. The impact of maternal alcohol use on offspring behaviour remained significant in their analyses, but maternal smoking in pregnancy did not. A cleverly designed study of exposure to parental smoking (rather than prenatal smoking) reported some provocative findings (Keyes et al. 2008). Adolescents adopted in infancy were no more likely to have behavioural problems if their parents smoked than if they did not, but among adolescents who had been brought up by their biological parents, the resulting effects of exposure included substance use, disruptive behaviour disorders, delinquency and aggressive attitudes.

Taken together, these studies suggest that a shared genetic vulnerability among women who smoke in pregnancy and their children with behaviour problems may be part of the story linking exposure to long-term behavioural effects. However, sorting out genetic versus environmental explanations is not straightforward, and a very likely scenario is that genetic vulnerability and exposure to tobacco smoke and family environment in its broadest sense interact in a complex causal pathway. Indeed, we have recently found that the effect of exposure seems to be modified by both sex and a susceptibility gene for aggression (Wakschlag et al. 2009). Exposed boys with one variant of the gene were at increased risk of conduct problems, but girls with a different variant were also at increased risk. Disentangling the effects of genes, exposure and environment requires more research, and the long-term impacts of maternal smoking during pregnancy will remain controversial.

The important message from research on both cognition and behavioural problems is that fetal exposure to maternal cigarette smoke is certainly a marker for heightened developmental risk beyond its well-established perinatal consequences. Mechanisms by which these are linked remain unclear. Regardless of mechanism, however, it is important to stress that this increased risk is for vulnerability rather than definitively condemning a child to long-term problems. Postnatal environmental factors that often go hand in hand with antenatal exposure have been clearly demonstrated to affect the likelihood that such vulnerability will develop into serious impairment. Responsive, warm parenting, an enriched intellectual environment, protection from further exposure to environmental tobacco smoke, and appropriate treatment for parental psychopathology will enhance the chances that exposed children are able to achieve their developmental potential.

REFERENCES

Agrawal A, Knopik VS, Pergadia ML, et al. (2008) Correlates of cigarette smoking during pregnancy and its genetic and environmental overlap with nicotine dependence. *Nicotine Tob Res* **10**: 567–578.

Ahlsten G, Cnattingius S, Lindmark G (1993) Cessation of smoking during pregnancy improves foetal growth and reduces infant morbidity in the neonatal period. A population-based prospective study. *Acta Paediatr* **82**: 177–181.

Appleton PL, Pharoah POD (1998) Partner smoking behaviour change is associated with women's smoking reduction and cessation during pregnancy. *Br J Health Psychol* **3**: 361–374.

Barker DJ (1999) Fetal origins of cardiovascular disease. *Ann Med* **31** Suppl 1: 3–6.

Batstra L, Hadders-Algra M, Neeleman J (2003) Effect of antenatal exposure to maternal smoking on behavioural problems and academic achievement in childhood: prospective evidence from a Dutch birth cohort. *Early Hum Dev* **75**: 21–33.

Batty GD, Der G, Deary IJ (2006) Effect of maternal smoking during pregnancy on offspring's cognitive ability: empirical evidence for complete confounding in the US National Longitudinal Survey of Youth. *Pediatrics* **118**: 943–950.

Beaty T, Maestri NE, Hetmanski JB, et al. (1997) Testing for interaction between maternal smoking and TGFA genotype among oral cleft cases born in Maryland 1992–1996. *Cleft Palate Craniofac J* **34**: 447–454.

Breslau N, Chilcoat HD (2000) Psychiatric sequelae of low birth weight at 11 years of age. *Biol Psychiatry* **47**: 1005–1011.

British Medical Association (2004) *Smoking and Reproductive Life. The Impact of Smoking on Sexual, Reproductive and Child Health.* London: BMA.

Brook JS, Brook DW, Whiteman M (2000) The influence of maternal smoking during pregnancy on the toddler's negativity. *Arch Pediatr Adolesc Med* **154**: 381–385.

Brooks DR, Mucci LA, Hatch EE, Cnattingius S (2004) Maternal smoking during pregnancy and risk of brain tumors in the offspring. A prospective study of 1.4 million Swedish births. *Cancer Causes Control* **15**: 997–1005.

Button TMM, Maughan B, McGuffin P (2007) The relationship of maternal smoking to psychological problems in the offspring. *Early Hum Dev* **83**: 727–732.

Chen A, Pennell ML, Klebanoff MA, et al. (2006) Maternal smoking during pregnancy in relation to child overweight: follow-up to age 8 years. *Int J Epidemiol* **35**: 121–130.

Copeland L (2003) An exploration of the problems faced by young women living in disadvantaged circumstances if they want to give up smoking: can more be done at general practice level? *Fam Pract* **20**: 393–400.

Cunningham J , Dockery DW, Speizer FE, et al. (1994) Maternal smoking during pregnancy as a predictor of lung function in children. *Am J Epidemiol* **139**: 1139–1152.

Dejin-Karlsson E, Hanson BS, Ostergren PO, et al. (1996) Psychosocial resources and persistent smoking in early pregnancy—a population study of women in their first pregnancy in Sweden. *J Epidemiol Community Health* **50**: 33–39.

de la Chica RA, Ribas I, Giraldo J, et al. (2005) Chromosomal instability in amniocytes from fetuses of mothers who smoke. *JAMA* **293**: 1212–1222.

D'Onofrio BM, Van Hulle CA, Waldman ID, et al. (2008) Smoking during pregnancy and offspring externalizing problems: an exploration of genetic and environmental confounds. *Dev Psychopathol* **20**: 139–164.

Dubois L, Girard M (2006) Early determinants of overweight at 4.5 years in a population-based longitudinal study. *Int J Obes* **3**: 610–617.

Gilman SE, Martin LT, Abrams DB, et al. (2008) Educational attainment and cigarette smoking: a causal association? *Int J Epidemiol* **37**: 615–624.

Goldenberg RL (1994) The prevention of low birthweight and its sequelae. *Prev Med* **23**: 627–631.

Graham H, Der G (1999) Patterns and predictors of smoking cessation among British women. *Health Promot Int* **14**: 231–239.

Hanna EZ, Faden VB, Dufour MC (1994) The motivational correlates of drinking, smoking, and illicit drug use during pregnancy. *J Subst Abuse* **6**: 155–167.

Huijbregts SC, Seguin JR, Zoccolillo M, et al. (2007) Associations of maternal prenatal smoking with early childhood physical aggression, hyperactivity–impulsivity, and their co-occurrence. *J Abnorm Child Psychol* **35**: 203–215.

Huijbregts SC, Seguin JR, Zoccolillo M, et al. (2008) Maternal prenatal smoking, parental antisocial behavior, and early childhood physical aggression. *Dev Psychopathol* **20**: 437–453.

Hutchinson J, Pickett KE, Green J, Wakschlag LS (2010) Smoking in pregnancy and disruptive behaviour in 3-year-old boys and girls: an analysis of the UK Millennium Cohort Study. *J Epidemiol Community Health* **64**: 82–88.

Jauniaux E, Burton GJ (2007) Morphological and biological effects of maternal exposure to tobacco smoke on the feto-placental unit. *Early Hum Dev* **83**: 699–706.

Kallen K (1997a) Maternal smoking and urinary organ malformations. *Int J Epidemiol* **26**: 571–574.

Kallen K (1997b) Maternal smoking during pregnancy and limb reduction malformations in Sweden. *Am J Public Health* **87**: 29–32.

Keyes M, Legrand LN, Iacono WG, McGue M (2008) Parental smoking and adolescent problem behavior: an adoption study of general and specific effects. *Am J Psychiatry* **165**: 1338–1344.

Kiernan K, Pickett KE (2006) Marital status disparities in maternal smoking during pregnancy, breastfeeding and maternal depression. *Soc Sci Med* **63**: 335–346.

Kodl MM, Wakschlag LS (2004) Does a childhood history of externalizing problems predict smoking during pregnancy? *Addict Behav* **29**: 273–279.

Lambe M, Hultman C, Torrang A, et al. (2006) Maternal smoking during pregnancy and school performance at age 15. *Epidemiology* **17**: 524–530.

Lassen K, Oei TPS (1998) Effects of maternal cigarette smoking during pregnancy on long-term physical and cognitive parameters of child development. *Addict Behav* **23**: 635–653.

Linnet KM, Dalosgaard S, Obel C (2003) Maternal lifestyle factors in pregnancy risk of attention deficit hyper-activity disorder and associated behaviors: review of the current evidence. *Am J Psychiatry* **160**: 1028–1040.

Martin LT, McNamara M, Milot A, et al. (2008) Correlates of smoking before, during, and after pregnancy. *Am J Health Behav* **32**: 272–282.

Martin RP, Dombrowski SC, Mullis C, et al. (2006) Smoking during pregnancy: association with childhood temperament, behavior, and academic performance. *J Pediatr Psychol* **31**: 490–500.

Maughan B, Taylor C, Taylor A, et al. (2001) Pregnancy smoking and childhood conduct problems: a causal association? *J Child Psychol Psychiatry* **42**: 1021–1028.

Maughan B, Taylor A, Caspi A, Moffitt TE (2004) Prenatal smoking and early childhood conduct problems: testing genetic and environmental explanations of the association. *Arch Gen Psychiatry* **61**: 836–843.

McFarlane J, Parker B, Soeken K (1996) Physical abuse, smoking, and substance use during pregnancy: prevalence, interrelationships, and effects on birth weight. *J Obstet Gynecol Neonatal Nurs* **25**: 313–320.

Milner AD, Rao H, Greenough A (2007) The effects of antenatal smoking on lung function and respiratory symptoms in infants and children. *Early Hum Dev* **83**: 707–711.

Montgomery SM, Ekbom A (2002) Smoking during pregnancy and diabetes mellitus in a British longitudinal birth cohort. *BMJ* **324**: 26–27.

Monuteaux MC, Blacker D, Biederman J, et al. (2006) Maternal smoking during pregnancy and offspring overt and covert conduct problems: a longitudinal study. *J Child Psychol Psychiatry* **47**: 883–890.

Office for National Statistics (2006) *Statistics on Smoking: England, 2006*. London: The Information Centre, NHS.

Oken E, Huh SY, Taveras EM, et al. (2005) Associations of maternal prenatal smoking with child adiposity and blood pressure. *Obes Res* **13**: 2021–2028.

Paarlberg KM, Vingerhoets AJJM, Passchier J, et al. (1999) Smoking status in pregnancy is associated with daily stressors and low well-being. *Psychol Health* **14**: 87–96.

Paneth N (1995) The problem of low birth weight. *Future Child* **5**: 19–34.

Peacock JL, Cook DG, Carey IM, et al. (1998) Maternal cotinine level during pregnancy and birthweight for gestational age. *Int J Epidemiol* **27**: 647–656.

Pickett KE, Wakschlag LS, Rathouz PJ, et al. (2002) The working-class context of pregnancy smoking. *Health Place* **8**: 167–175.

Pickett KE, Wakschlag LS, Dai L, Leventhal BL (2003) Fluctuations of maternal smoking during pregnancy. *Obstet Gynecol* **101**: 140–147.

Pickett KE, Rathouz PJ, Kasza K, et al. (2005) Self-reported smoking, cotinine levels, and patterns of smoking in pregnancy. *Paediatr Perinat Epidemiol* **19**: 368–376.

Pickett KE, Wood C, Adamson J, et al. (2008) Meaningful differences in maternal smoking behaviour during pregnancy: implications for infant behavioural vulnerability. *J Epidemiol Community Health* **62**: 318–324.

Pickett KE, Kasza K, Biesecker G, et al. (2009a) Women who remember, women who do not: a methodological study of maternal recall of smoking in pregnancy. *Nicotine Tob Res* **11**: 1166–1174.

Pickett KE, Wilkinson RG, Wakschlag LS (2009b) The psychosocial context of pregnancy smoking and quitting in the Millennium Cohort Study. *J Epidemiol Community Health* **63**: 474–480.

Pritchard CW (1994) Depression and smoking in pregnancy in Scotland. *J Epidemiol Community Health* **48**: 377–382.

Resnick MB, Gueorgguieva RV, Carter RL, et al. (1999) The impact of low birth weight, perinatal conditions, and sociodemographic factors on educational outcome in kindergarten. *Pediatrics* **104**: e74.

Rogers JM (2008) Tobacco and pregnancy: overview of exposures and effects. *Birth Defects Res C Embryo Today* **84**: 1–15.

Roza SJ, Verhulst FC, Jaddoe VWV, et al. (2009) Maternal smoking during pregnancy and child behaviour problems: the Generation R Study. *Int J Epidemiol* **38**: 680–689.

Salihu HM, Wilson RE (2007) Epidemiology of prenatal smoking and perinatal outcomes. *Early Hum Dev* **83**: 713–720.

Salihu HM, Aliyuh MH, Pierre-Louis BJ, Alexander GR (2003) Levels of excess infant deaths attributable to maternal smoking during pregnancy in the United States. *Matern Child Health J* **7**: 219–227.

Sasco AJ, Vainio H (1999) From in utero and childhood exposure to parental smoking to childhood cancer: a possible link and the need for action. *Hum Exp Toxicol* **18**: 192–291.

Sellström E, Arnoldsson G, Bremberg S, Hjern A (2008) The neighbourhood they live in: does it matter to women's smoking habits during pregnancy? *Health Place* **14**: 155–166.

Sen B, Swaminathan S (2007) Maternal prenatal substance use and behavior problems among children in the U.S. *J Ment Health Policy Econ* **10**: 189–206.

Silberg JL, Parr T, Neale MC, et al. (2003) Maternal smoking during pregnancy and risk to boys' conduct disturbance: an examination of the causal hypothesis. *Biol Psychiatry* **53**: 130–135.

Slotkin TA (1998) Fetal nicotine or cocaine exposure: which one is worse? *J Pharmacol Exp Ther* **285**: 931–945.

Stocks J, Dezateux C (2003) The effect of parental smoking on lung function and development during infancy. *Respirology* **8**: 266–285.

Svanes C, Jarvis D, Chinn S, et al. (2004) Parental smoking in childhood and adult obstructive lung disease: results from the European Community Respiratory Health Survey. *Thorax* **59**: 295–302.

Thue E, Schei B, Jacobsen G (1995) Psychosocial factors and heavy smoking during pregnancy among parous Scandinavian women. *Scand J Prim Health Care* **13**: 182–187.

US Surgeon General (2001) *Smoking and Women's Health. A Report of the Surgeon General.* Rockville, MD: US Department of Health and Human Services.

Von Kries R, Toschke AM, Koletzko B, Slikker WJ (2002) Maternal smoking during pregnancy and childhood obesity. *Am J Epidemiol* **156**: 954–961.

Wakefield M, Gillies P, Graham H, et al. (1993) Characteristics associated with smoking cessation during pregnancy among working class women. *Addiction* **88**: 1423–1430.

Wakschlag LS, Hans SL (2002) Maternal smoking during pregnancy and conduct problems in high-risk youth: a developmental framework. *Dev Psychopathol* **14**: 351–369.

Wakschlag LS, Pickett KE, Cook E, et al. (2002) Maternal smoking during pregnancy and severe antisocial behavior in offspring: a review. *Am J Public Health* **92**: 966–74.

Wakschlag LS, Pickett KE, Middlecamp MK, et al. (2003) Pregnant smokers who quit, pregnant smokers who don't: does history of problem behavior make a difference? *Soc Sci Med* **56**: 2449–2460.

Wakschlag LS, Leventhal BL, Pine DS, et al. (2006a) Elucidating early mechanisms of developmental psychopathology: the case of prenatal smoking and disruptive behavior. *Child Dev* **77**: 893–906.

Wakschlag LS, Pickett KE, Kasza KE, Loeber R (2006b) Is prenatal smoking associated with a developmental pattern of conduct problems in young boys? *J Am Acad Child Adolesc Psychiatry* **45**: 461–467.

Wakschlag LS, Kistner EO, Pine DS, et al. (2009) Interaction of prenatal exposure to cigarettes and MAOA genotype in pathways to youth antisocial behavior. *Mol Psychiatry* (epub ahead of print) doi: 10.1038/mp.2009.22.

Wang X, Wypij D, Gold DR, et al. (1994) A longitudinal study of the effects of parental smoking on pulmonary function in children 6–18 years. *Am J Respir Crit Care Med* **149**: 1420–1425.

Weaver K, Campbell R, Mermelstein R, Wakschlag L (2008) Pregnancy smoking in context: the influence of multiple levels of stress. *Nicotine Tob Res* **10**: 1065–1073.

Zalacain M, Sierrasesumaga L, Larrannaga C, Patinno-Garcia A (2006) Effects of benzopyrene-7,8-diol-9,10-epoxide (BPDE) in vitro and of maternal smoking in vivo on micronuclei frequencies in fetal cord blood. *Pediatr Res* **60**: 180–184.

12
MANAGEMENT OF THE EFFECTS OF PRENATAL DRUGS IN CHILDREN OF DRUG-ABUSING PARENTS

Faye Macrory and Michael Murphy

The high prevalence of drug and alcohol use by adults in the USA and Europe exposes millions of children to parental drug and alcohol use disorders (Compton et al. 2007). Attempts to eradicate drugs from Western societies have been largely unsuccessful, and drugs and alcohol continue to be attractive to many young people, often initially in a so-called recreational setting, and inevitably resulting in pregnancies affected by substance use (Macrory and Emmerson 2007). Those active in the care of pregnant women and their infants, whether in the maternity, neonatal, paediatric or other involved services, need to be fully aware of the short- and longer-term implications of drug and alcohol use on both child health outcomes and parenting.

Parental drug and alcohol use can and does have a significant impact on parenting capacity, with obvious implications for child welfare. Characterized by secrecy and denial, there are a range of barriers to accessing services, with parents often falling through gaps in agency provision, resulting in a failure to fully meet children's needs (Kroll and Taylor 2003). Working with parental substance misuse presents professionals across disciplines with a range of practice dilemmas in assessment, intervention, and ensuring both the 'visibility' of children and effective interagency working.

This chapter aims to explore the physical, psychological and social outcomes of pre- and postnatal exposure of children to parental drug and alcohol use. We will examine interventions currently employed to alleviate some of the effects of that exposure on children and to protect them from further harm, and will then go on to explore the potentially difficult decision-making processes about safeguarding children or protecting them by removal from the family home. We will also offer an insight into some of the personal dilemmas encountered by parents, children and the practitioners who work with them.

It is important to note at an early stage that children and parents who are caught up in substance-misuse problems experience all the normal desires, conflicts and difficulties of family life. What they also find is that drug and alcohol problems can exaggerate family difficulties and introduce new conflicts of interest, which they then find difficult or impossible to cope with.

Although occasionally problematic for the individual user, the experimental or recreational use of drugs does not always negatively impact on family life. It is the long-term, dependent and often chaotic misuse of drugs and alcohol that is far more destructive to the family: "a compulsion or desire to continue taking a drug or drugs in order to feel good or avoid feeling bad" (SCODA 1997). In the longer term, dependence can thus impact on parenting, affecting mood, behaviour, emotional availability and overall health. The combination of these factors has a huge potential to radically impact on the parents' response to the child and to the wider family's lifestyle.

These tensions and potential conflicts of interest will be explored within the current political and personal context. Many authors (Harbin and Murphy 2000, Kroll and Taylor 2003, Kearney et al. 2005, Barnard 2007) have commented on the significant similarities from a child's point of view between the impact of drugs and alcohol. Other research from Britain and the USA (Murphy et al. 1991, Forrester and Harwin 2008) suggests that harm from familial alcohol misuse may actually exceed harm from drug misuse. As problematic substance misuse rarely sits in isolation from other complexities these must necessarily form part of the debate.

It is not possible to provide definitive answers but we explore the issues surrounding the difficult and sometimes painful part of the responsibilities that professionals must carry and navigate when working in this minefield of multiple needs. We also hope to offer some practice guidance to support professionals to make decisions in the best interests of children and their families.

The UK context

The multiple and complex issues involved in working with families who have substance misuse problems have long been evident. While the Government response to the issue in the UK has taken some time to emerge, there is now a growing volume of policy documents committed to delivering integrated and focused frontline services. We know that between 250 000 and 350 000 children are affected by parental drug misuse in the UK and up to 1.3 million children are living with parents who misuse alcohol (O'Kane 2009). The evidence also shows that parental substance misuse "causes serious harm to children at every age from conception to adulthood", one of six key messages from *Hidden Harm*, a report from the UK government's Advisory Council on the Misuse of Drugs (2003).

That report revealed perhaps for the first time the true extent of the impact of parental problematic drug use in the UK, representing approximately 2–3% of under-16-year-olds in England and Wales and 4–6% of the same age-group in Scotland. The complexity of the situation also means it is not possible to determine the precise effects on any individual child. However, a large proportion of the children of problem drug users are clearly being disadvantaged and damaged in many ways, and few will escape entirely unharmed. Subsequently in 2008 the government published a new four-year drug strategy that for the first time included a strand on improving family life around substances (Home Office 2008).

The first report of the Families at Risk Review, *Reaching Out: Think Family* (Cabinet Office 2006), also provided a rigorous analysis of what we mean by families at risk, i.e. a shorthand for families with multiple and complex problems such as unemployment, poor mental health and substance misuse. The focus includes those who already have complex and ongoing problems as well as those who are at risk of developing them.

The English context has also been radically affected by the deaths of Victoria Climbié (Laming 2003) and Baby Peter (OFSTED 2008, Laming 2009). However, it should be noted that significant substance misuse was not the most obvious problem in either of these families. In the Scottish context, however, there have been a worrying number of high-profile deaths of young children in families with chronic substance-misuse problems (O'Brien et al. 2003) where the male carer was convicted of the death of their child.

Management in pregnancy

The change of title of the seventh Report of the Confidential Enquiries into Maternal Deaths in the UK, from *Why Mothers Die* to *Saving Mothers' Lives* more aptly reflects the purpose of this continuing, crucial, component of maternity service provision in the UK (Lewis 2007). In recent years, the Enquiry has expanded its remit to cover wider public health issues, and its findings and recommendations in this area have played a major part in helping the development of other, broader, policies to help reduce inequalities for the poorest families and for socially excluded women. Without this current report, for example, it would not be known that, even in the UK in the 21st century, the most deprived pregnant women have a risk of dying that is seven times higher than that of the broad majority of other pregnant women (Lewis 2007).

Ninety-three of the women whose deaths were assessed for the period 2003–2005 had problems with substance misuse. Of these, 52 were drug addicts, another 32 were occasional drug users, and the remaining women were alcohol dependent. Seven died in early pregnancy before they could access maternity care. It is noteworthy that the majority of deaths due to, or associated with, substance misuse occurred more than 42 days after delivery. For women who are recruited by drug and alcohol services into treatment while pregnant, it is a matter of concern that these treatments are largely directed at stabilizing the substance misuse during the pregnancy and that, after delivery, particularly if the child is removed from the woman's care, many of these women disengage themselves or are discharged from treatment. Therefore, further efforts are required to retain substance-misusing women in treatment programmes after pregnancy (Lewis 2007).

Good maternal health and high-quality maternity care throughout pregnancy and after delivery have a marked effect on the health and life chances of newborn babies, on their prospects for healthy development and on their resilience to problems encountered later in life (Department for Education and Science 2004, Department of Health 2007).

The maternity standard of the National Service Framework for Children, Young People and Maternity Services (Department of Health 2004) sets out the need for flexible services. This highlights in particular the serious impact that physical, emotional and/or sexual abuse, neglect and domestic abuse/violence, parental mental ill health and substance-misuse problems have on every aspect of a child's health, development and well-being.

The high cost of these problems to individuals and to society underpins the statutory responsibility of all health organizations in the UK to make arrangements to safeguard and promote the welfare of children under the Children Act (2004). The difficult issues involved in the crossover between parental substance misuse and the safeguarding of children have been obvious in the USA and in many other developed countries for the last 25 years. Murphy et al. (1991) revealed the significant link between parental substance misuse and child-care court proceedings in Boston, Massachusetts. Dore et al. (1995) discussed the impact on child-care case loads of the increasing use of crack cocaine by poor urban mothers. In a study from Canada, Walsh et al. (2003) reported a twofold increase in exposure to physical or sexual abuse for children with a parent who had substance-misuse problems, this risk increasing incrementally from father only, to mother only, to both parents affected by substance misuse. That study did not include the additional increased likelihood of exposure to neglect. In a study of children brought into care because of child maltreatment, Besinger et al. (1999) discovered that parental substance misuse was a factor in 79% of the sample.

Whilst national governments have sought, although usually unsuccessfully, to reduce the supply of drugs into communities, international child-care systems have been caught within a very difficult dichotomy in attempting to support children of substance-misusing parents. The dilemma lies between deciding whether to keep them within their own families (in spite of some poor outcomes for some children) or to take a more punitive approach by using court and care systems to place them in alternative care (Dore et al. 1995). Parents' responses to this dichotomy are sometimes logical from an individual, but not an organizational, viewpoint. Thus Lam et al. (2004) claim that "mothers who abuse drugs and are not engaged in treatment services may be especially vulnerable to being separated from their children." Yet more research indicates that becoming a parent may lead some mothers not to go into treatment because of increased demands from child care (McMahon et al. 2002) or because of stigma and fear of child removal (Kearney et al. 1994).

In 1985, Dr Mary Hepburn established the Glasgow Women's Reproductive Health Service (UK) for women who were at most risk of the negative impacts of social deprivation, poverty and drug misuse. This community-based service continues to offer sympathetic, supportive and non-judgemental help, which through a multidisciplinary approach addresses the whole range of problems, both medical and non-medical, encountered by the women and their families.

As a consultant midwife since 2001, Faye Macrory leads the Manchester Specialist Midwifery Service. This provides a city-wide service to women and their families where drug/alcohol use and mental health is problematic, and also supports and coordinates care for pregnant women who test positive for the human immunodeficiency virus (HIV). The team currently consists of five specialist midwives and a secretary. Service provision is firmly rooted in the sphere of public health, and embraces all aspects of a vulnerable, socially excluded lifestyle. The service involves close collaboration across a wide range of health and social care agencies in addressing the complex issues associated with mental health, domestic abuse/violence, sexual abuse, prostitution and HIV. Training is also provided to all relevant agencies.

Prentice (2007) is clear that a specialist midwife is ideally placed to coordinate the involvement of acute hospital trusts, community midwives, general practitioners, mental health and drug services, social services and sometimes the police. The aim during pregnancy is to engage the client with these multiple agencies, to help bring a degree of order to their lifestyles and to reduce the harm associated with substance misuse. Abstinence and detoxification are not necessarily the priority as the financial, psychological, social and domestic problems associated with drug misuse are often of greater importance than the physical and medical concerns.

The antenatal care for women with drug and/or alcohol problems has exactly the same aims as for any woman, namely to keep her in good health and to give her baby the best start in life. However, achieving these aims is often complicated by the pharmacological effects of the drugs and the ongoing complexities of the accompanying lifestyle. With opiate use, stability is a key priority. Encouraging women to be completely drug-free for the first time in many years by the time of delivery leaves them vulnerable both to overdose and to being unable to cope with the demands of a new baby. Methadone maintenance treatment introduces a routine, health-care opportunities and engagement with services that optimizes consistent parenting.

Lewis (2007) reminds us that while there are examples of truly outstanding integrated care, it is far more usual to find a lack of integration between community midwifery and specialist midwives and hospital-based obstetric care. An increasing number of maternity services within the UK have appointed specialist midwives to coordinate care for substance-misusing women and to promote interagency care planning. Funding is also often jointly commissioned with local drug and alcohol strategy teams, leading to shared responsibility and improved communication. Lewis recommends that integration be achieved in each maternity service, ideally by joint service provision between addiction services and maternity services for these vulnerable women, or, where that is not possible, by joint discussion of care plans between services to improve the information held by each.

International perspectives

Since the 1980s, practice in the UK has offered public health and harm-reduction initiatives rather than just crime control. In some parts of the USA policy and practice remain quite punitive, but since the early 1990s maternal drug research emerging from the UK has challenged conventional studies and practice in North American countries (Macrory and Boyd 2007). Although it is an ongoing challenge, Canada has adopted harm reduction as a national drug strategy. Among other initiatives, Fir Square opened in 2003 as the first programme in Canada to provide women-centred harm-reduction care for pregnant substance-using mothers and their infants in a hospital setting.

Although some harm-reduction programmes do exist in the USA (see Chapter 13), US federal law and some states reject harm-reduction approaches and continue to support punitive approaches to women suspected of maternal drug use. In fact, since the 1980s the regulation of mothers and challenges to women's reproductive autonomy have increased in the USA (Macrory and Boyd 2007).

The European Collaborating Centres in Addiction Studies maternal health monograph (Baldacchino et al. 2003) attempts to identify the common issues across the sociocultural context of European countries. It explores both the recognition of the problem and the policies and practices in the maternal health care of individuals with a drug-abuse problem

(Ghodse 2003). It is quite evident that while there are common features and similarities of views, there are also differences even in the same country between practitioners in the field as to what should be the most appropriate intervention. While everyone seems to agree with counselling, support and social care, not everyone shares the same view on prescribing, dosage, abstinence and the role of substitute prescribing.

It seems clear that, without appropriate training and education, staff may adopt an approach to care based on a moral view and personal opinion, rather than one where understanding and respect for the individual can lead to more effective engagement and improved outcomes.

Immediate postnatal management and neonatal withdrawal

All first-time parents will experience considerable change and challenge when the normal problem of looking after yourself, either as a single adult or within a couple, is superimposed upon the problem of caring for a highly dependent child with multiple needs (Klee et al. 2002). Usual caring resources may prove to be insufficient as the infant may demand much more than young adults are able to give. However, when a parent is additionally dealing with significant substance dependence, the early weeks in their new baby's life are crucially important. The combination of a parent struggling with drug/alcohol dependence and the intensive demands of a newborn baby is extremely stressful, particularly if the infant is dealing with the effects of drug withdrawal. As Klee et al. (2002) point out, "The withdrawing baby is harder to comfort and can seem rejecting and the mother often needs reassurance that her mothering skills are not at fault."

Neonatal drug withdrawal is a common problem in populations where there is a ready availability of drugs taken for therapeutic, recreational or addiction purposes by pregnant women (Kuschel 2007). The clinical picture of infants withdrawing from in utero substance exposure has been termed neonatal abstinence syndrome (NAS), the assessment and management of which can pose difficulties for staff and families. The first reports of NAS were published in 1979 and guidelines for care were developed in the USA (Macrory and Boyd 2007). There is, however, a lack of prospective studies and few research studies specifically assessing the merits of one management approach over another, with most reports predominantly describing experience with infants exposed to opioids such as heroin, morphine and methadone (see Chapter 8). A study carried out by Theis et al. (1997) suggests that a morphine derivative appears to be the most effective therapy when treating opioid withdrawal in infants.

Increasingly, pharmacological treatment of NAS is not considered essential but rather is used as part of a general management strategy of comforting as well as sedation. Other causes of irritability need to be excluded before assuming that all the symptoms are due to NAS. A short course of treatment or even one dose of opiate can enable the infant to regain its normal pattern of sleeping and feeding.

Breastfeeding is now widely recommended as an effective intervention in reducing the need for the infant to receive treatment for NAS. A recent study by Dryden et al. (2009) found that breastfeeding for more than 72 hours significantly reduced the need for treatment of NAS. Apart from the benefits of breast milk and the way that breastfeeding soothes agitated infants, researchers noted that small traces of the drugs taken by the mother are excreted into the breast milk, thus lessening the infant's withdrawal symptoms. However, women should be informed that they must *never* give the infant any of their own medication because of the risk of sudden death.

At its most extreme in the days immediately after the birth, the 'relational fit' (Hackett 2003) of parent to child may also be problematic. Alison (2000) noted, "Those babies experiencing withdrawal symptoms in the newborn period were most likely to have the poorest social outcomes, presumably because these were the babies of mothers who had continued drug taking right up until the birth." There were 75 child protection conferences held for 25 of the children in their study, and the majority of the initial conferences were held as a result of an incident or because of concerns about neglect. Alison also found that the use of drugs was associated with increased referral to child-care departments and increased levels of contact with child-care practitioners even at relatively low levels of drug use.

Impact of drug taking on the child

Five factors need to be taken into account in assessing the impact of parental drug taking on the child's welfare: (1) substance dependence itself; (2) partner conflict; (3) parenting style and capacity; (4) impact on family routine and lifestyle; (5) response of the child-care system. Not all will impact directly on the child, but each factor may combine with other factors to increase the impact of substance-misuse problems on the health and social well-being of the parent and child.

Substance dependence may impact on the adult user as an individual. Chaotic use of substances is likely to increase the risk of health problems (up to and including death through overdose), unemployment, arrest, incarceration and, at many levels, alienation from extended family and friends (Barnard 2007, Murphy et al. 2007). These consequences for the individual parent often indicate significant loss for the child (Kearney et al. 2005, Murphy and Ingham 2007).

The use of substances generally has been a source of conflict between partners for hundreds of years (Gordon 1989). Where one partner uses substances in a dependent or chaotic fashion, this can significantly impact on the quality and viability of the couple's relationship. In partnerships where both partners are dependent, the relationship can be similarly negatively affected, and furthermore, with joint dependency, simultaneous drug treatment and change can become overwhelming for the couple and the whole family. In the British child-care system we have become increasingly concerned about the co-occurrence of substance misuse with significant domestic violence and/or child abuse (Cleaver et al. 1999, 2007). Although many children can maintain a level of resilience in the face of a substance problem that occurs alone, it becomes far more difficult when that problem is interlaced with significant partner or family violence (Velleman and Templeton 2006).

In the wake of the Victoria Climbié (Laming 2003) and Baby Peter cases in the UK (Laming 2003, 2009; OFSTED 2008), we are also concerned at the frequency with which new and unknown partners are introduced into the lives of vulnerable children. Where substance misuse and domestic violence are present within a relationship, it may be even more difficult for the original parent to protect the child.

Parenting style and ability is a complex phenomenon that is influenced by an individual's experience of parenting, their view on the role of a parent, and their current and functional capability to undertake a parenting role (Cleaver et al. 1999, Harbin and Murphy 2000, Hackett 2003). A significant substance dependency can interfere with a parent's 'normal' parenting style. In this way significant drug use exaggerates normal parenting dilemmas – how to prioritize their infant's needs while still meeting their own and their partner's needs. A substance dependency always complicates this dilemma by increasing the parent's needs. Where resources, both financial and psychological, are finite, this increase in parental need can often only be met at the expense of the child's needs (Mahoney and Makechnie 2001, Kearney et al. 2005).

According to Velleman and Templeton (2006), the impact of substance use on family routine and lifestyle is related not to the type or style of substance use but rather to the quality and consistency of that routine and lifestyle. "If cohesion and harmony can be maintained in the face of substance misuse then there is a high chance that the child will not go on to have problems." Nair et al. (2003) claim that it is the combination of risk factors that predicts maternal stress and child mistreatment, and if the number of these factors can be kept low or reduced, child maltreatment is far less likely to occur.

At the same time as the parents are struggling to come to terms with the demands of the new baby, with any problems with NAS, and with their own substance dependence, the child-care system can also be struggling to know how to respond to that family situation. Uncertainty on the part of professionals in responding to the family's needs will exacerbate the problems.

Parenting assessments and interventions

Substance misuse affects parents, their children and whole families. The central challenge for assessment is to determine the extent to which a parent's drug taking, in the longer term, reduces their ability to parent so that their child's life becomes damaged beyond effective repair, or the child suffers significant harm. When is this point reached? How can this be effectively assessed and managed? These are the issues that all professionals working in the community need to bear in mind whether they are involved with parents or their children or both (Weir and Douglas 1999). Beck-Sander (1999) (in discussing ways to reduce conflict between services) suggests that a fundamental caveat of all risk-management work is that not all risks posed by parents to their children can be prevented. At best, risks can only be reduced. It is not even feasible to aim to identify all risks – and any service adopting this aim would be doomed to failure, with workers becoming overcautious in a vain attempt to avoid any possible harm occurring. Beck-Sander goes on to say that, as risk is sometimes unpredictable, harm may still occur, and, in this event, workers would be vulnerable to scapegoating, as this would be seen as a service failure. Such unrealistic, risk-averse services would then have such high expectations of partner agencies as to make interagency cooperation unworkable. Calder (2003) agrees that risk avoidance in child care is impossible to achieve, and so risk management and risk reduction is the preferred goal.

The task of risk management is therefore to carefully weigh up the harms and benefits in a calculation to reduce potential conflict between services and effectively protect the child.

What may appear a 'reasonable risk' (i.e benefit outweighs harm) to one service may appear unreasonable (i.e. harm outweighs benefit) to another (Beck-Sander 1999). Risk assessment in itself presents an enormous challenge because of the highly variable course of associated adult problems including mental illness and substance misuse, and the balance of risk may need frequent reevaluation.

Weir and Douglas (1999) also remind us that staff working with children and families need to understand precisely how a particular parent's mental health problem affects his or her parenting ability when they are quantifying the impact of adult mental health problems on individual children. Hart and Powell (2006) state that the questions they pose below could and should be as readily considered for parents with substance-misuse problems when making an assessment of parenting capability. Broadly speaking, Weir and Douglas suggest that the following concerns should be addressed.

• When does an adult's mental health/substance misuse problem pose a conflict of interest within a family?
• When do these factors pose risks for the safety and well-being of their child?
• How does parenting capacity become impaired in these circumstances?
• What is a child's capacity to tolerate the changed and often detrimental care that he or she may receive?
• How can those risks be assessed, and how can they be managed?
• Who decides when those risks become acceptable?
• What services need to be available to meet the needs of both adults and children in these circumstances?
• How do professionals working in these circumstances need to be trained and supported?
• What can be done to bridge the gulf between the professionals who are trying to meet the respective needs of children and parents?
• How can the different agencies involved ensure consistent practice and good communication between each other?

While it can be very difficult to separate out the effects of specific parental mental disorder, the severity of parental illness is an important predictor of difficult behaviour in their children. A high level of psychosocial disadvantage is also of great importance (Sameroff and Seifer 1990). In understanding risk and protective factors, many disciplines are in agreement about the nature of risk factors that predispose children and adolescents to problem behaviours, and the protective factors that may mitigate against negative outcomes (Velleman and Templeton 2006). It is certainly the case that children exposed to more than one adult-oriented problem will often find the road to resilience more difficult (Cleaver et al. 1999, 2007). Children who experience ante-/postnatal complications (including NAS or fetal alcohol syndrome), who live in extreme poverty or in constant conflict, and who are exposed to multiple traumatic events are known to be at significant risk for developing substance misuse and mental health disorders in later life (Table 12.1).

As Weir and Douglas (1999) state, the combination of a parent with severe mental health problems with or without substance-misuse problems and a child who may be in need of protection demands an almost impossibly high level of skill in risk assessment and decision making. The stakes are high, with severe injury to the child or loss of liberty of the adult,

TABLE 12.1
Parental drug misuse: potential risk and resilience factors for children living within drug- or alcohol-abusing families

Area	Risk factors	Resilience factors
Environmental/contextual	High drug availability to parent Low socio-economic status Family association with other drug users Family association with delinquency	Protective social networks High socio-economic status
Family factors	Multiple substance users in household Poor parental monitoring Parental rejection Poor disciplinary practices Family conflict/divorce Domestic violence Low parental expectations Chaotic lifestyle Family disruption including unemployment	Non-using adult within family Supportive wider family Protective older siblings Cohesive and stable family unit High-quality parent–child attachment High level of parental supervision and stimulating home environment Predictable family routine
Parental history	Early onset of risky parental behaviour, smoking, drinking Early onset of illicit drug use Rapid escalation in substance misuse Multiple drug use by parents Parental resistance to treatment	Absence of early loss or separation Late onset of risky behaviour and substance misuse Early engagement with treatment
Maternal factors	Mental health problems Strain/stress Depression Aggression Impulsivity/hyperactivity Antisocial personality Sensation seeking	Absence of coincident mental health problems High self-esteem Low impulsivity Easy temperament
Educational	Poor parental school performance Low educational aspirations Poor parental commitment to formal education Absence, truancy and drop-out Little formal educational support	Supportive educational placement Good teacher relations High parental education aspirations Educational success

or both, the possible outcomes of professional error. Even with regular, good-quality supervision, staff may be asked to manage situations for which they do not have sufficient personal or professional training or experience. Where lives are at stake, can we be sure that the present system is good enough?

When assessing the impact of parental substance misuse on child well-being there are three key elements to the assessment (Fig. 12.1). As Murphy and Harbin (2003) point out, "The job of the assessment is to discover the impact of the particular style and type of substance use on the parenting capacity of adults in that particular family, and then to gauge that combined impact on the development and safety of individual children within that family."

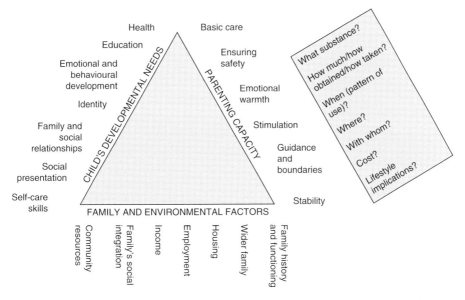

Fig. 12.1. Key elements in the assessment of the impact of parental substance misuse on a child's well-being.

The first element is to assess the substance issue – what is the relationship of this parent to their substance(s) of choice? What do they use, how, how much, when, with whom, how do they obtain it, and what are the lifestyle implications of that relationship? A study by Pilowsky et al. (2001) of intravenous drug users in the USA found that parents who were able to minimize the risk factors in their drug use were far more likely to retain care of their children than those parents who engaged in high-risk drug practices.

The second key component of the assessment is to track that relationship with substance across to parenting capacity, capability and style. How does that relationship impact upon the parent's ability to provide basic care, safety, emotional warmth, stimulation, guidance and stability (Department of Health 2000)? Alternatively, because opiate misuse is so closely associated with child neglect (Forrester 2000, Stevenson 2007), how does that relationship with substance impact on the parent's capacity to provide for the child's basic needs, to supervise (particularly around safety) and to be emotionally available to the child? Significant substance dependence will always have some impact on parenting capacity, but some dependent parents do manage to maintain and operate some levels of parenting capacity and availability.

Lastly and most importantly, how does the relationship with substance misuse and the subsequent effect on parenting capacity actually impact on the child's development and developmental needs, e.g. health, education, emotional and behavioural development, identity, family and social relationships, social presentation and self-care skills (Department of Health 2000)? Where some level of parenting capacity is maintained (often through

TABLE 12.2
UK thresholds in child care

1. Universal – a child for whom universal services will be sufficient

2. Targeted services for vulnerable children

3. Child in need (Children Act 1989) requiring specialist provision

4. Section 47 inquiry – child protection inquiry or investigation to see if significant harm has occurred

5. Child protection plan – child in need of safeguarding/protective services, by an interagency group

6. Care proceedings – separation from birth family and placed in residential or foster care

7. Adoption – final separation from birth family and permanent placement with alternative family

a non-dependent partner or extended family member), there may be less impact on the child's development; however, when the impact on the child's development is high, this is when thresholds for more intrusive intervention should come into operation and the likelihood of significant harm to the child should be assessed by a formalized child protection investigation (Table 12.2; see below).

Statutory and legal interventions

THE PROBLEM OF NUMBERS

With 250 000–350 000 children affected by parental drug dependence in the UK, there is a predictable dilemma for child-care systems. The safeguarding and care system in Britain is set up to deal with very small numbers of children who may suffer significant developmental delay or harm. The use of drugs on its own is not, in itself, a criterion for inclusion in the safeguarding or care system, but the impact of drug misuse on parenting and subsequent impact on child development can be grounds to include children in either system (Murphy et al. 1991, Forrester 2000, Forrester and Harwin 2008). It is not possible for the majority of children who are brought up in substance-misusing households to be included in the safeguarding or care system – if they were, these systems would collapse under sheer weight of numbers. This poses the questions, which children are going to be included in statutory child protection and care systems, and how are the majority of other children going to be protected and supported?

THE PROBLEM OF THRESHOLDS

To manage the problem of numbers requires a range of service provision dependent on the needs of an individual child and family. Exceeding a specific threshold of need (Table 12.2) will result in the provision of a more intensive intervention to protect the child and family. For example,

• at threshold 1, services are delivered to all children in the community

• at threshold 7, a very small number of children are permanently removed from their families to be brought up by another adoptive family.

How do the practitioners in the child-care system collectively measure the right level of response to a particular child and parent in each situation? In the UK at each threshold stage the decision-making mechanisms can be slightly different. At threshold 2 the Common Assessment Framework will try to determine the services required for individual children who are seen as vulnerable. At threshold 3 a multidisciplinary 'Child in Need' interagency meeting should be called to discuss how best to provide a package of specialist services to children in a particular family. For example, a single parent with an opiate addiction, who is relatively stable in treatment services, may be struggling to care for a child with a significant disability. Alternatively, a couple with significant opiate dependency but already well supported by their extended family may need extra support services while they engage in a community detoxification programme.

At thresholds 4 and 5, a child protection inquiry will be followed by an interagency child protection conference and (at threshold 5) a child protection plan, resulting in a core group of practitioners working intensively with the family. This will usually happen when substance-misuse problems are chaotic and are leading to significant family violence/abuse and child neglect.

Example: In the Smith family, chaotic use of cocaine and amphetamine has exaggerated the volatile nature of the parents' relationship. The children are now witnessing significant violence on a daily basis and are showing a strongly negative response to it.

Thresholds 6 and 7 are usually only reached where the impact on parenting and child well-being is so severe that the child is considered to be suffering significant harm, as defined under the Children Act 1989, and requiring removal from the family home.

Example: Jonathan is a 12-month-old child brought up in a family where the drug and alcohol use has become increasingly chaotic. He is showing significant developmental delay and has been locked in his room for long periods of time. He also suffered major burns in a recent house fire when he had been left alone and where neighbours had to break open his door to rescue him.

The ongoing challenge of assessment in substance-misusing families is to attempt to discover the appropriate level of intrusion into individual families (Murphy and Harbin 2003, Hart and Powell 2006). Only a very small proportion of children brought up in substance-misusing families will be taken into care or adopted, with the majority continuing to be supported within their family and community. The question is, how can we collectively establish what level of support or intrusion an individual child or family warrants in order to ensure the child's needs are being met?

INTERAGENCY WORKING

The key to working with children, parents and families where substance misuse is an issue is interagency collaboration, but this may be difficult to achieve (Kearney et al. 2000, Murphy and Oulds 2000, Kroll and Taylor 2003, Cleaver et al. 2007). As well as including all relevant child-care staff and agencies, it is crucial to also include adult substance misuse and adult mental health services that may be working with the individual parent. However, substance and mental health practitioners may employ a very adult-oriented approach to a family's problems, while child-care staff may have a more child-centred focus, and this can lead to significant differences in perspective (Kearney et al. 2000, Murphy and Oulds 2000, Cleaver et al. 2007).

Collaboration should include the collecting and sharing of information, and joint assessment and decision-making about appropriate thresholds and which services and treatments should be provided to both adults and children to try to improve the family's situation. Cleaver et al. (2007) state that the following are crucial to effective interagency collaboration.

- Understanding and respecting the roles and responsibilities of other services
- Good communication across agency boundaries
- Regular contacts and meetings
- Common priorities
- Interagency training
- Knowing what services are available and whom to contact
- Clear guidelines and procedures
- Low staff turnover.

However, research has indicated that these crucial components may be very difficult to achieve (Forrester 2000, Hart and Powell 2006, Forrester and Harwin 2008). Interagency collaboration across the child-care/adult substance treatment divide is beset with multiple structural problems that seem resistant to recent organizational change (Murphy and Oulds 2000, Cleaver et al. 2007). Hallett and Birchall (1992) suggest a four-level typology of co-ordination that involves

1. Collaboration between frontline staff
2. Systematic coordination at planning meetings and child protection conferences
3. Programme coordination with procedures and protocols at all levels
4. Central policy coordination at government level.

It is clear that structural blockages to collaboration can occur at any level. Hart and Powell (2006) discovered in their research in two localities that collaboration at level 1 was quite reasonable, but at level 3 there was a complete lack of procedures and protocols. Forrester (2000) in his research in a local area in London discovered real problems at level 2: "In the 34 most recent case conferences involving substance using parents, only four specialist substance use workers were invited [to the child protection conference]. It is certainly of concern that only two of these workers attended."

It is clear that collaboration at all four levels needs individual, agency and government commitment. It is hoped that the increasing awareness of the need to collaborate will drive positive change.

Building resilience in children and parents (see Table 12.1)
What information is available to inform us how well children respond to different types of treatment and intervention? Forrester and Harwin (2006, 2008) undertook a review of 100 families (186 children) who were referred to four Children and Families agencies in England. Their study identified the factors that were (a) linked with early care interventions, and (b) associated with health and well-being two years after referral. They found that early admission into a drug treatment programme, having a supportive extended family, and the

absence of alcohol-related violence were all associated with more positive outcomes. Conversely, resistance to treatment, late intervention and the presence of alcohol-related violence predicted poorer outcomes for the children concerned.

Velleman and Templeton (2006) outlined the different ways in which children and their parents can develop resilience in the face of their substance-related problems. These include the maintenance of predictability and family routine, positive couple relationships, and, for children, positive relationships with older siblings, the presence of significant other caring adults and success in other arenas, including the school setting. The following approaches have proved useful in helping parents and children to successfully overcome some of the early difficulties in child care associated with substance misuse.

Early and committed entry by parents into treatment has been seen as a key to positive change in child care in families for two decades (Murphy et al. 1991, Forrester and Harwin 2008). Hepburn (2002) stresses the need to treat the mother as a mother first and someone who has a drug problem second: "The challenge for service providers therefore is to provide maternity care which is appropriate to the women's needs and which the women will want to use." In this way the whole treatment programme must concentrate on promoting the joint health and social care of parent and child, and developing a relational fit between mother and child, often in suboptimal social circumstances. In this way Hepburn recommends that treatment services utilize the normal wishes of pregnant and new mothers to control or change aspects of their lifestyle that they acknowledge as being harmful to their child.

Punishment, prosecution or demeaning treatment are also not helpful in obtaining good outcomes for the child (Macrory and Boyd 2007), and Miles et al. (2006) outline how changes in staff perception of mothers and improved working relationships can create significant improvements in outcomes for children and their mothers. In a similar way, although resistance to entry into treatment (Forrester and Harwin 2006) is seen to have a negative impact on child care, entry into treatment (usually involving detoxification or substitute prescribing) is associated with improvements in the welfare of parent and child (Klee and Jackson 1998, McKeganey 2002, Forrester and Harwin 2008). Kearney et al. (2005) and Harbin (2006) claim that there is a need to involve the child fully in the treatment process, particularly if parents repeatedly enter into treatment and relapse.

It is also the case that children who are brought up in substance-misusing families will strive very hard to be resilient, seeking out those children and adults (related and non-related) who can offer stability, optimism in them and belief in their future (Gilligan 2000, Doyle 2006, Velleman and Templeton 2006). This often includes older siblings, family friends and extended family. When children are older they do benefit from direct services (Kearney et al. 2005, Wheeler 2006). In the early stages, it is important that younger children have access to those resilience figures who can offer them the predictability of care that will help them to develop well.

Although substance-misusing parents can be notoriously hard to access (Murphy et al. 1991, Kroll and Taylor 2003, Barnard 2007), if the services that are on offer are seen to be useful, suitable or hopeful (Murphy and Harbin 2006, Murphy et al. 2007), drug-using parents can be very eager users of child-care services. In some family services there was a strong sense that if the project and community workers were prepared to work with "people like us" then they should also work hard for them.

- *Parent:* "If they're prepared to work with us, I'm prepared to work with them."

For others there was a strong sense that they were desperate to participate in a service that might help.

- *Parent:* "This is what I was looking for to do, to see which steps to go forward, 'coz I was at a loss with [the child's] behaviour. Just going round in circles. Every weekend was getting worse."

By offering a concurrent service to children and parents it is possible to encourage the parent (as a parent not an individual) into treatment (Murphy et al. 2007) while at the same time offering a service that helps the child to be resilient. In this way parent and child can benefit in ways that can positively impact on their self-esteem and their relationships with each other (Murphy et al. 2007)

In some ways the stigma of being a drug-using parent can convince the adult that child-care services have little to offer. Outreach work to overcome stigma and access hard-to-reach populations (Macrory 2002) is essential to include parents with substance problems in all services.

External family support

For a significant number of substance-misusing families, extended family care, usually with grandparents, will offer some help towards stability, or an alternative home (Klee and Jackson 1998, Elliott and Watson 2000, Hogan and Higgins 2001, Kearney et al. 2005). However, research also indicates that where grandparents do provide an alternative home, they frequently find it difficult to get the support they need from child-care services. Although kinship care may have some complex dilemmas (Kroll 2007), for individual children the benefits of extended family care can be significant.

Family breakdown

There is a crucial dilemma around the temporary or permanent removal of children from their birth families because of significant drug or alcohol problems. While some children respond by making excellent progress in their care placements (Phillips 2004, Harwin and Forrester 2008), other children may not. The task of re-forming the bond between birth parent and child once a child has been away from home for more than six months can be extremely complex (Bullock et al. 1998). Permanent foster care and adoption should be seen as the right choice if drug problems have been very chronic, for a significant period of time, with no sign of engagement with drug-treatment services or change in lifestyle. Early, realistic, multi-agency prebirth strategy meetings can be used to assess the risks to the child and set realistic goals to be met by the parents, with criteria for success and failure, so that the child may be protected early and removed from the family if required. For the small number of children taken early into permanent care, the long-term outcomes appear positive (Forrester and Harwin 2006). It should be pointed out, however, that although alternative care placements can have beneficial results, further difficulties can emerge (Phillips 2004) that stem from the early experiences of deprivation and neglect and the effects of intrauterine exposure to drugs (see Chapter 8). As a result, children within the care system will require very experienced foster carers or adoptive parents who are aware of the potential long-term problems.

It is also the case that child-care systems seem slower to respond to chronic alcohol problems than to chronic drug problems, even when the impact on children can be as great or more exaggerated (Forrester and Harwin 2006, 2008; Murphy et al. 2007). This can lead to children living in very neglectful or abusive family situations for far longer than is good for their long-term well-being. As recently as September 2009, Martin Narey, the Chief Executive of the UK children's charity Barnado's, has called for less effort to be directed at "fixing families that can't be fixed" and for social workers to be braver about removing children at risk (*Observer* 2009). Acknowledging that his comments could be seen as "illiberal heresy", he went on to say, "I think if social workers were courageous and sought to intervene quickly, and were supported properly in that, we would see far fewer problems … it is by no means out of the ordinary to meet a child whose foster placements run into double figures. There comes a time where we have to accept that it is not working."

In the same article, Phillipa Stroud of the think-tank Centre for Social Justice reacted cautiously to Narey's comments: "If the model is to move children very quickly to adoption, not necessarily from birth but certainly under a year, then that is something we would support. We need far more early intervention to try to stop this disintegration of the family we are seeing, but we would like to see more working with these families. With child protection, all the legislation is actually in place: it's the implementation that is the issue."

Summary and conclusions

Parental substance misuse is an increasing problem in families with multiple needs. It is recognized that children living in dysfunctional environments, where there are drug and alcohol misuse, mental health problems, domestic abuse and financial disadvantage, do not fare well. As Dawe et al. (2008) remind us, there is no one simple solution. Governments must ensure that the needs of children and families with parental substance misuse are prioritized in policy documents. Treatment agencies and services should have an organizational commitment to the provision of family-focused services. Clinicians need to be given support and receive effective ongoing clinical supervision, and managers need to understand the complexity of the work in supporting families with multiple problems and needs. Those of us who work in the substance-misuse field also need to know how to work with psychological trauma in order to make sense of the often chaotic lives and histories of our client group. However, workers also need to recognize when thresholds for more intensive action are reached to protect children effectively from the drift of indecision.

Improvements in services are an investment in the health of future, as well as present, generations. Meaningful and effective interventions have the great potential to have a positive impact on physical and mental health, and on parenting in the long term, to reduce the need for children to be placed into care, and to help break the present, intergenerational, cyclical nature of substance misuse, mental illness, poverty and despair.

As Maya Angelou (quoted in Weir and Douglas 1999) eloquently states, "How is it possible to convince a child of its own worth after removing him from a family which is said to be unworthy, but with whom he identifies?"

REFERENCES

Advisory Council on the Misuse of Drugs (2003) *Hidden Harm. Responding to the Needs of Children of Problem Drug Users.* London: HMSO.

Alison L (2000) What are the risks to children of parental substance misuse? In: Harbin F, Murphy M, eds. *Substance Misuse and Child Care.* Lyme Regis, Dorset: Russell House, pp. 9–21

Baldacchino A, Riglietta M, Corkery J, eds (2003) *Maternal Health and Drug Abuse: Perspectives Across Europe.* Denmark: European Collaborating Centres in Addiction Studies.

Barnard M (2007) *Drug Addiction and Families.* London: Jessica Kingsley.

Beck-Sander A (1999) Relapse prevention: a model for psychosis. *Behav Change* **16**: 191–202.

Besinger B, Garland A, Litrownik A, Landsverk J (1999) Caregiver substance abuse among maltreated children placed in out of home care. *Child Welfare* **78**: 221–239.

Bullock R, Gooch D, Little M (1998) *Children Going Home: The Re-unification of Families.* Aldershot, Hampshire: Ashgate.

Cabinet Office (2006) *Reaching Out: Think Family. Analysis and Themes from the Families at Risk Review.* London: Cabinet Office, Social Exclusion Task Force.

Calder M (2003) *Risk and Child Protection. CareKnowledge Briefing Number 9.* London: OLM CareKnowledge.

Cleaver H, Unell I, Aldgate J (1999) *Children's Needs – Parenting Capacity.* London: HMSO.

Cleaver H, Nicholson D, Tarr S, Cleaver D (2007) *Child Protection, Domestic Violence and Parental Substance Misuse.* London: Jessica Kingsley.

Compton WM, Thomas YF, Stinson FS, Grant BF (2007) Prevalence, correlates, disability, and comorbidity of DSM-IV drug abuse and dependence in the United States. Results from the National Epidemiologic survey on alcohol and related conditions. *Arch Gen Psychiatry* **64**: 566–576.

Dawe S, Harnett P, Frye,S (2008) Think child, think family: how adult specialist services can support children at risk of abuse and neglect. *J Subst Abuse Treat* **22**: 381–390.

Department for Education and Skills (2004) *Every Child Matters: Change for Children.* London: DfES.

Department of Health (2000) *A Framework for the Assessment of Children in Need and Their Families.* London: The Stationery Office.

Department of Health (2004) *National Service Framework for Children, Young People and Maternity Services.* London: The Stationery Office.

Department of Health (2007) *Maternity Matters: Choice, Access and Continuity of Care in a Safe Service.* London: The Stationery Office.

Dore M, Doris J, Wright P (1995) Identifying substance misuse in maltreating families: a child welfare challenge. *Child Abuse Negl* **19**: 531–543.

Doyle C (2006) *Working with Abused Children.* Basingstoke, Hampshire: Palgrave.

Dryden C, Young D, Hepburn M, Mactier H (2009) Maternal methadone use in pregnancy: factors associated with the development of neonatal abstinence syndrome and implications for healthcare resources. *BJOG* **116**: 665–671.

Elliott E, Watson A (2000) Responsible carers, problem drug takers or both? In: Harbin F, Murphy M, eds. *Substance Misuse and Child Care.* Lyme Regis, Dorset: Russell House, pp. 27–38.

Forrester D (2000) Parental substance misuse and child protection in a British sample. *Child Abuse Rev* **9**: 235–246.

Forrester D, Harwin J (2006) Parental substance misuse and child care social work: findings from the first stage of a study of 100 families. *Child Fam Social Work* **11**: 325–335.

Forrester D, Harwin J (2008) Parental substance misuse and child welfare: outcomes for children two years after referral. *Br J Social Work* **38**: 1518–1535.

Ghodse H (2003) Foreword. In: Baldacchino A, Riglietta M, Corkery J, eds (2003) *Maternal Health and Drug Abuse: Perspectives Across Europe.* Denmark: European Collaborating Centres in Addiction Studies.

Gordon L (1989) *Heroes of Their Own Lives.* London: Virago.

Hackett S (2003) A framework for assessing parenting capacity. In: Calder M, Hackett S, eds. *Assessment in Child Care.* Lyme Regis, Dorset: Russell House, pp. 156–171

Hallett C, Birchall E (1992) *Coordination and Child Protection: A Review of the Literature.* London: HMSO.

Harbin F (2006) The roller coaster of change: the process of parental change from a child's perspective. In: Harbin F, Murphy M, eds. *Secret Lives: Growing with Substance.* Lyme Regis, Dorset: Russell House, pp. 80–94.

Harbin F, Murphy M, eds (2000) *Substance Misuse and Child Care.* Lyme Regis, Dorset: Russell House.

Harbin F, Murphy M, eds (2006) *Secret Lives: Growing with Substance: Working with Children Who Live with Substance Misuse.* Lyme Regis, Dorset: Russell House.

Hart D, Powell J (2006) *Adult Drug Problems, Children's Needs: Assessing the Impact of Parental Drug Use.* London: National Children's Bureau.

Hepburn M (2002) Providing care for pregnant women who use drugs. In: Klee H, Jackson M, Lewis S, eds. *Drug Misuse and Motherhood.* London: Routledge, pp. 250–260.

Hogan D, Higgins L (2001) *When Parents Use Drugs: Key Findings from a Study of Children in the Care of Drug Using Parents.* Dublin: Trinity College.

Home Office (2008) *Drugs: Protecting Families and Communities. The 2008–2018 Drugs Strategy.* London: The Stationery Office.

Kearney M, Murphy S, Rosenbaum M (1994) Mothering on crack-cocaine: a grounded theory analysis. *Social Sci Med* **38**: 351–361.

Kearney P, Levin E, Rosen G (2000) *Alcohol, Drug and Mental Health Problems: Working with Families.* London: Social Care Institute for Excellence.

Kearney J, Harbin F, Murphy M, et al. (2005) *The Highs and Lows of Family Life: Familial Substance Misuse from a Child's Perspective.* Bolton, Lancashire: Bolton Area Child Protection Committee.

Klee H, Jackson M (1998) *Illicit Drug Use, Pregnancy and Early Motherhood.* Manchester: Centre for Social Research on Health and Substance Abuse, Manchester Metropolitan University.

Klee H, Jackson M, Lewis S, eds. (2002) *Drug Misuse and Motherhood.* London: Routledge.

Kroll B (2007) A family affair? Kinship care and parental substance misuse: some dilemmas explored. *Child Fam Social Work* **12**: 84–93.

Kroll B, Taylor A (2003) *Parental Substance Misuse and Child Welfare.* London: Jessica Kingsley.

Kuschel C (2007) Managing drug withdrawal in the newborn infant. *Semin Fetal Neonatal Med* **12**: 127–133.

Lam WK, Wechsberg W, Zule W (2004) African-American women who use crack-cocaine: a comparison of mothers who live with and have been separated from their children. *Child Abuse Negl* **28**: 1229–1247.

Laming H (2003) *The Victoria Climbié Inquiry.* London: The Stationery Office.

Laming H (2009) *The Protection of Children in England: a Progress Report.* London: The Stationery Office.

Lewis G, ed (2007) *The Confidential Enquiry into Maternal and Child Death (CEMACH). Saving Mother's Lives: Reviewing Maternal Deaths to Make Motherhood Safer 2003–2005. The Seventh Report on Confidential Enquiries into Maternal Deaths in the United Kingdom.* London: Centre for Maternal and Child Enquiries.

Macrory F (2002) The drug liaison midwife: developing a model of maternity services for drug-using women from conception to creation. In: Klee H, Jackson M, Lewis S, eds. *Drug Misuse and Motherhood.* London: Routledge, pp. 239–249.

Macrory F, Boyd SC (2007) Developing primary and secondary services for drug and alcohol dependent mothers. *Semin Fetal Neonatal Med* **12**: 119–126.

Macrory F, Emmerson A, eds (2007) Drug abuse in pregnancy and effects on the newborn. *Semin Fetal Neonatal Med* **12**: 2 (editorial).

Mahoney C, MacKechnie S (2001) *In a Different World. Parental Drug and Alcohol Use.* Liverpool: Liverpool Health Authority.

McKeganey N, Barnard M, McIntosh J (2002) Paying the price for their parents' drug use: the impact of parental drug use on children. *Drug Educ Prevent Policy* **3**: 233–246.

McMahon T, Winkel J, Suchman N, Luthar S (2002) Drug dependence, parenting responsibilities, and treatment history: why doesn't mom go for help? *Drug Alcohol Depend* **65**: 105–114.

Miles J, Sugumar K, Macrory F, et al. (2006) Methadone exposed newborn infants: outcome after alterations to a service for mothers and infants. *Child Care Health Dev* **33**: 206–212.

Mullally S (2004) Foreword. In: *The Chief Nursing Officer's Review of the Nursing, Midwifery and Health Visiting Contribution to Vulnerable Children and Young People.* London: Department of Health.

Murphy J, Jellinek M, Quinn D, et al. (1991) Substance abuse and serious child mistreatment: prevalence, risk and outcome in a court sample. *Child Abuse Negl* **15**: 197–211.

Murphy M, Harbin F (2000) Background and current context of substance misuse and child care. In: Harbin F, Murphy M, eds. *Substance Misuse and Child Care.* Lyme Regis, Dorset: Russell House, pp. 1–8.

215

Murphy M, Harbin F (2003) The assessment of parental substance misuse and its impact on child care. In: Calder M, Hackett S, eds. *Assessment in Child Care*. Lyme Regis, Dorset: Russell House, pp. 353–361.

Murphy M, Harbin F (2006) What do we know about children and young people who grow up in substance misusing households? In: Harbin F, Murphy M, eds. *Secret Lives: Growing with Substance*. Lyme Regis, Dorset: Russell House, pp. 1–11.

Murphy M, Ingram S (2007) *The Manchester Highs and Lows*. Manchester: University of Salford.

Murphy M, Oulds G (2000) Establishing and developing cooperative links between substance misuse and child protection systems. In: Harbin F, Murphy M, eds. *Substance Misuse and Child Care*. Lyme Regis, Dorset: Russell House, pp. 111–112.

Murphy M, Harbin F, Halligan F, Murphy C (2007) *No Longer Alone. An Evaluation of the Holding Families Project. Final Report*. Manchester: University of Salford.

Nair P, Schuler M, Black M, et al. (2003) Cumulative environmental risk in substance abusing women: early intervention, parenting stress, child abuse potential and child development. *Child Abuse Negl* 27: 997–1017.

O'Brien S, Hammond H, McKinnon M (2003) *Report of the Caleb Ness Inquiry*. Edinburgh: Edinburgh City Council.

Observer (2009) More children should be taken into care at birth, says Barnardo's chief. 6 September 2009.

O'Kane A (2009) Safeguarding children: the role of addiction specialists. *SCANbites* 6(1): 7.

OFSTED (2008) *Joint Area Review Haringey Children's Services Authority Area (Baby Peter)*. London: OFSTED.

Philips R (2004) *Children Exposed to Parental Substance Misuse: Implications for Family Placement*. London: British Association for Adoption and Fostering.

Pilowsky DJ, Lyles CM, Cross SI, et al. (2001) Characteristics of injection drug using parents who retain their children. *Drug Alcohol Depend* 61: 113–122.

Prentice S (2007) Substance misuse in pregnancy. *Obstet Gynaecol Reproduct Med* 17: 272–277.

Sameroff AJ, Seifer R (1990) Early contributions to developmental risk. In: Rolf J, Mastern AS, Cichetti D, et al., eds. *Risk and Protective Factors in the Development of Psychopathology*. Cambridge: Cambridge University Press, pp. 52–66.

SCODA (1997) *Drug Using Parents: Policy Guidelines for Interagency Work*. London: Local Government Association.

Stevenson O (2007) *Neglected Children and their Families*. Oxford: Blackwell.

Theis JGW, Selby P, Ikizler Y, Koren G (1997) Current management of the neonatal abstinence syndrome: a critical analysis of the evidence. *Biol Neonate* 71: 345–356.

Velleman R, Templeton L (2006) Reaching out: promoting resilience in the children of substance misusers. In: Harbin F, Murphy M, eds. *Substance Misuse and Child Care*. Lyme Regis, Dorset: Russell House, pp. 12–27.

Walsh C, MacMillan H, Jamieson E (2003) The relationship between parental substance misuse and child maltreatment: findings from the Ontario Health Supplement. *Child Abuse Negl* 27: 1409–1425.

Weir A, Douglas A, eds. (1999) *Child Protection and Adult Mental Health: Conflict of Interest?* London: Butterworth-Heineman.

Wheeler E (2006) Using group work to support young people living with substance misuse. In: Harbin F, Murphy M, eds. *Secret Lives: Growing with Substance*. Lyme Regis, Dorset: Russell House, pp. 28–41.

13
PRENATAL AND POSTNATAL INTERVENTION STRATEGIES FOR ALCOHOL-ABUSING MOTHERS IN PREGNANCY

Ann P Streissguth and Therese M Grant

Historical perspective on fetal alcohol syndrome and early prevention/intervention efforts

When fetal alcohol syndrome (FAS) came to public awareness with the work of Lemoine et al. (1968) in Nantes, France, and Jones and Smith (1973) and Jones et al. (1973) in the USA, questions arose about the link between maternal alcohol abuse and this birth defect in children. In the late 1970s, in connection with a research study at Boston City Hospital, Rosett et al. (1976, 1977, 1978, 1981) developed a '5-Question Screening Interview' for pregnant alcohol-abusing women with the aim of quantifying their alcohol use and helping them have healthier babies, just as epidemiological studies were starting to demonstrate adverse offspring effects of prenatal alcohol exposure (Little 1977, Harlap and Shiono 1980, Kline et al. 1980).

THE PREGNANCY AND HEALTH PROGRAM AND OTHER FETAL ALCOHOL SYNDROME PREVENTION PROGRAMMES

By 1978, the National Institute of Alcohol Abuse and Alcoholism (NIAAA) was funding two FAS prevention programmes, including a community-wide one in Seattle addressing the problem of female alcohol abuse during pregnancy, the Pregnancy and Health Program (PHP; Little et al. 1980). Throughout its two years of operation, the main message was "When you're pregnant, the best drink is no drink at all." The community was alerted with posters, public service announcements on radio and television, and signs in all Seattle buses (Fig. 13.1). We developed a 24-hour, 7-day-per-week prenatal alcohol hotline, '5-HEALTH', staffed by professionals and highly trained volunteers, to which one in every 44 pregnant women in Seattle phoned in for help or information (Little et al. 1984).

Flyers were inserted into all purchases of alcoholic beverages at Washington State Liquor Stores, and made available at other public venues such as libraries. A team of professional colleagues were trained as trainers, who then educated 6300 similar professionals who might encounter a pregnant woman or her child (physicians, nurses, alcoholism

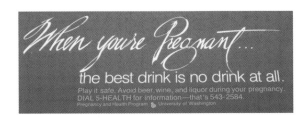

Fig. 13.1. Bus sign, Pregnancy and Health Program, Seattle (1979).

counsellors, social workers, psychologists and teachers). We distributed 220 000 informational brochures and posters from nearly 5000 locations in the area, and provided free evaluations for 151 children who were alcohol-exposed in utero, and made recommendations to their families. We screened at two Seattle hospital prenatal clinics for women drinking at risky levels ('risky drinking'), and found two simple questions that identified 92% of the women we believed to be at general risk in terms of pregnancy outcome: "Did you ever during the pregnancy drink five or more drinks on any occasion?" and "Did you ever feel you should cut down on your drinking?" We also provided risky-drinking mothers with feedback and up to three brief interventions, followed by referrals to alcohol counsellors, whom we had also trained (Little et al. 1985). A total of 304 pregnant women were personally seen and given information and/or treatment for alcohol problems as needed. For these women, entry into the programme was associated with a significant decrement in drinking, and this, in turn, was related to healthier infants at birth. Intervention in drinking during pregnancy was found to be feasible and to provide positive results (Little and Streissguth 1987).

Community surveys conducted on 474 residents in King County, Washington, before PHP (1979) and after PHP (1981) revealed a high level of awareness of the risks of drinking during pregnancy even before the programme began (Little et al. 1981, 1984). Initially, obstetricians were the only group surveyed who had less than 90% awareness; but by 1981 their awareness of the risks of drinking during pregnancy had risen from 76% to 96%. Belief in abstinence during pregnancy in the King County sample increased from 16% to 21% during PHP, while health professionals' belief in abstinence during pregnancy (other than doctors) increased from 43% to 56%. In another aspect of the study, we also obtained permission from local obstetricians (n=41 pre-PHP; n= 47 post-PHP) to survey over 300 of their patients. To our surprise, at the outset of PHP, more pregnant women (47%) believed in abstaining from alcohol during pregnancy than did their own obstetricians (12%) (Little et al. 1983). These data validated the importance of direct public education.

Although a comprehensive model programme had been established for detecting and helping babies born to risky-drinking mothers, there was not enough lead time to incorporate the programme into the ongoing health-care delivery system before a new federal administration was installed, federal funding ended, and the programme came to an abrupt halt. Although the basic ingredients of a comprehensive community FAS prevention programme were outlined, it was not until a decade later that it was possible to develop another demonstration–intervention programme, this time targeting very-high-risk, alcohol-abusing mothers

218

picked up in hospital after delivery, the Parent–Child Assistance Program (PCAP), originally known as Birth-to-3. This second time, we had a better understanding of the importance of working very closely with the community to develop a programme that could fit into the existing public health structure and would continue after the termination of federal demonstration funds.

After these early prevention programmes were developed in conjunction with research projects in Boston and Seattle, there was little formal activity on the prevention front until May and Hymbaugh (1989) and Masis and May (1991) published an inexpensive, macro-level FAS prevention programme for Native Americans and Alaskan Natives that educated trainers in local communities across the USA in comprehensive prevention skills and provided technical assistance for developing local programmes. For little more than $300 000, May and Hymbaugh trained almost 2000 people in 92 Indian Health Service Units. Using 8-hour workshops and resource materials developed and provided by a central source, the prevention programme capitalized on local talent, enthusiasm and commitment.

INTERNATIONAL PROGRAMMES FOR UNDERSTANDING AND PREVENTING FETAL ALCOHOL SYNDROME

In 1980, the NIAAA funded the first International Workshop on Alcohol and Pregnancy, held May 2–4, in Seattle (Streissguth et al. 1981). The concept of 'fetal alcohol effects' (FAE) was introduced by Dr David W Smith, in addition to classic FAS. He noted, "One finds every gradation, from FAS to milder effects of alcohol on the developing fetus" (Smith 1981). A surprising degree of similarity was apparent in the facial photographs of patients from around the world displayed at this meeting; although the words used to describe them varied considerably from country to country, everyone felt the need to describe some sort of a continuum. From Sweden, Olegård et al. (1979), who had begun diagnosing newborn infants in the mid-1970s, reported a prevalence of 1 per 600 infants with "full FAS" and 1 per 300 with "partial FAS" (defined as having some specific features of FAS, but not all). From Germany, Majewski (1981) reported on 108 children with what he called "alcohol embryopathy", a term arrived at by rating each patient on a point system of symptom severity. He found that the degree of embryopathy was related to the stage of maternal alcoholism, and that, among sibling pairs, the younger one tended to be more severely affected than the elder. A similar finding with respect to decreasing birthweight among later siblings of alcoholic mothers was made in France by Dehaene et al. (1981). Darby et al. (1981) reported on eight Seattle children who were diagnosed with FAS in early infancy by David Smith. Of these, four had been diagnosed at birth, and the mothers of all four were dead by the time of the follow-up examination between 4 and 6 years later, possibly a reflection of advanced stages of alcoholism. Silva et al. (1981) demonstrated that women from the favelas (shanty towns) of São Paulo, Brazil who drank pinga (sugar cane alcohol) heavily during pregnancy had more babies with FAE (including short palpebral fissures, microcephaly and small size for gestational age) than comparable women from the same impoverished environment who drank moderately or not at all.

In Finland, the first diagnosis of a child with FAS was made in 1979, and by 1983 Finnish researchers had begun a major campaign to counsel women in antenatal clinics to reduce

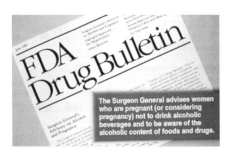

Fig. 13.2. US Surgeon General's Advisory on Alcohol and Pregnancy (1981).

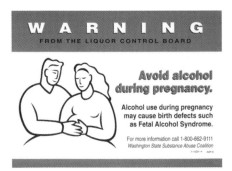

Fig. 13.3. Washington State warning sign (1993).

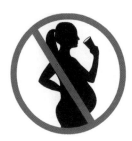

Fig. 13.4. Warning label on alcohol beverage containers in France (2006).

their drinking during pregnancy. Thus began a series of studies on the children of these mothers (e.g. Halmesmäki 1988, Autti-Rämö 2000), which concluded that decreasing alcohol use in the first trimester was more efficacious in terms of offspring development than decreasing alcohol use later in pregnancy. Among the 41 children located at 12 years, eight of the mothers were dead and four had been in prison. Studies were now showing the toll of maternal alcoholism on the mothers as well as their offspring.

In the USA during this period, public policy continued to move forward, but not without controversy. In 1981, following the publication of a summary paper reviewing the available evidence at the time (Eckardt et al. 1981), abstinence was officially recommended by the Surgeon General (Fig. 13.2): "Women who are, or plan to become, pregnant are advised to abstain; health professionals who care for them are urged to ask routinely about alcohol consumption and enter this information into the medical record" (US Department of Health and Human Services 1981). Then in 1988, after an initial failed attempt in the early 1980s, the USA became the first country to introduce mandatory warning labels on all alcoholic beverage containers, when the US Congress approved Public Law 100-690, the Alcoholic Beverage Labelling Act. The label reads, "According to the Surgeon General, women should not drink alcoholic beverages during pregnancy because of the risk of birth defects." Finally, cities and states in the USA began to post warning signs about not drinking during pregnancy, beginning with New York City in 1988. In 1993, Washington State adopted a state ordinance: three warning signs were approved, and each venue selling alcohol by

220

container or by glass was required by law to post two such signs (Fig. 13.3). Similar practices were then adopted by many other states and cities (Streissguth 1997).

France followed suit in 2004 with a recommendation that women should not drink during pregnancy: "La consommation de boissons alcooliques pendant la grossesse, même en faible quantité, peut avoir des consequences graves sur la santé de l'enfant." In 2006 it became the first European country to mandate bottle labelling (Fig. 13.4). The Irish Medical Association has petitioned the government to introduce a major awareness campaign with explicit health warnings on alcohol products following a study reporting that 63% of women surveyed admitted drinking alcohol during pregnancy, with 7% drinking six or more units per week; 81% of more than 1000 respondents in a survey by the Food Safety Authority of Ireland agreed that alcoholic beverages should carry warning labels (Gantly 2010). Italy has recently launched an advertising campaign in the Veneto region: "Mama Beve, Bimbo Beve" (when Mum drinks, baby drinks too) (Squires 2010). The European Alcohol Policy Alliance (www.eurocare.org) has announced that alcohol is the leading cause of birth defects and developmental disorders, and Scottish MEP Alyn Smith has called for bottle labelling to be mandated across the European Union (Moss 2010).

According to Gantly (2010), more than 20 countries have now recognized the need for mandatory labelling. South Africa introduced it in 2007, after several studies revealed the highest prevalence of FAS yet reported in the world, namely 40.5–46.4 per 1000 in a study of children aged 5–9 years and their mothers in several wine-growing areas of the Western Cape Province (May et al. 2000, 2005). In 2009, Russia introduced an awareness campaign aimed at children, teenagers, and pregnant and nursing women, including warning labels for beer, wine and liquor (Medetsky 2009). The Republic of Korea gives a choice of three different labels, each with specific warnings such as "women who drink while they are pregnant increase the risk of congenital anomalies" (Gantly 2010). The World Health Organization recommends that pregnant women should avoid drinking alcohol throughout their pregnancy (Squires 2010).

Studies of adolescents and adults with fetal alcohol syndrome/effects and their mothers

To obtain information on the long-term implications of FAS and FAE, our Seattle team examined 61 adolescents and adults who had been diagnosed earlier by dysmorphologists in and around Seattle, on Indian Reservations of the south-western USA, and in Vancouver, Canada, and reviewed their medical records. The findings had important public health implications: 31% of these patients had never been cared for by their biological mothers, and among those who were initially cared for by their mothers, the average age at which they stopped living with their mothers was 3.5 years. A surprising 69% of the biological mothers were known to be deceased (Streissguth et al. 1991a).

We now know that women get drunk faster, become addicted quicker, and die of alcohol-related disorders after fewer years of drinking than do men (Schenker 1997, Wagnerberger et al. 2008). Separate treatment facilities for women are now recognized as essential. Yet, according to Califano (2007), in the most recent year for which data were available (1989) less than 14% of all women and only 12% of pregnant women in the USA who needed substance-abuse treatment received it. Separate treatment opportunities for women with alcohol problems are an important component of a country's efforts to prevent FAS.

By 1988, there were numerous programmes throughout the USA and Canada involving public education, professional training, and services to educate women about the risks associated with drinking during pregnancy. They centred on the common theme of abstinence during pregnancy: "No Alcohol for Our Baby", "For Baby's Sake, Don't Drink", "A Pregnant Woman Never Drinks Alone" (Robinson and Armstrong 1988).

In Sweden, which has free medical care and a tradition of full prenatal care for all women, FAS prevention programmes were quickly built into existing, widely used, district maternal and child health clinics throughout the country. District social services offices monitored child welfare and provided finances, housing and psychological support as needed, to 99% of all Swedish women (Olegård 1988). Each regional clinic included a paediatrician, an obstetrician, a child psychologist and a coordinator responsible for continuing education of professionals. Confidentiality rules, which they believed had perpetuated secrecy and prevented sharing of critical information, were changed to permit professionals and authorities to exchange information in the interest of the unborn child: a huge step forward. Emphasis was placed on providing midwives with plenty of time to discuss alcohol use and abuse patterns with women at their first prenatal visit, and on the availability of suitable alcohol treatment programmes. As a result of these initial programmes, Olegård (1988) reported that the estimated incidence of FAS in Sweden had dropped from 1 in 600 infants in the mid-1970s to 1 in 2400 by the mid-1980s. More recently, Haver et al. (2001) have described the successful treatment of 120 women in special woman-oriented inpatient and outpatient treatment programmes in Sweden.

A decrease in FAS incidence was also documented in Roubaix, France (Dehaene et al. 1991, Dehaene 1995), where systematic diagnoses of newborn infants with FAS had been ongoing since 1977, and special community programmes for their mothers had been developed (Titran 1993).

Changes in alcohol use by pregnant women across time in Seattle
In 1974–75 and 1980–81, we studied two cohorts of pregnant women (approximately 1500 in each cohort) who were interviewed before the sixth month of pregnancy by specially trained nurse–interviewers not part of the clinic staff (Streissguth et al. 1983).

The number of women who reported any alcohol use around the time of the first prenatal visit dropped from 81% in 1974–75 to 42% in 1980–81. The number of binge drinkers (≥5 drinks on any occasion) prior to pregnancy recognition was 19% and 17% for the two studies respectively, not a significant difference. However, the number of binge drinkers during pregnancy decreased from 12.2% to 7.5% (highly significant).

Between 1989 and 2004 we carried out three more screening studies in the Seattle area, this time of over 12 000 women in hospital following delivery (Grant et al. 2009). As in our earlier study, we again found a substantial decrease in any alcohol use during pregnancy (from 30% to 12%) across almost all demographic groups. We also found that the rate of binge drinking during pregnancy fell to 3%, 4% and 1% respectively in the three studies. However, we found that binge drinking in the month or so before women knew they were pregnant increased significantly over this time period (among all racial categories except Native American). This latest study calls for increased attention to the concept of stopping alcohol use when you *plan* to have a baby, rather than after you know you are pregnant, in order to avoid offspring exposure prior to pregnancy recognition.

Postnatal interventions and prevention of intergenerational alcohol abuse

In northern France, the neonatologist Phillipe Dehaene began diagnosing FAS in newborn infants in the early 1980s (Dehaene et al. 1981), beginning his ongoing documentation of the birth prevalence of FAS in Roubaix (Dehaene et al. 1991). Maurice Titran, a paediatrician, helped organize an early social/rehabilitative programme for mothers of young children with FAS/FAE and other problems, called the 'Tuesday Group', which is still ongoing. The objective was to promote parental competence and behaviour in order to increase the mothers' capacity to successfully nurture their children (Titran 1993). These families had high rates of medical and social problems including poverty, violence, exclusion and alcohol abuse. The programme operates through CAMSP (Centre d'Action Médico-Sociale Précoce in Roubaix), which provides day care and residential care as needed for such children. The mothers call their group ESPER ('hope' in English), an acronym from the French words 'Écoute, Santé, Parents, Enfants, Respect'. Mothers and pregnant women meet weekly as a group with the same professionals, primarily targeting families with transgenerational alcoholism. The key concept is continuously accessible support. In a study of 22 white families assessed seven years after their participation ended (mandatory when children were age 6), Dumaret et al. (2009a) found that alcohol abuse, violence and child neglect had decreased significantly. All but two of the maternal grandmothers were alcoholic, 14 mothers had FAS/FAE and eight of their children had FAS/FAE. IQ tests administered to mothers and children revealed an 18-point IQ difference between mothers with and without FAS/FAE and between children with and without FAS/FAE. Familial alcohol problems predicted school failure even in the absence of FAS/FAE. Three-quarters of the families (n=18) lived below the poverty level. Special education and institutionalization were higher for children with FAS/FAE, but accumulation of alcohol problems in the family still predicted school failure, even in the absence of FAS/FAE (Dumaret et al. 2009b).

In 1996, the French government began ongoing clinical studies to identify children with FAS/FAE in the French province of Réunion Island in the Indian Ocean. Lesure (1988) had originally reported a rate of FAS/FAE of 6 per 1000 births, and this was confirmed by Maillard et al. (1999). As in Roubaix, the identification of numerous babies with FAS encouraged the setting-up of prevention programmes (Lamblin et al. 2008) as well as active groups of mothers and pregnant women with alcohol problems, and professionals working together, focused around the CAMSP programmes.

It is now clear that the prevention of future infants with FAS requires continuing postnatal intervention with the birth mother following the birth of an exposed index child, and especially following the birth of a child with FAS. High-risk mothers will still need continued help with their lives and their sobriety as they resume life with a newborn baby. They need to continue decreasing alcohol and substance use, engage in successful contraception, and build healthy, meaningful lives for themselves and their children before having future pregnancies. They cannot do this alone, so we developed a specialized programme in Washington State to meet their complex needs (Grant et al. 2005a,b; 2007).

The Parent–Child Assistance Program

The Parent–Child Assistance Program (PCAP), originally known as Birth-to-3 because it is a three-year programme, is an intensive home-visitation intervention that works with very-high-risk mothers who abused alcohol or drugs heavily during pregnancy and are estranged from the usual community service providers. PCAP is an advocacy/case management model that offers personalized support over three years, a period of time long enough for the process of gradual and realistic change to occur. The primary aim of the intervention is to prevent future alcohol- and drug-exposed births among high-risk mothers who have already delivered at least one exposed child. To achieve this aim, highly trained and well-supervised PCAP case managers, with a caseload of 16, work with clients for three years beginning during pregnancy or within six months after the birth of an index child (Grant et al. 2003).

RECRUITING HIGH-RISK MOTHERS

When PCAP first began, we recruited women in hospital, the day after they delivered their babies. We had already developed a one-page Hospital Screening Questionnaire (HSQ; Streissguth et al. 1991b) that we had used successfully to screen over 7000 immediately postpartum mothers. The HSQ is a confidential self-report instrument distributed to each mother in hospital. It asks about demographic characteristics, and use of any alcohol, binge alcohol (≥ 5 drinks on one occasion), illicit drugs and cigarettes during two time periods, the 'month or so before pregnancy' and 'during this pregnancy'. The HSQ can be scored with the Binge Alcohol Rating Criteria (Barr and Streissguth 2001). Women who acknowledge binge drinking, or who acknowledge illicit drug use, are invited to participate in PCAP if they are not already effectively engaged with community service providers. Now, after many years of operation, PCAP receives most referrals directly from service providers and so hospital screening is unnecessary. We strive to enrol substance-abusing women as early in pregnancy as possible, so we no longer use the postpartum HSQ to identify potential participants. However, in starting PCAP in a new community, the HSQ would still be useful to routinely identify women who are not known to community service providers and are in need of help, especially those who come to the hospital to deliver without receiving prenatal care.

THE CLIENTS

Most of the mothers in PCAP experienced as children many of the same devastating circumstances their own children are now experiencing, and the same circumstances we find in mothers of children with FAS: chronic familial substance abuse, poverty, violence and neglect. The typical PCAP client was born to substance-abusing parents. She was physically and/or sexually abused as a child, she did not complete high school, and began to use alcohol and drugs herself as a teenager. She is now in her late 20s, has been in jail more than once, and has been through drug treatment and relapsed. She does not use birth control or plan her pregnancies, and now has three or more children, with at least one in the foster

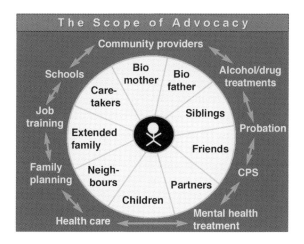

Fig. 13.5. The Parent–Child Assistance Program's 'wheel of support'.

care system. Her current partner is abusive, her housing situation is unstable, and her main source of income is welfare.

THE MODEL

The critical component of the PCAP model is the personalized, caring support over three years, a period of time long enough for the process of gradual and realistic change to occur. The model draws on concepts of relational theory, which emphasizes the importance of positive interpersonal relationships in women's growth, development and definition of self (Miller and Rollnick 1991), and in their addiction, treatment and recovery (Finkelstein 1993). The model puts into operation the idea that paraprofessionals with some shared history and life experiences can play a unique and therapeutic role in two ways, by helping clients become connected to another person in a trusting, healthy relationship for perhaps the first time in their lives, and by bridging the gap between high-risk families and the services they need but are unlikely to obtain without help.

HOW ADVOCACY WORKS

PCAP intervention activities are conducted by paraprofessional advocates who receive intensive initial and ongoing training and are clinically supervised by a professional in social work, mental health or chemical-dependency treatment. The model uses a case-management approach to help mothers reduce the spectrum of risk behaviours associated with substance abuse, and to increase protective factors to enhance the health and social well-being of the mothers and their children. PCAP does not provide direct substance-abuse treatment or clinical services. Instead, the programme offers consistent home visitation, and links women and their families with a comprehensive array of existing community resources, with an emphasis on alcohol/drug treatment, family planning, housing, health care, parenting and legal resources (Fig. 13.5). Advocates/case managers visit client homes frequently during the first six weeks, and thereafter work with clients and their service providers approximately once a week or so, depending on client needs. They transport clients and their children to important appointments, and work actively within the context of the extended family. According to state law, case managers are mandated reporters of child abuse and neglect and abandonment. They monitor the safety of the child in the current home setting, and continue to stay in contact with the client and the child when they are separated. Case managers trace clients who are missing, and stay in touch with the clients' family members. Clients are never asked to leave the programme because of relapse or setbacks.

GOAL SETTING FOR VULNERABLE FAMILIES

> "I never knew what goals were until I had an advocate."
>
> PCAP client

PCAP is organized around helping mothers reach the goals that are meaningful for them. Because these mothers often have difficulty conceptualizing and expressing their goals, we have developed a special protocol to facilitate this process. Case managers use a card-sort assessment strategy called the 'Difference Game' (Grant et al. 1997a) to help their clients identify major problems and goals in their lives, and to develop the specific, incremental steps they will need to take to reach those goals. This involves sorting a set of 31 cards with various items and identifying those that would 'make a difference' in their lives. PCAP Case managers help their clients organize their thoughts and articulate their concerns and goals. They facilitate development of a step-by-step plan that addresses concerns of providers, yet is realistic for the client, and does not impose impossible expectations. For example, one way they help their clients implement their plans is to arrange meetings or conference calls (with the client present) to bring the client's service provider network together to help the client cope with her problems (equivalent in British practice, completion of Children's Assessment Framework, see Chapter 12).

> "There were times when I felt like I was going to relapse and my advocate would be there for me, and she'd keep checking on me, and I'd get through it. I've learned so much about myself and being responsible again and being a good mother. It was all what she taught me – she changed my life for me."
>
> PCAP client

PROFESSIONAL TRAINING OF ADVOCATES

Comprehensive ongoing training of providers is essential to a successful paraprofessional programme. Formal training sessions on relevant topics are conducted by professionals at the beginning of the project and throughout the programme (Grant et al. 1999). PCAP directors arrange training sessions with representatives from key provider agencies (e.g. Child Protective Services, Planned Parenthood). It is important for case managers to work within, and with knowledge of, the other services in their area. For details of the PCAP case manager training – including therapeutic aspects of the intervention; establishing the relationship; identifying client goals; assessment and planning; role modelling; teaching basic skills; strengthening the mother–infant dyad; interfacing with the child welfare system; strategies for helping mothers enter and complete treatment; and strategies for helping mothers choose a family planning method – and a case study demonstrating the use of the Difference Game with a client, see Grant et al. (2007). Advocates/case managers at each site have a weekly individual supervision session on each client, as well as a weekly group staffing meeting to collectively discuss their problems with clients, as well as their successes, and to learn from each other (Grant et al. 2002).

> "I look forward to the staff meetings, particularly when I'm stuck on a particular client. I need a lot of positive reinforcement and I get a lot of that at the staff meetings."
>
> PCAP case manager

PCAP case management is not delivered according to a specific model of behavioural intervention. Instead, case managers develop a positive, empathic relationship with their clients, offer regular home visitation, and help the women address a wide range of environmental problems. A foremost task is to assist clients in obtaining alcohol and drug treatment and staying in recovery. Advocates connect women and their families with existing community services and teach them how to access those services themselves; coordinate services among this multidisciplinary network; assist clients in following through with provider recommendations; and ensure that the children are in safe home environments and receiving appropriate health care.

When we ask former clients what made the programme work for them, we consistently hear "persistence".

> "My case manager never gave up on me. She kept believing in me until I finally started to believe in myself."
>
> PCAP client

MEASURED OUTCOMES AND COST EFFECTIVENESS

Future alcohol- and drug-exposed births can be prevented in one of two ways: by helping women avoid alcohol and drug use during pregnancy, or by helping them avoid pregnancy if they are using alcohol or drugs. To evaluate our progress in PCAP, we compared PCAP intervention findings from two different cohort experiences in Washington State: the original demonstration (1991–1995) and the Seattle/Tacoma replications (1996–2003) (Grant et al. 2005a). Compared with the original demonstration programme, outcomes at the replication sites were either improved (alcohol/drug treatment completed; abstinence from alcohol/drugs; subsequent delivery unexposed to alcohol or drugs) or maintained (regular use of contraception and use of a reliable method; number of subsequent deliveries during the programme).

In studying mothers completing the three-year PCAP replication programmes (Grant et al. 2005a), we found that 65% of the 78 enrolled prenatal binge drinkers were no longer at present risk of having another alcohol- or drug-exposed pregnancy, either because they were using a reliable contraceptive method (31%), or because they had abstained from alcohol/drugs for at least six months (23%), or both (12%). On the basis of subsequent local birth rates and the estimated incidence of FAS among heavy drinkers, we estimate that PCAP prevented at least one and up to three new cases of FAS. The cost of the PCAP programme is approximately $15 000 per client over the three years, including intervention, administration and evaluation. If PCAP prevented just one new case of FAS, the estimated lifetime cost savings are equivalent to the cost of the PCAP intervention for 102 women (Grant et al. 2005a). A 2004 independent economic analysis by the Washington State Institute for Public Policy found an average net benefit of $6197 per client among selected well-researched home-visiting programmes, including PCAP, for at-risk families in the USA (Aos et al. 2004).

Between July 2005 and July 2008, we had 240 graduates from PCAP: 91% had completed alcohol/drug treatment or were in progress; 84% were abstinent from alcohol and drugs for six months or more; 82% of the index children were living with their own families; and 72% of the mothers had attended or completed a high school diploma, college or work training. Changes during the programme were as follows: 62% using a reliable family planning method vs 9% at enrolment; 74% in permanent housing vs 38% at enrolment; 46% now receiving state funds vs 71% at enrolment; 37% now employed vs 2% at enrolment. At the present time, PCAP serves 675 families in nine Washington counties and operates programmes in provinces throughout Canada.

INTERVENTION WITH WOMEN WHO THEMSELVES HAVE FETAL ALCOHOL
SPECTRUM DISORDERS

Whilst neuropsychological deficits and other adverse outcomes associated with prenatal alcohol exposure have been well documented for over 30 years, interventions for adults with FASD have not been systematically developed and evaluated. In 1999 PCAP expanded its eligibility criteria to enrol a sample of women with FASD. In 2001 we conducted a 12-month pilot study to examine more specifically how these women could be helped within the existing framework of PCAP (Grant et al. 2004). A total of 19 clients, either with FASD (n=11) or who were prenatally exposed to heavy alcohol use and had suspected FASD (n=8), were enrolled in the study. Their average age was 22 years, most were unmarried (16/19) and poorly educated (nine had a 9th grade education or less), and all but one had been physically or sexually abused as children. Among the 15 who were mothers, the mean number of children was 2.3 (range 1–6); on average, only half of the children were living with their biological mothers. All reported many unmet basic service needs. Without special community care, the quality of life and levels of psychiatric distress of adults with FASD living unrecognized in our communities are very poor (Grant et al. 2005b). Mothers with FASD are among the most difficult mothers with whom we have worked.

Adults and adolescents with FASD also have a high rate of suicide attempts (Lemoine and Lemoine 1992). In a separate study, we found that adults with FASD who had attempted suicide differed from those without suicide attempts in terms of more mental health disorders, substance abuse disorders, histories of trauma or abuse, financial stress and unstable social support (Huggins et al. 2008).

The cognitive deficits of people with FASD necessitate specific strategies to increase their connection to community services and to improve the quality of services they receive. Our community intervention for mothers with FASD consisted of delivering the standard PCAP model enhanced in two ways: (1) by modifying PCAP in order to accommodate the

228

special cognitive needs of clients with FASD; and (2) by educating community service providers about FASD so they could better accommodate our clients' needs (Grant et al. 2004, 2007).

A public health approach to fetal alcohol syndrome
First published in 1996 by the Institute of Medicine (Stratton et al. 1996) in conjunction with the NIAAA, and recently updated by the US Department of Health and Human Services (2009), the public health approach to FAS has involved three activities.

Universal prevention activities promote general knowledge and social conditions that reduce substance abuse and promote healthy pregnancy practices. Warning signs, public health messages, bottle labels, newspaper articles and so forth continue to inform each new generation about the risks of drinking during pregnancy. An excellent example is the work of Kaskutas and Graves (1994) who found that it took three different types of warnings before a pregnant woman really changed her behaviour regarding alcohol use in pregnancy. Another is the work of Dufour et al. (1994), who used data from the 1985 US Health Promotion and Disease Prevention survey and the 1990 US National Health Inventory Survey. The samples included over 8100 men and 10 000 women between the ages of 18 and 44 years in 1985 and over 9000 men and 13 000 women in 1990. These respondents were selected to represent the total US non-institutionalized population aged from 18 to 44 years. Dufour and colleagues found a statistically significant increase between 1985 and 1990 in the number of respondents able to correctly identify FAS as a birth defect. However, in 1990, the same survey found that 60% of those who had heard of FAS thought that it referred to an alcohol-addicted baby, and only 29% could correctly identify it as a birth defect.

Selective prevention interventions involve screening instruments, training health-care professionals, working with family members of a pregnant woman abusing alcohol, developing biomarkers, brief interventions and referrals (Rosett et al. 1983; Little et al. 1984, 1985; Chang et al. 2005; Floyd et al. 2007; O'Connor and Whaley 2007).

Indicated preventions are applied to individuals at highest risk for adverse outcomes; that is, women or couples with alcohol- or substance-abuse problems, and those who have already given birth to a child with FAS. Our PCAP is such an example, and has already been applied to that highest-risk group of all, mothers who have both alcohol problems and FAS (Grant et al. 1997b, 2004; Ernst et al. 1999).

Collaborative public health approaches for preventing alcohol-exposed pregnancies
Preventing alcohol-exposed pregnancies requires many steps. Countries contemplating the broader problem of reducing alcohol-exposed pregnancies would do well to consider steps that we have found useful in the USA and in Washington State, involving many types of public health actions. However, implementation in countries with an existing universal health-care system should be easier (see 'Hidden Harm' in Chapter 12).

Government warnings regarding "no safe level of alcohol use during pregnancy" are an effective first step, warranted by the compelling animal and human research published in the past 35 years. At the national level, bottle-labelling of all alcohol-containing beverages can be an important step, as well as point-of-purchase warning signs at all local venues where alcohol is sold in any form.

The commission of national funds for research and policy implementation, increased funding for female alcohol problems (for example, protocols for how to detoxify a pregnant woman), and development of guidelines for routine screening for alcohol use and abuse during pregnancy are all important.

Enlisting the support of professional organizations can also be extremely important. At the national level, in 1999 the American Medical Association endorsed universal alcohol screening for all patients over the age of 14 years, and the American College of Obstetricians and Gynecologists (2004) outlined the ethical rationale for using a consolidated alcohol protocol including universal screening, brief intervention and referral to treatment. The American Academy of Pediatrics (2000) endorsed the Surgeon General's recommendation for abstinence during pregnancy, and additionally recommended federal legislation requiring the inclusion of health and safety messages in all print and broadcast alcohol advertisements as well as providing information about FAS and not drinking during pregnancy in marriage licences.

Coordinating efforts with parent organizations and advocacy organizations can be extremely effective in raising public awareness, providing hope and help to families of people with FAS, and developing and raising funds for needed programmes. One such advocacy organization with international connections is NOFAS (the National Organization on Fetal Alcohol Syndrome). There is now a NOFAS-UK, with its own website (see Table 14.3, p. 247).

Finally, an essential component of each evidence-based research demonstration programme is the ultimate incorporation of successful strategies into the ongoing public health programming of the country. Comprehensive prevention efforts are more cost-effective for countries than managing the costs to society, families and children of raising future generations of alcohol-effected children.

ACKNOWLEDGEMENTS

This work was supported by the Substance Abuse and Mental Health Services Administration (H86 SPO2897 to APS), the Substance Abuse and Mental Health Services Administration (SPO9423 to TMG), the National Institute on Drug Abuse (3R01 DA05365 to APS), the National Institute on Alcohol Abuse and Alcoholism (AA01455 to APS), the National Institute on Alcohol Abuse and Alcoholism (H84 AA03736 to Ruth E Little), and the Washington State Department of Social and Health Services, Division of Alcohol and Substance Abuse (0965-69005 to TMG).

REFERENCES

American Academy of Pediatrics, Committee on Substance Abuse and Committee on Children with Disabilities (2000) Fetal alcohol syndrome and alcohol-related neurodevelopmental disorders. *Pediatrics* **106**: 358–361.

American College of Obstetricians and Gynecologists Committee on Ethics (2004) ACOG Committee Opinion No. 294, May 2004. At-risk drinking and illicit drug use: ethical issues in obstetric and gynecologic practice. *Obstet Gynecol* **103**: 1021–1031.

Aos S, Lieb R, Mayfield J, et al. (2004) *Benefits and Costs of Prevention and Early Intervention Programs for Youth.* Olympia, WA: Washington State Institute for Public Policy.

Autti-Rämö I (2000) Twelve-year follow-up of children exposed to alcohol in utero. *Dev Med Child Neurol* **42**: 406–411.

Barr HM, Streissguth AP (2001) Identifying maternal self-reported alcohol use associated with fetal alcohol spectrum disorders. *Alcohol Clin Exp Res* **25**: 283–287.

Califano JA (2007) *High Society: How Substance Abuse Ravages America and What to Do About It.* New York: Public Affairs.

Chang G, McNamara TK, Orav EJ, et al. (2005) Brief intervention for prenatal alcohol use: a randomized trial. *Obstet Gynecol* **105**: 991–998.

Darby BL, Streissguth AP, Smith DW (1981) A preliminary follow-up of 8 children diagnosed fetal alcohol syndrome in infancy. *Neurobehav Toxicol Teratol* **3**: 157–159.

Dehaene P (1995) *Que C'est Je? La Grossesse et l'Alcool.* Paris: Presses Universitaires de France.

Dehaene P, Crépin G, Delahousse G, et al. (1981) [Epidemiological aspects of fetal alcohol syndrome: 45 cases.] *Presse Med* **10**: 2639–2643 (French).

Dehaene P, Samaille-Villette C, Boulanger-Fasquelle P, et al. (1991) [Diagnosis and prevalence of fetal alcoholism in maternity.] *Presse Med* **20**: 1002 (French).

Dufour MC, Williams GD, Campbell KE, Aitken SS (1994) Knowledge of FAS and the risks of heavy drinking during pregnancy, 1985–1990. *Alcohol Health Res World* **18**: 86–92.

Dumaret AC, Constantin-Kuntz M, Titran M (2009a) Early intervention in poor families confronted with alcohol abuse and violence: impact on families' social integration and parenting. *Fam Society J Contemp Soc Serv* **90**: 11–17.

Dumaret AC, Cousin M, Titran M (2009b) Two generations of maternal alcohol abuse: impact on cognitive levels in mothers and their children. *Early Child Dev Care* (epub ahead of print).

Eckardt MJ, Harford TC, Kaelber CT, et al. (1981) Health hazards associated with alcohol consumption. *JAMA* **246**: 648–666.

Ernst CC, Grant TM, Streissguth AP, Sampson PD (1999) Intervention with high-risk alcohol and drug-abusing mothers: II. 3-year findings from the Seattle Model of Paraprofessional Advocacy. *J Community Psychol* **27**: 19–38.

Finkelstein N (1993) Treatment programming for alcohol and drug-dependent pregnant women. *Int J Addict* **28**: 1275–1309.

Floyd RL, Sobell M, Velasquez MM, et al. (2007) Preventing alcohol-exposed pregnancies: a randomized controlled trial. *Am J Prev Med* **32**: 1–10.

Gantly D (2010) Groups want explicit warnings on alcohol. *Irish Medical Times* January 15.

Grant TM, Ernst CC, McAuliff S, Streissguth AP (1997a) The Difference Game: facilitating change in high-risk clients. *Fam Soc* **78**: 429–432.

Grant T, Ernst C, Streissguth A, Porter J (1997b) An advocacy program for mothers with FAS/FAE. In: Streissguth A, Kanter J, eds. *The Challenge of Fetal Alcohol Syndrome: Overcoming Secondary Disabilities.* Seattle: University of Washington Press, pp. 102–112.

Grant TM, Ernst CC, Streissguth AP (1999) Intervention with high-risk alcohol and drug-abusing mothers: I. Administrative strategies of the Seattle Model of Paraprofessional Advocacy. *J Commun Psychol* **27**: 1–18.

Grant T, Streissguth A, Ernst C (2002) Benefits and challenges of paraprofessional advocacy with mothers who abuse alcohol and drugs and their children. *Zero to Three* **23**: 14–20.

Grant T, Ernst CC, Pagalilauan G, Streissguth A (2003) Postprogram follow-up effects of paraprofessional intervention with high-risk women who abused alcohol and drugs during pregnancy. *J Commun Psychol* **31**: 211–222.

Grant T, Huggins J, Connor P, et al. (2004) A pilot community intervention for young women with fetal alcohol spectrum disorders. *Commun Ment Health J* **40**: 499–511.

Grant TM, Ernst CC, Streissguth AP, Stark K (2005a) Preventing alcohol and drug exposed births in Washington State: intervention findings from three parent–child assistance program sites. *Am J Drug Alcohol Abuse* **31**: 471–490.

Grant TM, Huggins JE, Connor PD, Streissguth AP (2005b) Quality of life and psychosocial profile among young women with fetal alcohol spectrum disorders. *Ment Health Aspects Dev Disabil* **8**: 33–39.

Grant T, Pedersen JY, Whitney N, Ernst C (2007) The role of therapeutic intervention with substance abusing mothers: preventing FASD in the next generation. In: O'Malley KD, ed. *ADHD and Fetal Alcohol Spectrum Disorders (FASD).* New York: Nova Science Publishers, pp. 69–93.

Grant TM, Huggins, JE, Sampson, PD, et al. (2009) Alcohol use before and during pregnancy in western

231

Washington, 1989–2004: implications for the prevention of fetal alcohol spectrum disorders. *Am J Obstet Gynecol* **200**: 278.e1–278.e8.

Halmesmäki E (1988) Alcohol counselling of 85 pregnant problem drinkers: effect on drinking and fetal outcome. *Br J Obstet Gynecol* **95**: 243–247.

Harlap S, Shiono PH (1980) Alcohol, smoking, and incidence of spontaneous abortions in the first and second trimester. *Lancet* **ii**: 173–176.

Haver B, Dahlgren L, Willander A (2001) A 2-year follow-up of 120 Swedish female alcoholics treated early in their drinking career: prediction of drinking outcome. *Alcohol Clin Exp Res* **25**: 1586–1593.

Huggins JE, Grant T, O'Malley K, Streissguth AP (2008) Suicide attempts among adults with fetal alcohol spectrum disorders: clinical considerations. *Ment Health Aspects Dev Disabil* **11**: 33–41.

Jones KL, Smith DW (1973) Recognition of the fetal alcohol syndrome in early infancy. *Lancet* **ii**: 999–1001.

Jones KL, Smith DW, Ulleland CN, Streissguth AP (1973) Pattern of malformation in offspring of chronic alcoholic mothers. *Lancet* **i**: 1267–1271.

Kaskutas L, Graves K (1994) Relationship between cumulative exposure to health messages and awareness and behavior-related drinking during pregnancy. *Am J Health Promot* **9**: 115–124.

Kline J, Shrout P, Stein Z, et al. (1980) Drinking during pregnancy and spontaneous abortion. *Lancet* **ii**: 176–180.

Lamblin D, Maillard T, Provost C, Ricquebourg M (2008) [Fetal alcohol spectrum disorder prevention in Reunion Island.] *Arch Pediatr* **15**: 513–515 (French).

Lemoine P, Lemoine P (1992) [Outcome of children of alcoholic mothers (study of 105 cases followed to adult age) and various prophylactic findings.] *Ann Pediatr* **39**: 226–235 (French).

Lemoine P, Harrousseau H, Borteyru JP, Meneut JC (1968) [Children of alcoholic parents : anomalies observed in 127 cases.] *Ouest Med* **21**: 476–482 (French).

Lesure JF (1988) L'embryofoetopathie alcoolique a l'Ile de la Reunion: un drame social. *Rev Pediatr* **24**: 265–271.

Little RE (1977) Moderate alcohol use during pregnancy and decreased infant birth weight. *Am J Public Health* **67**: 1154–1156.

Little RE, Streissguth AP (1987) Reducing fetal alcohol effects: the Seattle pregnancy and health program. In: Majewski F, ed. *Die Alkohol-Embryopathie*. Frankfurt/Main: Umwelt & Medizin Verlagsgesellschaft, pp. 197–203.

Little RE, Streissguth AP, Guzinski GM (1980) Prevention of fetal alcohol syndrome: a model program. *Alcohol Clin Exp Res* **4**: 185–189.

Little RE, Grathwohl HL, Streissguth AP, McIntyre C (1981) Public awareness and knowledge about the risks of drinking during pregnancy in Multnomah County, Oregon. *Am J Public Health* **71**: 312–314.

Little RE, Streissguth AP, Guzinski GM, et al. (1983) Change in obstetrician advice following a two-year community educational program on alcohol use and pregnancy. *Am J Obstet Gynecol* **146**: 23–28.

Little RE, Young A, Streissguth AP, Uhl CN (1984) Preventing fetal alcohol effects: effectiveness of a demonstration project. *CIBA Found Symp* **105**: 254–274.

Little RE, Streissguth AP, Guzinski GM, et al. (1985) An evaluation of the pregnancy and health program. *Alcohol Health Res World* **10**: 44–53, 71, 75.

Maillard T, Lamblin D, Lesure, Fourmaintraux A (1999) Incidence of fetal alcohol syndrome on the southern part of Reunion Island. *Teratology* **60**: 51–52 (letter).

Majewski R (1981) Alcohol embryopathy: some facts and speculations about pathogenesis. *Neurobehav Toxicol Teratol* **3**: 129–144.

Masis KB, May PA (1991) A comprehensive local program for the prevention of fetal alcohol syndrome. *Public Health Rep* **106**: 484–489.

May PA, Hymbaugh KJ (1989) A macro-level fetal alcohol syndrome prevention program for Native Americans and Alaska Natives: description and evaluation. *J Stud Alcohol* **50**: 508–518.

May PA, Brooke L, Gossage JP, et al. (2000) Epidemiology of fetal alcohol syndrome in a South African community in the Western Cape Province. *Am J Public Health* **90**: 1905–1912.

May PA, Gossage JP, Brooke LE, et al. (2005) Maternal risk factors for fetal alcohol syndrome in the Western cape province of South Africa: a population-based study. *Am J Public Health* **95**: 1190–1199.

Medetsky A (2009) State will require labels on alcohol. *The Moscow Times* 18 December.

Miller WR, Rollnick S (1991) *Motivational Interviewing: Preparing People to Change Addictive Behavior.* New York: Guilford Press.

Moss L (2010) Call for EU-wide warnings on alcohol. *Scotland on Sunday* 21 March.

O'Connor MH, Whaley SE (2007) Brief intervention for alcohol use by pregnant women. *Am J Public Health* **97**: 252–258.

Olegård R (1988) The prevention of fetal alcohol syndrome in Sweden. In: Robinson GC, Armstrong RW, eds. *Alcohol and Child/Family Health.* Vancouver: University of British Columbia, pp. 73–82.

Olegård R, Sabel KG, Aronsson M, et al. (1979) Effects on the child of alcohol abuse during pregnancy. Retrospective and prospective studies. *Acta Paediatr Scand Suppl* **275**: 112–121.

Robinson GC, Armstrong RW, eds (1988) *Alcohol and Child/Family Health.* Vancouver: University of British Columbia.

Rosett HL, Ouellette EM, Weiner L (1976) A pilot prospective study of the fetal alcohol syndrome at the Boston City Hospital. Part I. Maternal drinking. *Ann N Y Acad Sci* **273**: 118–122.

Rosett HL, Ouellette EM, Weiner L, Owens E (1977) The prenatal clinic: a site for alcoholism prevention and treatment. In: Seixas FA, ed. *Currents in Alcoholism, vol. 1.* New York: Grune & Stratton: pp. 419–430.

Rosett HL, Ouellette EM, Weiner L, Owens E (1978) Therapy of heavy drinking during pregnancy. *Obstet Gynecol* **51**: 41–46.

Rosett HL, Weiner L, Edelin KC (1981) Strategies for prevention of fetal alcohol effects. *Obstet Gynecol* **57**: 1–7.

Rosett HL, Weiner L, Edelin KC (1983) Treatment experience with pregnant problem drinkers. *JAMA* **249**: 2029–2033.

Schenker S (1997) Medical consequences of alcohol abuse: is gender a factor? *Alcohol Clin Exp Res* **21**: 179–181.

Silva VA, Laranjeira RR, Dolnikoff M, et al. (1981) Alcohol consumption during pregnancy and newborn outcome: a study in Brazil. *Neurobehav Toxicol Teratol* **3**: 169–172.

Smith DW (1981) Fetal alcohol syndrome and fetal alcohol effects. *Neurobehav Toxicol Teratol* **3**: 127.

Squires N (2010) Italy launches foetus in cocktail glass poster to stop women drinking. *Telegraph* 26 May.

Stratton K, Howe C, Battaglia F, eds (1996) *Fetal Alcohol Syndrome: Diagnosis, Epidemiology, Prevention, and Treatment.* Washington, DC: Institute of Medicine, National Academy Press.

Streissguth AP (1981) Summary and recommendations. Epidemiologic and human studies on alcohol and pregnancy. *Neurobehav Toxicol Teratol* **3**: 241–242.

Streissguth AP (1997) *Fetal Alcohol Syndrome: A Guide for Families and Communities.* Baltimore: Paul H Brookes.

Streissguth AP, Noble EP, Randall CL, et al. (1981) Fetal alcohol syndrome research: selected papers from the fetal alcohol syndrome workshop, Seattle, Washington, 1980. *Neurobehav Toxicol Teratol* **3**: 69.

Streissguth AP, Darby BL, Barr HM, et al. (1983) Comparison of drinking and smoking patterns during pregnancy over a 6-year interval. *Am J Obstet Gynecol* **145**: 716–724.

Streissguth AP, Aase JM, Clarren SK, et al. (1991a) Fetal alcohol syndrome in adolescents and adults. *JAMA* **265**: 1961–1967.

Streissguth AP, Grant TM, Barr HM, et al. (1991b) Cocaine and the use of alcohol and other drugs during pregnancy. *Am J Obstet Gynecol* **164**: 1239–1243.

Titran M (1993) Témoignage: le groupe du Mardi. *Arch Public Health* **51**: 135–139.

US Department of Health and Human Services (1981) Surgeon General's advisory on alcohol and pregnancy. *FDA Drug Bulletin* **11**: 9–10.

US Department of Health and Human Services (2009) *Reducing Alcohol-Exposed Pregnancies. A Report of the National Task Force on Fetal Alcohol Syndrome and Fetal Alcohol Effect.* Atlanta, GA: Centers for Disease Control and Prevention.

Wagnerberger S, Schafer C, Schwarz E, et al. (2008) Is nutrient intake a gender-specific cause for enhanced susceptibility to alcohol-induced liver disease in women? *Alcohol Alcoholism* **43**: 9–14.

14

COGNITIVE AND BEHAVIOURAL INTERVENTIONS TO AMELIORATE THE EFFECTS OF FETAL ALCOHOL SPECTRUM DISORDERS IN CHILDREN AND ADOLESCENTS: PROMOTING POSITIVE OUTCOMES

Wendy O Kalberg and Julie Gelo

Positive outcomes for children are defined from a variety of points of view: the family perspective, the child's perspective, and various professional perspectives. Outcome is defined based on our own unique philosophical underpinnings, educational background, expertise, expectations and experience.

This chapter is written by an adoptive parent of children with fetal alcohol spectrum disorders (FASDs), Julie Gelo, and a professional working with children who have FASD, Wendy Kalberg. As a backdrop for this chapter, we would like to introduce our beliefs about 'improving outcomes' for children with FASD.

From our blended perspective, we believe that (1) we all want to feel a sense of membership in a group; (2) all individuals are capable of learning and developing skills; and (3) regardless of a diagnosis, each of us is a unique individual.

To this end, we believe we can improve outcomes in quality of life for children with FASD in the following ways: (1) provide necessary support for children so that they can have a sense of membership in a group; (2) support them to develop a positive sense of self; and (3) help provide support or environmental modifications that enable them to move toward a greater sense of competence and, ultimately, a greater level of independence. This includes academic goals as well as functional and life goals.

Emphasis will be placed on the need to maintain an holistic approach and to work together as a team to help promote successful programming for children with FASD within multiple levels of the service delivery system. This will include specific strategies for intervention in school to improve cognitive, language and organizational skills as well as targeted behavioural interventions.

The holistic approach to treatment for the child and caregiver clearly shows the potential for decreasing the compassion fatigue or emotional stress in the parent by helping to maintain the parent–child relationship. This approach also serves as a way to break the cycle of abuse and alcoholism so intimately intertwined with each case of FASD. The tragedy of transgenerational repetition of alcohol/substance abuse is a legacy of FASD. Only a therapeutic approach that involves systems that empower the parent–child or parent–adolescent relationship can loosen this compulsion to repeat and continue the vicious cycle.

When a child is diagnosed with FASD it can be a frightening and unique challenge. This chapter was written to help professionals in the journey of supporting children with FASD. It contains information about the body of research that substantiates cognitive and behavioural deficits and thereby informs the need for interventions. Guidelines and suggestions for interventions that may help ameliorate the cognitive and behavioural deficits of FASD are presented. In addition, reviews of the empirically proven school interventions are provided for the reader. Please note that this chapter is only an introduction to the challenge of providing cognitive and behavioural interventions to ameliorate the effects of prenatal alcohol exposure and resultant FASD among affected children and individuals.

Empirically proven areas of potential deficit

Despite ongoing efforts to prevent maternal drinking during pregnancy, prenatal alcohol exposure continues to be the leading nongenetic cause of learning disability (Stratton et al. 1996). In addition, there is converging evidence from large longitudinal studies that suggests that mild to moderate prenatal alcohol exposure can produce dose-dependent effects on neurocognitive functioning (Greene et al. 1991, Jacobson et al. 1993, Sampson et al. 1997). There is a body of literature describing the neurocognitive deficits associated with heavy prenatal alcohol exposure and fetal alcohol syndrome (FAS), as well as reports focusing on neurocognitive deficits in the absence of the full syndrome (see also Chapters 6 and 7). Researchers have reported that children with prenatal alcohol exposure perform less competently than age-matched controls on a wide range of tests, including those measuring intellectual functioning, academic achievement, attention, memory, problem solving, visual construction, social behaviour and fine motor skills.

INTELLECTUAL FUNCTIONING

Numerous researchers have consistently found intellectual deficits in children with FAS, with the average IQs of these children falling in the range of borderline to mild learning disability (Streissguth et al. 1991, Mattson et al. 1997). Given that subtest scores provide useful information pertinent to defining behavioural phenotypes, researchers have conducted 'profile analyses' of subtest scores from standardized test batteries (Mattson et al. 1997, Adnams et al. 2001). Results from these analyses show that children with FAS score lower than controls on all subtests. Mattson et al. (1998) also concluded that there was no significant discrepancy between verbal and nonverbal abilities.

EXECUTIVE FUNCTIONING (see also Chapter 7)

There is converging evidence that alcohol-affected individuals show difficulty with complex tasks that involve holding and manipulating information in working memory. Tests measuring executive control skills typify such complex tasks. Kodituwakku et al. (2001a) demonstrated that some tests measuring executive control functioning (tests sensitive to orbitofrontal lobe functioning) are consistent and reliable predictors of behavioural problems in alcohol-affected individuals. Mattson et al. (1998) reported that children diagnosed with FAS and alcohol-related neurodevelopmental deficits are equally impaired in neurocognitive functioning.

Notwithstanding notable advances in delineating a profile of cognitive strengths and weaknesses and associated neural substrates in children with prenatal alcohol exposure, a set of core deficits that is unique to the disorder has not yet been established. There is evidence, however, that executive dysfunction among individuals with prenatal alcohol exposure is at the root of their behavioural and learning problems. Kodituwakku et al. (2001a) found that set-shifting difficulties (modification of behaviour in response to changing environmental conditions) accounted for about 50% of the variance in parent-rated problems in alcohol-exposed children. Similarly, classroom behaviours that Carmichael-Olson et al. (1992) found most significant in alcohol-exposed children were related to executive control functioning (e.g. does not persist with tasks, slow to settle down, trouble with organization). Researchers have also reported that executive dysfunction in alcohol-exposed children interferes with their ability to learn effectively. Mattson et al. (1996) found that alcohol-exposed children showed response inhibition problems on a verbal learning test. Similarly, Carmichael-Olson et al. (1998) noted impulsivity and disorganization in alcohol-affected adolescents on a visual learning test. Therefore, it is reasonable to target executive dysfunction in alcohol-exposed children when developing individualized intervention programmes for them.

As noted above, deficits in executive functioning appear to be associated with reported behavioural problems in children with prenatal alcohol exposure. Two primary neurocognitive processes are involved in achieving a goal in an efficient manner: working memory and response inhibition. Working memory allows a person to hold temporal information in active memory, e.g. what has been done and what needs to be done. Response inhibition is required to suppress habitual responses irrelevant to the task. Executive function can be further divided into two categories: cognition-based and emotion-related. Abilities subsumed under cognition-based executive function include conceptual planning, conceptual set-shifting, and rapid generation of verbal and nonverbal responses. In emotion-related executive function, action selection is based on rewards and punishments (i.e. positive and negative reinforcement) obtained in the past in similar situations (Rolls et al. 1994). Both animal and human research shows that the dorsolateral region of the prefrontal cortex plays a critical role in cognition-based executive function and the orbitofrontal cortex in emotion-related executive function (Dias et al. 1996).

Researchers have obtained evidence that individuals with prenatal alcohol exposure are impaired in both cognition-based and emotion-related executive function (Kodituwakku et al. 2001b). Children with prenatal alcohol exposure perform less competently than controls on tests of planning (Kodituwakku et al. 1995, Mattson et al. 1999), conceptual set-shifting (Coles et al. 1997), verbal and nonverbal fluency (Schonfeld et al. 2001), and fluid reasoning (Kodituwakku et al. 1995). Kodituwakku et al. (2001b) found that people with prenatal alcohol exposure were markedly impaired in emotion-related learning compared with controls, as measured by visual discrimination reversal. Deficient performance on this test and on a test of conceptual set-shifting (Wisconsin Card Sorting Test) was found to be associated with parent-rated behavioural problems in the participants of the study. Furthermore, researchers have obtained evidence that children with FAS and alcohol-exposed children without FAS (e.g. those with alcohol-related neurodevelopmental deficits) are equally impaired on tests of executive control functioning (Mattson et al. 1999, Kodituwakku et al. 2001).

Executive function has been the focus of a number of additional studies (Rapport et al. 2001, Aragon et al. 2008). Alcohol-exposed children demonstrated marked difficulty in complex working-memory-related tasks and shifting sets in both cognitive- and emotion-based tasks, planning ability, cognitive flexibility, selective inhibition, auditory and visual sustained attention, and concept formation and reasoning (Carmichael-Olson et al. 1998, Mattson and Riley 1998, Mattson et al. 1999, Connor et al. 2000, Kodituwakku et al. 2001b, Coles et al. 2002, Willford et al. 2004, Burden et al. 2005, Rasmussen 2005). This increasing evidence points to executive dysfunction at the root of the behavioural and learning problems among prenatally alcohol-exposed individuals. Behavioural and learning deficits, therefore, may be remediable given an individualized plan that begins with a thorough understanding of the child's neurocognitive strengths and challenges and how those deficit areas might be supported through environmental, curricular and positive behavioural supports.

ATTENTION AND CONCENTRATION

Although there is some consensus among researchers that attention and executive control functioning are 'core deficits' in children with FASD, there is less agreement as to what skills are mostly deficient. Streissguth et al. (1998) found that adolescents with prenatal alcohol exposure were more impaired on tests assessing 'focused' and 'sustained' elements than those assessing 'encoding' and 'shifting' elements of attention. In contrast, Coles et al. (1997) found that children with prenatal alcohol exposure were impaired only on shift and encode elements. In a subsequent study of sustained attention in alcohol-affected children, Coles et al. (2002) found a significant modality by group interaction. That is, the alcohol-exposed group had more difficulty with sustaining attention when processing visual stimuli than when processing auditory stimuli.

COGNITIVE PLANNING

Look-ahead puzzles are often used to measure cognitive planning abilities. Kodituwakku et al. (1995, 2001a,b) reported that alcohol-exposed children were markedly impaired on planning ability, as assessed by the Progressive Planning Test, a look-ahead puzzle. However, using the California Tower Test, Mattson et al. (1999) obtained less pronounced deficits in planning with alcohol-affected children. Many researchers have utilized the Wisconsin Card Sorting Test to assess the shifting aspect of attention (Lezak 1995). As noted above, researchers have found variable levels of impairments in the shift element of attention in alcohol-exposed children. However, on most laboratory tasks that measure response inhibition, children with prenatal alcohol exposure do not exhibit impulsivity (Coles et al. 1997, Kodituwakku et al. 2001).

LEARNING AND MEMORY

There is consistent evidence that children with prenatal alcohol exposure perform less competently than controls on learning and memory tasks that involve conscious effort of encoding and retrieval. Mattson and colleagues (Mattson et al. 1996, Mattson and Roebuck 2002) have reported that children with heavy prenatal alcohol exposure obtained lower scores than controls on verbal and nonverbal list learning tasks such as the California Verbal Learning Test for Children. Verbal memory deficits in children with prenatal alcohol exposure have also been documented with other methods of testing such as story recall (Streissguth et al. 1989).

Numerous reports exist in the literature on spatial learning, specifically place learning, with alcohol-exposed children. Using a spatial recall task, Uecker and Nadel (1998) found a general spatial memory deficit in alcohol-exposed children. Streissguth et al. (1994) have found that prenatal alcohol exposure was associated with deficient performance on a visually guided maze-learning test. Place-learning difficulties in alcohol-exposed children have been demonstrated with a virtual Morris water task (a computerized version of a task, often used in animal studies, in which the participant is required to learn the position of a platform in a virtual water tank) (Hamilton et al. 2003).

There is also accumulating evidence that alcohol exposure does not produce impairments in recognition memory or procedural memory (Carmichael-Olson et al. 1998, Mattson and Riley 1998). On tests of memory and learning, children with prenatal alcohol exposure demonstrate normal rates of acquisition and retention of relatively simple information, but they show difficulty in learning relatively complex information.

VERBAL FLUENCY

Impaired verbal fluency has also been found in children with FASD (Mattson and Riley 1998, Kodituwakku et al. 2006). Letter fluency is a complex task that involves a number of operations simultaneously: rapidly generating words by phonemic similarity, checking responses to ensure that they meet the test constraints, and keeping a record of responses already produced in working memory. Letter fluency can be contrasted with category fluency, in which subjects are required to rapidly generate exemplars from a semantic category (e.g. animals, fruit and vegetables). Replicating previous findings, Kodituwakku et al. (2006) reported that children with FASD displayed greater difficulty in letter fluency than in category fluency.

MOTOR PERFORMANCE

Neuropsychological and experimental studies of motor performance of alcohol-exposed children show deficient manual dexterity and disturbance of balance (Mattson et al. 1998, Roebuck et al. 1998b). One study (Kalberg et al. 2006) reported that children with FAS showed significantly discrepant development between their fine-motor and gross-motor development as measured by the Vineland Adaptive Behavior Scales, with significantly lower fine-motor scores. Because the children were matched on several factors, including communication age-equivalent scores, this finding suggests that the fine-motor delays in children with FAS do not necessarily parallel the cognitive/language delays, but may be related to specific neurobehavioural deficits that affect fine motor skills.

SENSORY PROCESSING

Sensory processing has long been associated with FASD but with little research to substantiate the issue. Franklin et al. (2008) conducted a study looking at the potential co-occurrence of sensory processing and problem behaviours among children with FASD. Their findings suggest that sensory processing may contribute to an affected child's ability to adapt their behaviour to various expectations of their environments. This substantiates the need for sensory supports in the school, home and community environments of children affected with FASD. In another study, the relationship between sensory processing, sensorimotor abilities, and home and school functioning were explored (Jirikowic et al. 2008). Correlations were significant between sensory processing and sensorimotor measures and some aspects of academic performance.

SOCIAL IMPAIRMENTS

Social impairments in children with prenatal alcohol exposure are also well documented in the literature. Caregivers and teachers have consistently reported social difficulties among children with prenatal exposure (Roebuck et al. 1999). These studies explored social abilities while controlling for cognitive ability and found social deficits are seen regardless of the cognitive functioning of the child. Issues with understanding social cues, difficulty communicating in social contexts, lack of consideration for the rights and feelings of others, and difficulty accepting the limits set by authority figures are all seen in children prenatally exposed to alcohol (Streissguth et al. 1996, Roebuck et al. 1999, Schonfeld et al. 2005).

The current literature on empirically proven intervention programmes (Table 14.1) With reported rates of FASD increasing and armed with the information about the known deficits seen in affected children, there is a growing demand for appropriate interventions for affected children. However, it has been historically difficult to meet the needs of this population within the service delivery system. Often children with the complex and diffuse difficulties of FASD do not fit into the eligibility categories defined by the special educational system, yet the behavioural and learning issues associated with prenatal alcohol exposure are evident and those deficits stand in the way of success for these children within their schools, homes and communities (Carmichael-Olson et al. 1992, Kalberg and Buckley 2006, Kalberg et al. 2006).

Systematic outcome studies of intervention programmes are now beginning to be reported in the literature. Several of those intervention projects are outlined below.

LANGUAGE AND LITERACY TRAINING

An intervention trial targeted at building basic literacy skills in a cohort of affected children in the Republic of South Africa was recently completed and found to be successful (Adnams et al. 2007). In this study, although no significant gains were found in FAS children versus controls on general scholastic measures, there were significant improvements in specific categories of language and early literacy (syllable manipulation, letter sound knowledge, written letters, word reading and non-word reading, and spelling).

This pilot study investigated the efficacy of a classroom language and literacy intervention in children with FASD in the Western Cape Province of South Africa. For the language and early literacy study, 40 9-year-old children identified as having FASD and 25 typically developing controls were recruited. The children with FASD were randomly assigned to either a language and early literacy intervention group or an FASD control group. Prior to intervention and after nine school-term months of treatment, general scholastic tests, teacher and parent questionnaires, classroom observations and specific language and literacy tests were administered to the participants. Despite cognitive and classroom behavioural difficulties, the children with FASD, from a vulnerable environment, demonstrated significant cognitive improvements with interventions in specific areas targeted. Although some other intervention trials have been conducted, this is the only known targeted intervention in a classroom setting.

SOCIO-COGNITIVE HABILITATION

A team at Emory University in Atlanta, Georgia, USA, with a long history of research on FAS and the neurocognitive deficits seen in children prenatally exposed to alcohol, have recently begun to assess potential interventions for children with FAS and FASD. One such intervention focused on improving behaviour and numeracy in children aged 3–10 years through parent workshops and interactive maths tutoring with the children. Their programme included workshops for parents targeted at improving their knowledge about the effects of prenatal alcohol exposure on learning and behaviour. Resources to support the affected child's education and behavioural management techniques were also presented, including case management of needed medical regimens. Finally, focused maths interventions were developed (Kable et al. 2007). The results of the programme showed gains in parental knowledge of learning and behavioural issues associated with FASD, fewer problem behaviours as assessed using the Achenbach Child Behavior Checklist (Achenbach and Edelbrock 1986), and significantly greater competence in maths ability among the group who received direct maths instruction.

SOCIAL SKILLS TRAINING

One promising systematic outcome study involves social skills training targeted at social engagement and interaction among children with FASD (O'Connor et al. 2006). This programme tested specific techniques for assisting children with FASD to follow the steps of appropriate social engagement and interaction. Social skills that were taught in the treatment settings included introducing oneself to the group, how to exchange information, where to make friends, how to join a group that is already at play, how to be a good sport, how to praise others, how to react to teasing, how to handle situations when unjustly accused of bad behaviour by an adult, being a good winner, how to avoid conflict, and how to resolve conflict.

Ninety-six children completed the study. Criteria for enrolment in the study were social skills deficits (≥ 1 SD below the mean) as measured by the socialization domain of the Vineland Adaptive Behavior Scales (Sparrow et al. 1984), and a verbal IQ ≥ 70 on the Kaufman Brief Intelligence Test (Kaufman and Kaufman 1990). The study compared the effect of parent-assisted children's friendship training (Frankel and Myatt 2003) on a

TABLE 14.1
Summary of empirically proven interventions for children with fetal alcohol spectrum disorders (FASD) and their families

Intervention (reference)	Improvements/benefits
Language and literacy training (Adnams et al. 2007)	Improved language and literacy skills (syllable manipulation, letter sound knowledge, written letters, word reading and non-word reading, and spelling). Supported academic foundations in language development – verbal abilities.
Socio-cognitive habilitation (Kable et al. 2007)	Behavioural improvements. Increased competence in maths. Increased parental understanding of FASD.
Social skills training (O'Connor et al. 2006)	Increased ability to engage in socially appropriate ways. Better social pragmatics.
Neurocognitive habilitation through self-regulation strategies (Alert Program®: How Does Your Engine Run?) (Bertrand 2009)	Increased ability to self-regulate.
Behavioural consultation (Bertrand 2009)	Increased sense of self-efficacy. Increased engagement in self-care. Increased number of family needs met.
Family summer camp (National Organization on Fetal Alcohol Syndrome, Washington State, USA) (Gelo 2009)	More knowledge about and access to critical services. Improved ability to advocate for their rights. Decreased stress and increased feelings of competence, resilience, hope and healing, due largely to the support they were getting from the families they met at the camp.
Advocacy (Duquette et al. 2006)	Persistence in high school for a group of adopted adolescents with FASD through parent advocacy. Parental expectations that their children complete high school. Parents increased their knowledge of FASD and helped create a safe and supportive academic and social environment at their child's school, appropriate accommodations and programmes. They also provided emotional and academic support at home.

treatment group and a delayed-treatment control group with regard to the maintenance of social skills gained over a three-month period. Results indicated improvements in the children's social skills knowledge and social skills along with a decrease in problem behaviours. These gains were maintained over the three-month follow-up period. Additionally, questionnaires were given to parents to assess their knowledge about prenatal alcohol exposure and their satisfaction with the intervention: 92.5% of the parents reported that the information about prenatal alcohol exposure was useful, and 89.2% reported that they would recommend the training to family and friends.

NEUROCOGNITIVE HABILITATION THROUGH SELF-REGULATION STRATEGIES
Another innovative research project, carried out by Children's Research Triangle in Chicago, Illinois, evaluated a neurocognitive habilitation programme with welfare children who

were alcohol exposed or who were diagnosed as having FASD. This programme targeted self-regulation with the hope that, if children were better able to self-regulate, they would have better executive functioning abilities. The specific intervention combined a self-regulation programme and tools for improving executive functioning abilities such as memory, cause-and-effect reasoning, sequencing, planning and problem solving. At the core of the self-regulation component of the intervention were concepts adapted from the Alert Program® (Williams and Shellenberger 1994). The Alert Program® helps children understand their own arousal level using an engine metaphor. An individual's self-regulation is equated to the engine of a car: when the engine is moving slowly, the arousal level is low; when the engine is moving too quickly, the arousal level is too high; when the engine is running at a moderate speed, the engine is just right. Children were taught to identify their own engine speeds, and they were provided with strategies for bringing these to the desired speeds (desired levels of self-regulation). They were also taught how to monitor their sensory input in order to regulate their arousal state ("How is your engine running?").

The results of this study suggested that children with FASD who participated in a neurocognitive habilitation programme showed improvement in their executive functioning skills compared with children in the control group. Post-tests were used as outcome measures. The tests used as outcome measures were the Behavior Rating Inventory of Executive Function (Gioia et al. 2000) and the Roberts Apperception Test for Children (McArthur and Roberts 1982). Children learned the self-regulatory strategies and techniques, and, as a result, the parents reported improvement in the children's executive functioning skills (memory, cause and effect reasoning, sequencing, planning and problem solving). Thirty-six families completed the full intervention programme while 28 children comprised the control group. The control children received a full evaluation but were referred to existing community and school-based programmes that were considered the standard available services for that community (Bertrand 2009).

Supporting Behavioural Differences in Children with Fetal Alcohol Syndrome: Families Moving Forward

Behavioural consultation is currently being researched at the University of Washington through a groundbreaking project called Families Moving Forward (http://depts.washington.edu/fmffasd/index.html). This model provides behaviour consultation as a collaborative process between parents and trained support specialists in fortnightly visits to the home. These home-based services make intervention accessible to families. The model includes targeted school consultation, when the support specialist can accompany the parent to the school to meet with the school team at a time that is important for the child's school progress. The parent is usually the child's most important advocate across time.

To determine the programme's efficacy, the researchers evaluated their model by comparing their intervention group (n=26) with the randomized controls (n=26) who were receiving a community standard of care. Outcome measures were used and comparisons made between baseline and post-intervention. The following primary outcome measures were used: (1) parenting attitudes of efficacy and child-related stress as measured by the Parenting Sense of Competence Efficacy Scale (Johnston and Marsh 1989); (2) stress levels as measured by the Parenting Stress Index Child Domain score (Abidin 1995); (3) caregiver ratings of the child's disruptive behaviour using the Eyberg Child Behavior Inventory Problem score (Eyberg and Pincus 1999). In addition, the following outcome measures were used to assess group differences at follow-up: (1) perceived family needs met; (2) self-reported rating of change in parent self-care across the intervention period; (3) caregiver satisfaction with the provider's skill in caring for children with special health-care needs, measured using the Multidimensional Assessment of Parental Satisfaction (Ireys and Perry 1999).

The results of the study were promising. The caregivers of children with FASD in the intervention group showed a significantly improved sense of parenting self-efficacy right after treatment compared with the control group. A greater proportion of caregivers in the intervention group reported more engagement in self-care behaviours than parents in the community comparison group (19/26 vs 11/26). The intervention group reported that their family needs were more often met in comparison to the reporting of the control group. Finally, post-intervention caregiver report of perceived child behaviour revealed decreased numbers of challenging disruptive behaviour problems among the intervention group (Bertrand 2009).

General considerations for intervention
MAKING SURE THE FAMILY'S WISHES ARE AT THE CENTRE OF HELPING THE CHILD
A key ingredient in providing successful life strategies for a person with FASD is a strong support network. This network is centred on the family. From early intervention efforts through to adulthood, the family's role is key because families know their children best and hold hopes, wishes and desires for their children. The family's desired life outcome for their child is achieved by setting realistic yearly goals for the child (Giangreco et al. 2000). Family information must be at the centre of any discussion about what will best support their child. A professional's knowledge and skills can be helpful, but it is important to remember that professionals are temporary in the child's life. Professionals move in and out of children's lives; families are invested in their child for their entire life.

PROVIDING A FOUNDATION: GUIDELINES FOR SUPPORTING A CHILD WITH A FETAL ALCOHOL SPECTRUM DISORDER (Table 14.2)
Addressing the needs of a child with FASD means developing strategies that are tailored for that individual. The following guidelines are meant to help in your approach to supporting a child with FASD. They are not hard and fast 'rules' because each guideline will need to be adapted for each person. However, they do provide a strong and realistic basis for developing successful interventions for children with FASD. The guidelines are based on research findings and real-world experiences of families.

1. *Provide structure.*
A child with FASD needs a foundation. By providing structured daily routines and schedules, a child will have an easier time navigating through his or her day. A structured day allows children to focus and organize their personal and social routines.

2. *Use simple language and be concrete.*
A child with FASD will understand language that is direct and to the point. Avoid terms

TABLE 14.2
Specific behavioural interventions

Deficit area	Intervention	References
Executive function – Memory – Planning – Sequencing	Repetition Clear structure	Dias et al. (1996), Mattson and Riley (1998), Connor et al. (2000), Kodituwakku et al. (2001a,b), Rasmussen (2005)
Auditory memory	Repetition Reinforcement Concrete and clear Language and directions	Kodituwakku et al. (1995; 2001a,b; 2006), Mattson et al. (1996, 1998, 1999), Mattson and Roebuck (2002)
Attention/hyperactivity	Sensory support Structure Novelty	Coles et al. (1997, 2002), Streissguth et al. (1998), Mattson et al. (2006), Bertrand (2009)
Behavioural – Sensory regulation – Social pragmatics – Social–emotional	Sensory support Functional behavioural assessment Positive behavioural support (consistency) Social skills training	Koegel et al. (1996), Mattson and Riley (1998), Roebuck et al. (1999), Schonfeld et al. (2005), O'Connor et al. (2006), Bertrand (2009)

that are vague like 'time for bed'. Use instructions that are positive and help the child focus on a task, such as "You need to brush your teeth and put on your pyjamas." Be concrete with instructions; show the child how to do a task or use 'props' such as a checklist or picture card.

3. Be consistent.
Apply support consistently. Maintain routines, consequences and language so that a child will understand what it takes to succeed. Include everyone involved in the child's support in the routine so that the child's support is as similar as possible across settings. Sharing support strategies with school staff, family and anyone else who helps the child will increase consistency for the child.

4. Provide supervision.
Supervision will need to be provided more constantly and for longer for a child with FASD. Feedback needs to be immediate and positive (i.e. not punishing) so that the child can succeed.

BEHAVIOURAL SUPPORT
Behavioural consultation
A behavioural therapist or behavioural support professional offers services for caregivers and children. These services are a high priority and can provide flexible, ongoing and comprehensive support that is carefully targeted to the individual needs (and strengths) of children as well as their caregivers. Behavioural consultation can be provided at a clinic, in the schools or in the home. Behavioural consultation can reduce many treatment barriers

244

and generate practical intervention ideas based on a real understanding of the child at home, in the community and at school (Koegel et al. 1996).

Functional behaviour assessment

A functional behaviour assessment is also key to determining the necessary positive behaviour support that will help ameliorate the behavioural challenges that the child displays. Because there is a dearth of empirically tested intervention strategies available for affected children, a good functional behavioural assessment can be very helpful in creating and modifying an intervention programme (Shapiro and Kratochwill 2000). A functional behaviour assessment and intervention techniques can be linked in the following ways: (1) the data from the assessment can provide the information necessary to design a programme specific to the child's problems; (2) linking the assessment to the environmental conditions of the child's behaviour can help one understand the child's behaviour in relation to various environments; (3) ongoing assessments throughout the intervention period can be conducted so that necessary changes can be made to the programme based on the assessment results. The results of a functional behaviour assessment can be used to identify a profile of strengths and challenges and the potential conditions that maintain and support each child's positive behaviour. Functional behaviour assessment includes a variety of techniques and strategies to identify the causes and likely interventions intended to address problem behaviours. This information can be gathered through direct observations, interviews with parents, teachers, coaches, etc., and questionnaires (e.g. standardized behavioural questionnaires as well as criterion-referenced questionnaires). The questions that ideally should be answered as a result are the following: What helps this child? What gets in this child's way of being successful? What are this child's interests? In other words, what motivates this child to learn? And, what strengths does this child have?

ADVOCATING FOR CHILDREN WITH FETAL ALCOHOL SPECTRUM DISORDERS

Guidelines for working with school systems and social services

When a child diagnosed with FASD enters a school system or a social service system, this system can easily become a confusing and sometimes contradictory bureaucracy. The child will need an advocate who can work in partnership with the professionals to develop the best possible support system for the child's entire school career.

Advocacy is the process of influencing people and organizations to help provide the best outcomes for an individual or group of individuals. Advocates learn as much as they can about an issue (like FASD), learn where to go for help, and then develop partnerships with other people and organizations to succeed in their goals.

In the UK, advocacy models (their evaluation and cost) have been studied by Rapaport et al. (2005, 2006). It is widely acknowledged that advocacy outcomes are difficult to measure because of the wide variability of advocacy models and the unique and complex situations of each individual. Nevertheless, advocacy models are recognized as helpful in the attainment of services, assurance of individual rights, and the ultimate empowerment of the individual for whom the advocacy is promoted.

In a study by Duquette et al. (2006), persistence in high school for a group of adopted adolescents with FASD was explained in part by parents' support and advocacy as well as parental expectation that their children complete high school. These parents obtained information about FASD, and helped create a safe and supportive academic and social environment at their child's school including appropriate accommodations and programmes. In addition, they provided emotional and academic support at home.

Guidelines for advocacy

1. *Become informed.*
Educating yourself about the laws regarding special education, social security (the welfare and benefits system), and child protection and advocacy will give you a foundation of knowledge when working with school and social services professionals. You will also need to learn more about FASD and be prepared to help provide professionals with information on FASD and how it affects your child. A list of currently available internet-based resources is presented in Table 14.3.

2. *Gather information about your child.*
A child diagnosed with FASD faces a lifelong disability. It is a good idea to begin a file about your child as soon as you can. Keep records of past examinations, testing, reports and other documentation about your child. Keep a list of issues and concerns you have and update it often. This file can become a great resource for future meetings and other contacts with school or social services professionals.

3. *Learn where to go for help.*
Building a support network for you and your child will provide a foundation upon which you can build in the future. The first step is to find out what is available. FASD is the most common cause of learning disability (mental retardation) in the USA, and there are countless formal and informal organizations that exist to help support individuals and family members. It is the advocate's role to find them, ask questions, and begin assembling a network of support.

4. *Find other families and advocates.*
Part of developing a support network will be to seek out other families in similar situations. For many people, other families provide the best source of guidance about children with FASD. Support groups, both formal and informal, can share frustrations, hardships and triumphs regarding raising a child with a disability. Many family members are also advocates for others and can help mentor and instruct people in supporting children with FASD. Again, Table 14.3 has details of some online support groups for children with FASD.

5. *Stay positive.*
Parents will encounter obstacles and frustrations along the way. There will be misunderstandings, incompetence and prejudice when dealing with the 'outside' world. However, when parents find these barriers facing them, it is far better to remain in a positive frame of mind rather than become an adversary in the 'us against them' battle. By balancing the positive in a situation (for example, what is going well in school), common ground can more easily be found to deal with what is problematic (for example, what could be improved at school).

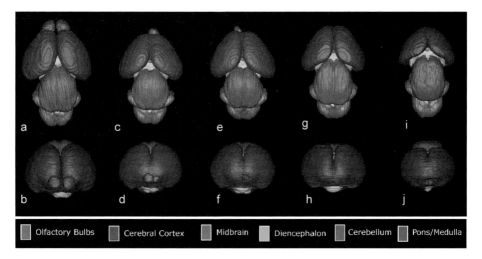

| Olfactory Bulbs | Cerebral Cortex | Midbrain | Diencephalon | Cerebellum | Pons/Medulla |

Fig. 3.11. Colour-coded magnetic resonance imaging reconstructions of control (a,b) and alcohol-exposed brains (c–j) illustrate increasing degrees of severity of holoprosencephaly in the latter. As viewed from the dorsal side (a,c,e,g,i), it is apparent that the major effect of alcohol-exposure is on the forebrain. Frontal views of the same brains (b,d,f,h,j) illustrate varying degrees of rostral union of the cerebral hemispheres and olfactory bulb deficiency or absence in the affected fetal brains. (Modified by permission from Godin et al. 2010).

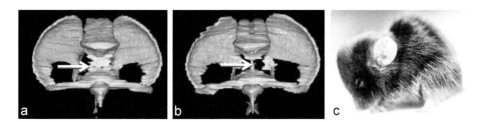

Fig. 3.16. Reconstructed magnetic resonance images of control (a) and alcohol-affected (b) ventricles, as seen in a posterior view, illustrate narrowing of the aqueductal isthmus (arrow) in the latter. Aqueductal stenosis is a causal basis for hydrocephaly, the condition evidenced by the enlarged head in the mouse in (c). Yellow = lateral ventricles; blue = mesencephalic (cerebral aqueduct) and fourth ventricle; orange = third ventricle.

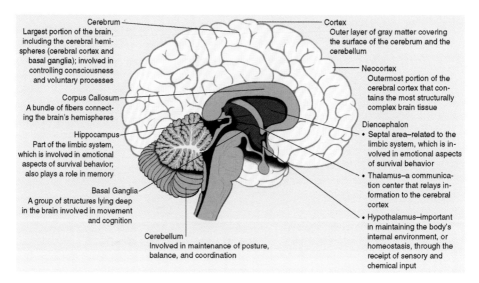

Cerebrum — Largest portion of the brain, including the cerebral hemispheres (cerebral cortex and basal ganglia); involved in controlling consciousness and voluntary processes

Cortex — Outer layer of gray matter covering the surface of the cerebrum and the cerebellum

Corpus Callosum — A bundle of fibers connecting the brain's hemispheres

Neocortex — Outermost portion of the cerebral cortex that contains the most structurally complex brain tissue

Hippocampus — Part of the limbic system, which is involved in emotional aspects of survival behavior; also plays a role in memory

Diencephalon
• Septal area—related to the limbic system, which is involved in emotional aspects of survival behavior

Basal Ganglia — A group of structures lying deep in the brain involved in movement and cognition

• Thalamus—a communication center that relays information to the cerebral cortex

• Hypothalamus—important in maintaining the body's internal environment, or homeostasis, through the receipt of sensory and chemical input

Cerebellum — Involved in maintenance of posture, balance, and coordination

Fig. 7.1. Areas of the brain that can be damaged in utero by maternal alcohol consumption. (Reproduced by permission from Mattson et al. 1994.)

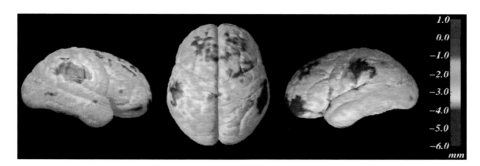

Fig. 7.2. Structural magnetic resonance imaging study that measured the difference in shape of the cerebrum in alcohol-exposed individuals and controls. Shape was quantified by measuring the distance from the centre of the brain to the surface (DFC) in millimeters. Areas highlighted in red reflect average differences of 4–6 mm in cortical thickness between alcohol-exposed individuals and controls. Negative values indicate that alcohol-exposed individuals have smaller DFC values than controls. Results illustrate that alcohol-exposed individuals have smaller brains than typically developing children, with narrowing in the inferior parietal region and some blunting in frontal areas. (Reproduced by permission from Sowell et al. 2002a.)

TABLE 14.3
Internet-based resources for information on fetal alcohol syndrome (FAS) and fetal alcohol spectrum disorders (FASDs)

National Organization on FAS
  http://www.nofas.org
  http://www.nofas-uk.org

FASD Center for Excellence
  http://fasdcenter.samhsa.gov

Teaching Students with FASDs
  http://education.alberta.ca/admin/special.aspx

Parenting Children Affected by Fetal Alcohol Syndrome – A Guide for Daily Living
  http://www.fasaware.co.uk/education_docs/daily_guide_for_living.pdf

FASD Support Network of Saskatchewan – FASD Tip Sheets
  http://www.skfasnetwork.ca

Special Needs Learning Website
  http://www.do2learn.com

Lett's Talk FASD: Parent-Driven Strategies in Caring for Children with FASD
  http://www.von.ca/FASD/index.html

Making A Difference: Working with Students with Fetal Alcohol Spectrum Disorders
  http://www.education.gov.yk.ca/pdf/fasd_manual_2007.pdf

Educational Advocacy Website
  http://www.wrightslaw.org

Transforming the Difficult Child, The Nurtured Heart Approach
  http://difficultchild.com

Also it is important to give yourself credit and make an effort to give yourself a break. Knowing that you are not alone, that others can and will help you, and that you deserve the support will go a long way in helping create the supports you want for your child.

DEVELOPING AND OFFERING A FAMILY SUMMER CAMP

One example of a resource that provides support for entire families is the FASD Family Summer Camp run by the National Organization on Fetal Alcohol Syndrome (Washington State).

This five-day camp provides a combination of family, child and parent activities. Parents receive 18 hours of workshop education and participate in eight hours of planned family activities. Children participate in recreational and skill-building activities as well as family activities. This camp is successful because of the ability to offer a very high adult-to-child ratio (1:3 minimum and 1:1 if needed), thanks to the dedication and passion of so many FASD Prevention Network staff, as well as trained volunteers and counsellors.

The balance between family, child and parent activities is the key to the programme's success. The camp provides children with disabilities recreational and outdoor opportunities that may not otherwise be available to them, or that they may be excluded from in their communities. They are placed into peer groups matched for developmental status and age.

247

There are also programmes for siblings and teenagers not affected by prenatal alcohol exposure.

Parent activities include workshops on parenting skills, understanding and advocating for their children's needs, and managing difficult behaviours. A specific networking opportunity for the fathers has been added. The camp environment allows parents to relax and take care of themselves while developing relationships with other caregivers. Camp activities focus on preventing the secondary disabilities of FASD (substance abuse, school failure, multiple home placements and involvement with the juvenile justice system), by strengthening and empowering children and families and increasing their capacity to succeed. Parental feedback on these camps has been very positive, as noted in Table 14.1.

Conclusion

Valuable research has been done in the past and new research is currently being conducted to identify promising intervention strategies for children with FASDs. The results of those studies can inform intervention teams and provide additional tools for the intervention tool box. However, the appropriateness of any given strategy for a child is dependent on the needs of that child.

In addition, the types and depth of services available for affected children vary greatly, depending on where the child lives and the range of service models available in that area. There are also many environmental factors that influence the services that are available. For example, some areas have access to centres of expertise in various disability areas such as autism spectrum disorders, some centres are focused on general disabilities, and some organizations have focused resources and efforts targeted at FASD. Rural areas typically have fewer specialized service personnel available to provide therapies. The issues of a given child are unique and complex, and the environment within which he or she resides may be continually changing.

In this chapter we have tried to build a bridge between empirically proven learning deficits in affected children and potential strategies to support children with those deficits. It is important for the reader to remember that all children are unique individuals and have their own life experiences and trajectories. To intervene appropriately, those unique factors must be assessed and reassessed to best meet the needs of the child intellectually, academically and behaviourally. The needs of any given child are dynamic and will change as the child's life and developmental course progress. Circumstances change, priorities of need change, and the interventions must be adjusted accordingly.

"Let us put our minds together and see what life we will make for our children."

Sitting Bull, Lakota Sioux, 1877

REFERENCES

Abidin RR (1995) *Parenting Stress Index, 3rd edn.* Odessa, FL: Psychological Assessment Resources.
Achenbach TM, Edelbrock CS (1986) *Child Behavior Checklist and Youth Self-Report.* Burlington, VT: Author.
Adnams CM, Kodituwakku PW, Hay A, et al. (2001) Patterns of cognitive–motor development in children with fetal alcohol syndrome from a community in South Africa. *Alcohol Clin Exp Res* 25: 557–562.

Adnams CM, Sorour P, Kalberg WO, et al. (2007) Language and literacy outcomes from a pilot intervention study for children with fetal alcohol spectrum disorders in South Africa. *J Stud Alcohol* **41**: 403–414.

Aragon AS, Kalberg WO, Buckley D, et al. (2008) Neuropsychological study of FASD in a sample of American Indian children: processing simple versus complex information. *Alcohol Clin Exp Res* **32**: 2136–2148.

Bertrand J (2009) Interventions for children with fetal alcohol spectrum disorders (FASDs): overview of findings for five innovative research projects. *Res Dev Disabil* **30**: 986–1006.

Burden MJ, Jacobson SW, Jacobson JL (2005) Relation of prenatal alcohol exposure to cognitive processing speed and efficiency in childhood. *Alcohol Clin Exp Res* **29**: 1473–1483.

Carmichael-Olson H, Burgess DM, Streissguth AP (1992) Fetal alcohol syndrome (FAS) and fetal alcohol effects (FAE): a life span view, with implications for early intervention. *Zero to Three* **13**: 24–29.

Carmichael-Olson H, Feldman JJ, Streissguth AP, et al. (1998) Deficits in adolescents with fetal alcohol syndrome: clinical findings. *Alcohol Clin Exp Res* **22**: 1998–2012.

Coles CD, Platzman KA, Raskind-Hood CL, et al. (1997) A comparison of children affected by prenatal alcohol exposure and attention deficit, hyperactivity disorder. *Alcohol Clin Exp Res* **21**: 150–161.

Coles CD, Platzman KA, Lynch ME, Freides D (2002) Auditory and visual sustained attention in adolescents prenatally exposed to alcohol. *Alcohol Clin.Exp Res* **26**: 263–271.

Connor PD, Sampson PD, Bookstein FL, et al. (2000) Direct and indirect effects of prenatal alcohol damage on executive function. *Dev Neuropsychol* **18**: 331–354.

Dias R, Robbins TW, Roberts AC (1996) Dissociation in prefrontal cortex of affective and attentional shifts. *Nature* **380**: 69–72.

Duquette C, Stodel E, Fullarton S, Hagglund K (2006) Persistence in high school: experiences of adolescents and young adults with fetal alcohol spectrum disorder. *J Intellect Dev Disabil* **31**: 219–231.

Eyberg SM, Pincus D (1999) *Eyberg Child Behavior Inventory and Sutter–Eyberg Student Behavior Inventory – Revised. Professional Manual.* Lutz, FL: Psychological Assessment Resources.

Frankel F, Myatt R (2003) *Children's Friendship Training.* New York: Brunner–Routledge.

Franklin L, Deitz J, Jirikowic T, Astley S (2008) Children with fetal alcohol spectrum disorders: problem behaviors and sensory processing. *Am J Occup Ther* **62**: 265–273.

Giangreco M, Cloninger CJ, Iverson VS (2000) *Choosing Outcomes and Accommodations for Children. A Guide to Educational Planning for Students with Disabilities, 2nd edn.* Baltimore: Paul H Brookes.

Gioia G, Isquith P, Guy S, Kenworthy L (2000) *Behavior Rating Inventory of Executive Function.* Odessa, FL: Psychological Assessment Resources.

Greene T, Ernhart CB, Ager J, et al. (1991) Prenatal alcohol exposure and cognitive development in the preschool years. *Neurotoxicol Teratol* **13**: 57–68.

Hamilton DA, Kodituwakku P, Sutherland RJ, Savage DD (2003) Children with fetal alcohol syndrome are impaired at place learning but not cued-navigation in a virtual Morris water task. *Behav Brain Res* **143**: 85–94.

Ireys HT, Perry JJ (1999) Development and evaluation of a satisfaction scale for parents of children with special health care needs. *Pediatrics* **104**: 1182–1191.

Jacobson SW, Jacobson JL, Sokol RJ, et al. (1993) Prenatal alcohol exposure and infant information processing ability. *Child Dev* **64**: 1706–1721.

Jirikowic T, Olson HC, Kartin D (2008) Physical and occupation therapy. *Pediatrics* **28**: 117–136.

Johnston C, Marsh EJ (1989) A measure of parenting satisfaction and efficacy. *J Clin Child Psychol* **18**: 167–175.

Kable JA, Coles CD, Taddeo E (2007) Socio-cognitive habilitation using the Math Interactive Learning Experience Program for Alcohol-Affected Children. *Alcohol Clin Exp Res* **31**: 1425–1434.

Kalberg WO, Buckley D (2006) FASD: What types of intervention and rehabilitation are useful? *Neurosci Biobehav Rev* **31**: 278–285.

Kalberg WO, Provost B, Tollison SJ, et al. (2006) Comparison of motor delays in young children with fetal alcohol syndrome to those with prenatal alcohol exposure and with no prenatal alcohol exposure. *Alcohol Clin Exp Res* **30**: 2037–2045.

Kaufman A, Kaufman N (1990) *Kaufman Brief Intelligence Test.* Circle Pines, MN: American Guidance Service.

Kodituwakku PW, Handmaker NS, Cutler SK, et al. (1995) Specific impairments in self-regulation in children exposed to alcohol prenatally. *Alcohol Clin Exp Res* **19**: 1558–1564.

Kodituwakku PW, Kalberg W, May PA (2001a) The effects of prenatal alcohol exposure on executive functioning. *Alcohol Res Health* **25**: 192–198.

249

Kodituwakku PW, May PA, Clericuzio CL, Weers D (2001b) Emotion-related learning in individuals prenatally exposed to alcohol: an investigation of the relation between set shifting, extinction of responses, and behavior. *Neuropsychologia* **39**: 699–708.

Kodituwakku P, Coriale G, Fiorentino D, et al. (2006) Neurobehavioral characteristics of children with fetal alcohol spectrum disorders in communities from Italy: preliminary results. *Alcohol Clin Ex Res* **30**: 1551–1561.

Koegel LK, Koegel RL, Dunlap G, eds (1996) *Positive Behavioral Support: Including People with Difficult Behavior in the Community.* Baltimore, MD: Brookes.

Lezak MD (1995) *Neuropsychological Assessment.* New York: Oxford University Press.

Mattson SN, Riley EP (1998) A review of the neurobehavioral deficits in children with fetal alcohol syndrome or prenatal exposure to alcohol. *Alcohol Clin Exp Res* **22**: 279–294.

Mattson SN, Roebuck TM (2002) Acquisition and retention of verbal and nonverbal information in children with heavy prenatal alcohol exposure. *Alcohol Clin Exp Res* **26**: 875–882.

Mattson SN, Riley EP, Delis DC, et al. (1996) Verbal learning and memory in children with fetal alcohol syndrome. *Alcohol Clin Exp Res* **20**: 810–816.

Mattson SN, Riley EP, Gramling L, et al. (1997) Heavy prenatal alcohol exposure with or without physical features of fetal alcohol syndrome leads to IQ deficits. *J Pediatr* **131**: 718–721.

Mattson SN, Riley EP, Gramling L, et al. (1998) Neuropsychological comparison of alcohol-exposed children with or without physical features of fetal alcohol syndrome. *Neuropsychology* **12**: 146–153.

Mattson SN, Goodman AM, Caine C, et al. (1999) Executive functioning in children with heavy prenatal alcohol exposure. *Alcohol Clin Exp Res* **23**: 1808–1815.

Mattson SN, Calarco KE, Lang AR (2006) Focused and shifting attention in children with heavy prenatal alcohol exposure. *Neuropsychology* **20**: 361–369.

McArthur D, Roberts G (1982) *Roberts Apperception Test for Children.* Los Angeles: Western Psychological Services.

O'Connor MJ, Frankel F, Paley B, et al. (2006) A controlled social skills training for children with fetal alcohol spectrum disorders. *J Consult Clin Psychol* **74**: 639–648.

Rapaport J, Manthorpe J, Moriarty J, et al. (2005) Advocacy and people with learning disabilities in the UK: how can local funders find value for money? *J Intellect Disabil* **9**: 299–319.

Rapaport J, Manthorpe J, Hussein S, et al. (2006) Old issues and new directions: perceptions of advocacy, its extent and effectiveness from a qualitative study of stakeholder views. *J Intellect Disabil* **10**: 191–209.

Rapport LJ, Van Voorhis A, Tzelepis A, Friedman SR (2001) Executive functioning in adult attention-deficit hyperactivity disorder. *Clin Neuropsychol* **15**: 479–491.

Rasmussen C (2005) Executive functioning and working memory in fetal alcohol spectrum disorder. *Alcohol Clin Exp Res* **29**: 1359–1367.

Roebuck TM, Mattson SN, Riley EP (1998a) A review of the neuroanatomical findings in children with fetal alcohol syndrome or prenatal exposure to alcohol. *Alcohol Clin Exp Res* **22**: 252–258.

Roebuck TM, Simmons RW, Mattson SN, Riley EP (1998b) Prenatal exposure to alcohol affects the ability to maintain postural balance. *Alcohol Clin Exp Res* **22**: 252–258.

Roebuck TM, Mattson SN, Riley EP (1999) Behavioral and psychosocial profiles of alcohol-exposed children. *Alcohol Clin Exp Res* **23**: 1070–1076.

Rolls ET, Hornak J, Wade D, McGrath J (1994) Emotion-related learning in patients with social and emotional changes associated with frontal lobe damage. *J Neurol Neurosurg Psychiatry* **57**: 1518–1524.

Sampson PD, Streissguth AP, Bookstein FL, et al. (1997) Incidence of fetal alcohol syndrome and prevalence of alcohol-related neurodevelopmental disorder. *Teratology* **56**: 317–326.

Schonfeld AM, Mattson SN, Lang AR, et al. (2001) Verbal and nonverbal fluency in children with heavy prenatal alcohol exposure. *J Stud Alcohol* **62**: 239–246.

Schonfeld AM, Mattson SN, Riley EP (2005) Moral maturity and delinquency after prenatal alcohol exposure. *J Stud Alcohol* **66**: 545–554.

Shapiro ES, Kratochwill TR (2000) *Behavioral Assessment in Schools. Theory, Research, and Clinical Foundations. 2nd edn.* New York: Guilford Press.

Sparrow S, Balla D, Cicchetti DV (1984) *The Vineland Adaptive Behavior Scales.* Circle Pines, MN: American Guidance Service.

Stratton KR, Howe CJ, Battaglia FC (1996) *Fetal Alcohol Syndrome. Diagnosis, Epidemiology, Prevention, and Treatment.* Washington, DC: National Academy Press.

Streissguth AP, Bookstein FL, Sampson PD, Barr HM (1989) Neurobehavioral effects of prenatal alcohol. Part III. PLS analyses of neuropsychologic tests. *Neurotoxicol Teratol* **11**: 493–507.

Streissguth AP, Randels SP, Smith DF (1991) A test–retest study of intelligence in patients with fetal alcohol syndrome: implications for care. *J Am Acad Child Adolesc Psychiatry* **30**: 584–587.

Streissguth AP, Barr HM, Olson HC, et al. (1994) Drinking during pregnancy decreases word attack and arithmetic scores on standardized tests: adolescent data from a population-based prospective study. *Alcohol Clin Exp Res* **18**: 248–254.

Streissguth AP, Barr HM, Kogan J, Bookstein FL (1996) *Understanding the Occurrence of Secondary Disabilities in Clients with Fetal Alcohol Syndrome (FAS) and Fetal Alcohol Effects (FAE). Final Report to the Centers for Disease Control and Prevention (CDC), August, 1996.* Seattle: University of Washington, Fetal Alcohol and Drug Unit (Technical Report No. 96-06).

Streissguth AP, Bookstein FL, Barr HM, et al. (1998) A fetal alcohol behavior scale. *Alcohol Clin Exp Res* **22**: 325–333.

Uecker A, Nadel L (1998) Spatial but not object memory impairments in children with fetal alcohol syndrome. *Am J Ment Retard* **103**: 12–18.

Willford JA, Richardson GA, Leech SL, Day NL (2004) Verbal and visuospatial learning and memory function in children with moderate prenatal alcohol exposure. *Alcohol Clin Exp Res* **28**: 497–507.

Williams MS, Shellenberger S (1994) *'How Does Your Engine Run?' A Leader's Guide to the Alert Program for Self-regulation.* Albuquerque, NM: Therapy Works.

15

FETAL TERATOGEN SYNDROMES: PSYCHIATRIC ASPECTS AND MANAGEMENT*

David J Bramble and Raja A S Mukherjee

Since the discovery that certain chemical compounds ingested prenatally could severely damage the physical development of fetuses, as exemplified by the case of thalidomide 50 years ago, the list of other extrinsic medicinal, recreational and industrial substances that could do this has steadily grown. Much of the research in this field has focused upon characterizing the specific physical abnormalities that are associated with exposure to specific compounds [e.g. cleft palate in the case of intrauterine valproic acid exposure (Kini 2006)] and screening new agents for these teratogenic effects using animal models. However, there is growing recognition that, in addition to the effects upon gross physical morphology and function, there are several chemical compounds, some of which are ubiquitous in human societies, that can also affect neurodevelopment (Chiriboga 2003, Glantz and Chambers 2006). These can lead to damage manifesting as abnormal central nervous system function both grossly, resulting in significant global intellectual impairment, and more subtly as specific developmental delays, such as dyspraxia or dyslexia, or common psychiatric disorders already accepted as having a strong neurobiological substrate such as attention-deficit–hyperactivity disorder (ADHD) and autism spectrum disorders (ASDs) (Mukherjee et al. 2005, Gray and Mukherjee 2007, Turk 2007). The impact upon the mental health of any child exposed to such compounds depends upon several factors beyond those directly attributable to the extent of the original damage or the period of neurodevelopment over which the exposure lasted; this is covered elsewhere (Chapter 3). The modern bio-psycho-social patho-aetiological model now commonly employed by mainstream mental health professionals serves to take into account as many factors as possible when attempting to understand why a particular child presents with the characteristic signs and symptoms of

---

*Note regarding terminology. The terms 'learning disability' and 'learning difficulty' are used with different meanings in different parts of the world. In the USA, 'learning disability' refers to all causes of disabilities of learning. In the UK, 'learning difficulty' would be used for this purpose. 'Learning disability' in the UK equates to the term 'mental retardation' in the USA. This is a term no longer used in many parts of the world due to its apparently stigmatizing nature; accordingly, the newer and more internationally accepted term of 'intellectual disability' is used in this chapter.

a particular psychiatric disorder, or combination of disorders, irrespective of his or her postnatal development. This review will focus upon the more common neurodevelopmental disorders and mental health problems encountered within the field of fetal teratogen syndromes (FTSs); it will describe their characteristic features, their usual presentations and the problems they pose; and it will provide broad suggestions for clinical interventions when they are indicated. While it will make reference to UK-based contexts, attempts to draw international correlates will also be made.

Specific associations
FETAL ALCOHOL SPECTRUM DISORDER AND ATTENTION-DEFICIT–HYPERACTIVITY DISORDER

The background and characteristic diagnostic features of fetal alcohol spectrum disorders (FASDs) have been discussed in Chapters 6 and 7. The high rates of psychiatric disturbance encountered in this group have been characterized by Streissguth et al. (1996, 1997) and several other workers and recently reviewed by Mukherjee et al. (2006). There would appear to be a particularly high association with ADHD, a condition that is conceptualized as being primarily a manifestation of impaired aspects of executive function underpinned by reduced dopaminergic activity. (DSM-IV diagnostic criteria for ADHD are reproduced in Table 15.1.) While there remain differences internationally in the conceptualization and diagnosis of ADHD (McGough and Barkley 2004), the association with FASD has been highlighted for many years (Oesterheld and Wilson 1997). Several studies have looked at ADHD as a diagnostic comorbidity, implying that it is a separate and distinct condition in its own right, rather than looking more closely at the associations made initially by Oesterheld and Wilson. Whilst many of these studies have been well-conceived (D'Onofrio et al. 2007), by being based on the presumption of separation of the conditions using phenomenological approaches, they leave many of the questions posed by Oesterheld and Wilson unanswered. Studies that have attempted to resolve these problems have relied upon small sample sizes, making wider generalizations difficult (Fryer et al. 2007).

Research in the general ADHD field is increasingly suggesting that, rather than basing diagnosis solely on psychopathological descriptive terms, a link to underlying brain function may be necessary (McGough and McCracken 2006). This may then allow differences between the various aetiological factors related to that brain damage to be identified, a strategy that may also be adopted and used in managing this group of individuals.

The common 'combined-type' presentation of ADHD is an individual who is pervasively physically overactive, has poor concentration skills and is likely to act impulsively, and these are all present to a disabling degree. Importantly, these features cannot be adequately explained by other factors such as general immaturity (intellectual disability) or the cognitive or behavioural effects of an underlying medical condition such as epilepsy. ADHD in its severe form has a prevalence rate in children of around 1%, but in the context of FASD this increases 10-fold, and in the full fetal alcohol syndrome (FAS) 40-fold. (For the distinction between FAS and FASD, see Chapter 6.) Further evidence would indicate that whilst many children with FASD may present with a combined type of ADHD, there are also a significant minority who are of the 'predominantly inattentive' subtype (O'Malley and

TABLE 15.1
The DSM-IV criteria for attention-deficit–hyperactivity disorder (ADHD)*

A. Either 1 or 2

1. Six or more of the following symptoms of inattention have been present for at least 6 months to a point that is disruptive and inappropriate for developmental level:

Inattention:

(a) Often does not give close attention to details or makes careless mistakes in schoolwork, work, or other activities.

(b) Often has trouble keeping attention on tasks or play activities.

(c) Often does not seem to listen when spoken to directly.

(d) Often does not follow instructions and fails to finish schoolwork, chores, or duties in the workplace (not due to oppositional behavior or failure to understand instructions).

(e) Often has trouble organizing activities.

(f) Often avoids, dislikes, or doesn't want to do things that take a lot of mental effort for a long period of time (such as schoolwork or homework).

(g) Often loses things needed for tasks and activities (e.g. toys, school assignments, pencils, books, or tools).

(h) Is often easily distracted.

(i) Is often forgetful in daily activities.

2. Six or more of the following symptoms of hyperactivity–impulsivity have been present for at least 6 months to an extent that is disruptive and inappropriate for developmental level:

Hyperactivity:

(a) Often fidgets with hands or feet or squirms in seat.

(b) Often gets up from seat when remaining in seat is expected.

(c) Often runs about or climbs when and where it is not appropriate (adolescents or adults may feel very restless).

(d) Often has trouble playing or enjoying leisure activities quietly.

(e) Is often "on the go" or often acts as if "driven by a motor".

(f) Often talks excessively.

Impulsivity:

(g) Often blurts out answers before questions have been finished.

(h) Often has trouble waiting one's turn.

(i) Often interrupts or intrudes on others (e.g. butts into conversations or games).

B. Some symptoms that cause impairment were present before age 7 years.

C. Some impairment from the symptoms is present in two or more settings (e.g. at school/work and at home).

D. There must be clear evidence of significant impairment in social, school, or work functioning.

E. The symptoms do not happen only during the course of a Pervasive Developmental Disorder, Schizophrenia, or other Psychotic Disorder. The symptoms are not better accounted for by another mental disorder (e.g. Mood Disorder, Anxiety Disorder, Dissociative Disorder, or a Personality Disorder).

Based on these criteria, three types of ADHD are identified: ADHD, Combined Type: if both criteria 1A and 1B are met for the past six months; ADHD, Predominantly Inattentive Type: if criterion 1A is met but criterion 1B is not met for the past six months; ADHD, Predominantly Hyperactive–Impulsive Type: if criterion 1B is met but criterion 1A is not met for the past six months.

*American Psychiatric Association (2000).

Storoz 2003); furthermore, the disabling symptom of inattention does not tend to attenuate with age (Streissguth 2007).

The presentation is often complicated by the fact that individuals with undiagnosed and untreated ADHD are also very likely to develop severe behavioural problems (including conduct disorder), to lead chaotic social lives, and to abuse alcohol and other drugs, all factors that can lead to FASD-affected women becoming inadvertently pregnant. Long-term follow-up studies of affected individuals in the USA have highlighted the high prevalence of these secondary disabilities, especially significant and disabling mental health problems and addiction to alcohol, as well as legal incarceration (Streissguth and O'Malley 2000). New mothers with FASD are also likely to experience difficulties in providing adequate care for their children, particularly if they are demonstrating neurodisabilities through intra-uterine alcohol exposure. Such children are thereby more likely to have developmental health problems that will render them more likely to repeat this pattern. Thus FASD can affect successive generations through an epigenetic route. These complex relationships and interactions continue to challenge clinicians working with affected children and their parents.

AUTISM AND FETAL TERATOGEN SYNDROMES

The traditional restricted view of what constitutes autism (i.e. delayed and distorted communication, impaired socialization and highly restricted imaginative development associated with strong resistance to change and rigid adherence to routines) has widened over recent years to include a broader range of symptoms, signs and developmental features that include unusual responses to sensory stimuli and impaired motor planning. This wider phenotype is referred to as autism spectrum disorder. Furthermore, the understanding of the different styles of social communication linked to the condition has been expanded and this helps to explain some of the differences seen between individuals with ASDs, some of whom originally may not have been considered to be classically autistic (Wing 1997). Through this expanding understanding, as well as through better diagnostic recognition techniques (Matson and Neal 2009), the general population prevalence of ASDs is estimated as being between 0.5% and 1.2% (Fombonne 2005, Baird 2006).

These key features of autism are also over-represented in FTS-affected children; for example, in children exposed to the anticonvulsant sodium valproate, rates of 20% have been reported (Dean et al. 2002, Kini 2006). These features are not explicable by other factors such as intellectual disability. For other teratogens, such as illicit drugs, the rates are less well defined. Studies in the FASD group are still the best reported; however, these studies are few in number and often have problems in their conceptualization. One recent study that compared the social and communication problems of two groups, one with ASD and the other with FASD, discovered that 34% of the FASD group also met criteria for autism (Bishop et al. 2007). Furthermore, people with ASDs are known to have high rates of mental health problems (up to 50%) of various types – behavioural problems (outwardly directed and self-injurious aggression), emotional problems (extremely disabling anxiety and depression), stereotypical and severe obsessional behaviour, and sleep problems (night-settling difficulties and disturbed sleep patterns) being the most prevalent (Tantam and Prestwood 1999). The combination of an ASD with an FTS will invariably add considerably to the overall disability for the affected individual and to the burden of care for their family. In the context of a full developmental work-up for a suspected FTS, the early detection of an ASD comorbidity would allow appropriate remedial educational, social, medical and other therapeutic measures to be taken. There is now a considerable literature that attests to the benefits of early intervention in enabling affected individuals to optimize their developmental potential and helping their families and carers to be able to manage them in the home setting for as long as possible (Matson and Minshawi 2006).

Diagnosis of mental health problems
The assessment of the underlying, specific teratogen-related syndromes is dealt with in previous chapters. Internationally, the best practice setting for the diagnosis of affected children, and particularly those with general developmental delays (intellectual disability), is in the context of a multidisciplinary assessment. Here the combination of paediatric, psychology, social work, speech and language therapy, physiotherapy and occupational therapy assessment results are collated. The final report is normally used to delineate the specialist health and educational input the affected child needs and what additional social support is required for the child's family. It is at this stage, most often in the case of preschool children, that specific and general intellectual disabilities and their associated comorbidities are detected. Often, however, people affected by prenatal teratogens show a broad range of intellectual impairments from an across-the-board IQ deficit to more specific difficulties with learning and intellectual functioning. Using FASD as an example, the average IQ has been shown to be shifted downwards by roughly 15 points. This does not, however, relate to functional ability, which is often more severely affected (Streissguth and O'Malley 2000). What is clear from wider neurodevelopmental work is that this group is particularly vulnerable to mental health disorders (Famy et al. 1998, Barr et al. 2006). Furthermore, later in life it would appear that they are also at greater risk of attempting suicide (Huggins 2008). Increasingly, mental health difficulties are also recognized with FTSs other than FASD. It is probably the case that much psychopathology tends to become slowly apparent as affected children grow older and their disabilities and differences compared with non-affected peers become more apparent and progressively more disabling. Thus early detection can be a useful strategy in the prevention of secondary disabilities (Chandrasena et al. 2009).

The role of child and adolescent mental health services
Internationally, each country has different strategies and methods by which disabled and potentially FTS-affected children will obtain diagnoses and management advice. Whether this is via paediatricians, dysmorphologists, clinical geneticists or psychiatrists, each centre has a method by which help is offered to a child. Using the UK as an example, referrals for mental health issues or behavioural and neurodevelopmental disorders often are received by child and adolescent mental health service (CAMHS) teams. These are the principal providers of secondary mental health services for children. Traditionally, they consist of multidisciplinary teams comprising psychiatrists, psychologists, nurses and various specialist therapists (psychotherapists, family therapists, occupational therapists, physiotherapists, and speech and language therapists).

256

Modern health-care planning requires that all children should be eligible for such services; however, given that many children with FTS have multiple physical needs as well as variable degrees of intellectual disability, affected families may find the specific help required difficult to obtain. Nevertheless, these services should be the first port of call for professionals requiring psychological or psychiatric intervention for their patients, pupils or clients when first-line measures (such as parent training courses and basic advice) fail. Given the high rates of ADHD, ASD and behavioural disorders in the group, the psychiatrist is likely to be the principal CAMHS professional involved, but will draw on the skills of colleagues as required. These services are potentially expensive resources but do offer the best practice provision for affected children to obtain help in a quick and timely manner.

Management of mental health problems: a model for professionals based upon neurodevelopmental strategies used in the UK

PRIMARY PREVENTION

As all of the major fetal teratogens are potentially avoidable, the roles of public education and pre-conception advice with high-risk women are most important here. These issues are discussed elsewhere in this volume (Chapters 2, 12 and 13). Government policies concerning the price, availability and legal proscription, especially as they apply to alcohol, tobacco and illicit substances, determine the thrust and remit of such measures, but specialist physicians (e.g. substance misuse psychiatrists), public health departments and primary care teams including general practitioners/family doctors are best placed to discuss the risks with women intending to become pregnant and especially those in high-risk groups. (For a description of effective preventative work with alcohol-dependent mothers, see Astley et al. 2000.)

Once a woman is confirmed to be pregnant, all relevant health-care personnel (midwives, general practitioners, obstetricians, etc.) should provide ongoing advice and monitor the continuing risk factors throughout the pregnancy.

EARLY DIAGNOSIS

The single biggest problem with FTS is that – other than for FAS as a full syndrome rather than FASD – there is no accepted easily identifiable pattern of facial or dysmorphic features unique to the condition. This makes recognition and management particularly difficult. Despite this, researchers have shown that early recognition can be beneficial in longer-term management. Appelbaum (1995) has shown that, for FASD at least, recognition is best made between 6 months and 3 years of age. Furthermore, the characteristic morphological features of FAS tend to fade with age (Spohr et al. 2007). Since early recognition is one factor seen as protective from secondary mental illness, the recognition, or at least highlighting of potential diagnosis, is vital for later management. This requires that young children showing the characteristic developmental delays and physical abnormalities associated with exposure to known teratogens should also be screened for emotional and behavioural problems as well as for specific neuropsychiatric conditions that are over-represented in the major teratogenic syndromes in order to prevent poorer long-term outcomes (Lockhart 2001). In particular, this should include ADHD and autism, two disorders that, if left undiagnosed

TABLE 15.2
Commonly used psychometric measures and tests

DSM-IV (American Psychiatric Association 1994) and ICD-10 (World Health Organization 1994): contain diagnostic criteria for all major mental health disorders

Strengths and Difficulties Questionnaire (Goodman 1999): a good screening instrument that includes items covering ADHD

Conners ADHD Questionnaires (Conners 1997): teacher and parent scales contain normative data for males and females in five age bands

Vineland Adaptive Behavior Scales (Sparrow et al. 1984): provide four dimensions of living skills with scoring against developmental norms

Developmental Behaviour Checklist for individuals with intellectual disability (Clarke et al. 2003): provides a behavioural score allowing measurement of outcome and change

Psychometry: includes broad IQ testing and specific tests of executive function

and unaddressed, can add considerably to the child's overall disability, as has been discussed previously.

One suggested model used in the UK is the Child Development Clinics. These are teams offering a full multidisciplinary developmental work-up, often (but not invariably) including psychometry such as IQ, executive function, working memory, communication and functional outcomes. For referred children, this contributes to an extremely informative type of assessment that has extremely strong heuristic value particularly in terms of planning for the child's educational and long-term needs. Furthermore, awareness in the UK by Child Development Clinic staff concerning the early features of ADHD and autism is generally increasing, and standardized assessment measures such as the Conners' ADHD questionnaires and the ADOS, DISCO and 3DI autism schedules are gaining popularity in this context. In this way early diagnosis can lead to early intervention and thus reduce the risk of developing secondary disabilities (Streissguth and O'Malley 2000, Matson and Neal 2009).

LATER DIAGNOSIS

Given that awareness by health professionals of the various FTSs is still at a relatively undeveloped stage (Gahagan et al. 2006), a large number of affected children and adults demonstrate the characteristic clinical features but remain undiagnosed. The prospects for older children and adolescents of receiving a late diagnosis and remedial help are probably far better than for those affected individuals who reach adulthood, especially in the UK, considering the lack of current adult neurodevelopmental specialists. However, even non-FTS-affected adults with undiagnosed ADHD or autism are currently unlikely to have their disorders diagnosed. A systematic review and clinical guidance document on ADHD pro-duced in 2008 by the National Institute for Health and Clinical Excellence, a body developed by the UK government to advise on evidence-based health practice similar to some of the roles of the Centers for Disease Control in the USA, recognizes the need for services for affected adults. Generally, if the FTS-affected adult has an associated intellectual disability, he or she is more likely to be referred to an FTS-aware clinician, usually in the context of adult intellectual disability mental health services. Unfortunately, for the majority who do not fall into this category, there is no specific service they can access.

SUMMARY OF PSYCHIATRIC ASSESSMENT AND INITIAL MANAGEMENT STRATEGIES
Assessment and diagnostic measures and tools commonly used in a psychiatric setting are listed in Table 15.2.

A general scheme for the psychiatric assessment of a patient with FTS in whom significant mental health problems are suspected is provided below. However, while this may be ideal, it may be extremely difficult at presentation to obtain all the information required, especially for children no longer in the family home. Relevant documentation, while extremely important, may be unavailable for complicated reasons such as maternal confidentiality, poor quality of historical documentation and loss of records.

Assessment process for individuals with suspected fetal teratogen disorders and comorbid psychiatric illness in clinic settings

1. Obtain background information (paediatric and obstetric notes, educational, communication and social services reports, developmental reports and growth charts)

2. Investigate suspected maternal fetal teratogen exposure

3. Establish whether parent(s) have ongoing alcohol or substance misuse habits, the severity of these and what help they are receiving for them

4. For adopted children, the age at which adoption occurred; and for all, the nature and the quality of care provided (in some settings birth and family details may be available from medical advisors in adoption and fostering)

5. Take full psychiatric, family and developmental histories including difficulties in areas related to the common comorbid conditions that have been discussed above

6. Examine the child for overt psychiatric morbidity, and establish approximate mental age or developmental quotient

7. Screening questionnaires for autism, ADHD and general morbidity (see Table 15.2)

8. Further information about key symptom areas (sleep patterns, ADHD and ASD symptoms, etc.)

9. Direct observation of the subject in key life environments (e.g. home and school)

10. Obtain paediatric opinion if outstanding physical conditions are discovered and physical investigations are required

11. Complete a diagnostic formulation and establish an agreed hierarchy of problem areas to address

12. Initiate treatment with full consent of participating individuals

Working with affected children with mental health problems

After the clinical assessment is completed, a hierarchical, problem-orientated diagnostic list is generated. Such a list should include information relating to level of intellectual function, aetiological causes, and presence of neurodevelopmental and psychiatric disorders. Normally, the most pressing, severe and disabling mental health disorder or behavioural difficulty should be considered first. While each individual assessment will highlight the areas to address, certain consistent patterns should be addressed. For example, in every case, the level of the patient's cognitive ability (approximate mental age) as well as the degree of any specific or general language or communication delays should be established so that any advice or reward system can be tailored in terms of its developmental appropriateness in order to enhance the likelihood of therapeutic success.

Generally, the types of difficulty presenting dictate the form of initial treatment required. In the case of unequivocal severe ADHD, for example, medication and psycho-educational advice should be provided. Common behavioural problems such as night-settling sleep problems should be addressed with behavioural advice by appropriately trained professionals or groups. Standard techniques to address oppositional and disruptive behaviour that require good language ability, such as problem-solving, solution-focused and anger-management strategies, should still be used, but may need to be modified in relation to each individual's language skills. For many in the FTS group this may be at a level lower than their general ability. Despite clinical evidence supporting these assertions it remains an area poorly researched and requiring lessons to be drawn from general developmental disabilities. This is an area that would warrant more detailed interventional research in the future (Chandrasena et al. 2009).

As highlighted by Streissguth and O'Malley (2000) in their study of individuals with FASD and their secondary disabilities, serious psychosexual difficulties are commonly encountered among cohorts of individuals with FASD. The combination of intrinsic difficulties relating to impulse control, empathy and emotional disinhibition coupled with a higher likelihood that affected individuals may themselves have experienced violence and abuse in their past histories, render them very likely to present such difficulties when they become sexually aware and active. Clinical evidence would suggest that these sexual presentations can range from inappropriate touching or public masturbation by a young person with intellectual disability, all the way to stalking, making obscene phone calls or committing incest as a more-able adult. Despite the seriousness of such problems they have received little research attention.

Treatment is therefore essentially pragmatic and commonly multimodal, aimed at reducing associated risk factors (e.g. treating ADHD-related impulsivity with medication, etc.) and limiting the opportunities for such behaviour to occur with appropriate levels of adult supervision. The use of external facilitators to overcome deficiencies in the child's decision-making abilities has been shown to be useful. Child friendship groups may also help affected individuals through effective peer support, such as providing helpful advice, to improve their overall capacity to function effectively in the social realm (Gray and Mukherjee 2007, Chandrasena et al. 2009). In the absence of such safeguards and ongoing risks, it can, in extreme cases, lead to the need to protect potential victims (often less-able peers) and to inform all relevant agencies of such individuals' propensities based on individual countries' responsibilities and professional requirements. Insight-orientated 'talking therapies' appear to be of limited usefulness (Shapiro 2009). Research into specific strategies that may be effective remains limited but clinical evidence would suggest that, often, behavioural approaches are best applied. More work is required to clarify this.

Prevention of secondary mental health morbidity

The work of Streissguth et al. (1999) has identified several factors that appear to be particularly beneficial in reducing the chances of young people with FASD developing secondary mental health problems. These include the early diagnosis of FTS; early detection and aggressive treatment of any emerging behavioural difficulties; being brought up in a loving, nurturing and stable home environment; eligibility for and obtaining benefits; involvement of special education and social services; and protection from exposure to violence.

Working with families

The interplay between the central nervous system damage, induced by any teratogen, and factors relating to the quality of the affected child's environment shapes the extent of developmental progress that any affected child may achieve. Early attachment behaviour and the influence of neglect in these groups cannot be discounted, but neither has sufficient work yet been undertaken to help extract the influence of biology from the environmental impact of potential abuse and neglect. Family factors have a variable influence upon this according to the specific teratogen involved and the circumstances that resulted in the child's intrauterine exposure to it. For example, clinical experience indicates that the child of a chronically alcoholic, single-parent mother is far more likely to suffer from the adverse effects of suboptimal parenting and other environmental risk factors (such as exposure to neglect and abuse) than a child exposed to the medicinal anticonvulsants prescribed for a mother with epilepsy in a stable family with no other difficulties.

These issues are not, however, always this simple. Evidence from other neurodevelopmental fields would suggest that in children with, for example, autism, attachment behaviour may not always be of a secure type, irrespective of parenting style. A study of parenting influence on attachment behaviour comparing children with ASD with normal controls and children without autism but with intellectual disability showed that children with ASD were rated as less securely attached than children in the other clinical and normal comparison groups (Rutgers et al. 2007). Furthermore, parents of the non-disabled control group reported higher levels of authoritative parenting than parents in the ASD group. Also, it was shown that, despite inadequate social support, parents of children with ASD often coped remarkably well with the challenges of raising such a child. This highlights that for a group where parental neglect may be an important factor, exploration of the parent–child relationships remains essential, and simple assumptions about causality of behaviour cannot easily be made. The research into the relationship between attachment behaviour and psychiatric outcomes in FTS-affected children clearly requires more detailed attention.

In order for any involvement with secondary level or 'specialist' clinical services to be successful, a child's basic needs have to be adequately addressed first (stable home, protection from adverse influences, adequate housing, adequate diet, etc.). In the case of children with FASD and exposure to illicit drugs, a disproportionate number are likely to be living within the 'looked-after' category or adoption and fostering systems of child care, depending upon each country's individual system's threshold for state child protection or care measures. In these circumstances the dedicated mental health team may be best placed to provide advice and support for foster carers and residential care workers, as well as working directly with children in collaboration with other statutory and voluntary services. However, for the most part, children will be treated in the context of their own (birth) families, and parents will be required to implement appropriate behavioural or family-therapy-based strategies as well as supervising the administration of any psychotropic medications.

Parental drug and alcohol exposure

The prevalence rates for alcohol and other substance misuse, particularly among women of childbearing age, have been steadily rising in the UK (BMA 2008, House of Commons 2009). There is also evidence of change in consumption levels worldwide (European Commission 2006, International Center for Alcohol Policies 2008). The low price and widening general availability of alcohol as well as a reduction in the social stigma attached to women drinking in public have all contributed to this. Mothers with alcohol- and substance-misuse problems are also likely to have other social, medical and psychological problems. When involving these women in any therapeutic programmes for their children, it is important that their own health and welfare needs are also supported by the appropriate adult services (e.g. adult drug and alcohol services and the probation service).

Parental drug misuse may also limit the pharmacological options available to the paediatrician or psychiatrist owing to the risk of diversion of controlled drugs such as methylphenidate or dexamphetamine. However, formulations of methylphenidate, such as the long-acting 'Concerta XL' osmotic delivery capsule that prevents extraction of the active medication, and atomoxetine, a non-stimulant drug, may be used as alternatives in these circumstances. Furthermore, once-a-day formulations such as these can improve compliance with medication in disorganized families. Parents who themselves have degrees of intellectual disability will also require help in their own right because any therapeutic work for the child requires that the child's needs are the primary focus of the CAMHS involvement and not those of the entire family. Adult intellectual disability teams are best placed to provide this support.

Adult services for individuals with fetal alcohol syndrome

As FTS is a developmental condition, it is important to realize that, whilst some areas of function may change over time, long-term follow-up studies have shown that persistent delays remain. For example, in the case of prenatal alcohol exposure the results for two such cohort groups have been reported (Streissguth et al. 1999, Spohr et al. 2007). They both show that changes, especially in some of the physical characteristics of the syndrome, do occur; however, other issues become more prevalent, namely secondary disabilities. As services that support children exposed to the psychological and cognitively damaging effects of teratogens develop and more affected children benefit from individually tailored care

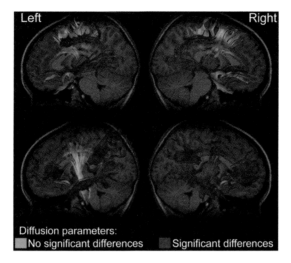

Fig. 7.3. Integrity of 10 white matter tracts in the cerebrum of children with prenatal alcohol exposure using diffusion tensor imaging tractography techniques. Diffusion tensor imaging allows measurement of white matter microstructure, which can be recreated in three dimensions through tractography. Of the 10 tracts studied, seven showed significant abnormalities in the alcohol-exposed group. These tracts included the genu and splenium of the corpus callosum, cingulum, corticospinal tracts, inferior fronto-occipital fasciculus, and inferior and superior longitudinal fasciculus. (Adapted by permission from Lebel et al. 2008.)

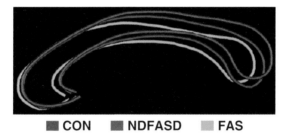

Fig. 7.4. Displacement of the corpus callosum, the major fibre tract between the two cerebral hemispheres, in children with prenatal alcohol exposure. The figure displays contours of the corpus callosum generated from structural magnetic resonance imaging. The area outlined in red is the shape and location of the corpus callosum of the control (non-alcohol-exposed) group; the contour in green represents that of the FAS group; and the contour in blue represents that of the alcohol-exposed children who did not meet criteria for FAS. Results illustrate the displacement of the isthmus and splenium (most posterior regions) in the inferior and anterior direction for alcohol-exposed children relative to non-exposed controls. (Adapted by permission from Sowell et al. 2001a.)
CON = control group (typically developing children with no history of alcohol exposure).
NDFASD = non-dysmorphic fetal alcohol spectrum disorder (children exposed to significant levels of alcohol in utero, but who did not meet full criteria for a diagnosis of FAS).
FAS = fetal alcohol syndrome (children who met full clinical criteria for FAS).

3

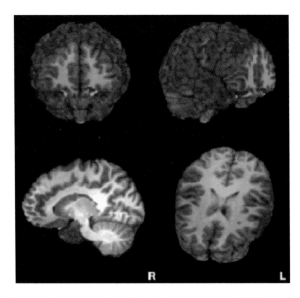

R   L

Fig. 7.5. Functional magnetic resonance imaging during a response inhibition task. Areas highlighted in blue indicate greater brain activation for alcohol-exposed children, whereas areas in orange reflect greater activation for control children during the task. During performance of the inhibition task, alcohol-exposed children showed greater activation in the right middle frontal and left superior frontal gyri (top views) and less activation in the right caudate nucleus (bottom views) relative to controls. (Reproduced by permission from Fryer et al. 2007b.)

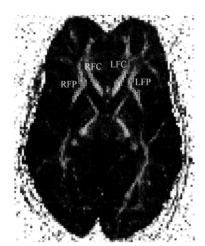

Fig. 8.2. Axial image showing white matter regions of interest. RFP = right frontal projection fibres; RFC = right frontal callosal fibres; LFC = left frontal callosal fibres; LFP = left frontal projection fibres. Cocaine-exposed children showed significantly higher average diffusion in LFC and RFC fibres. (Reprinted by permission from Warner and Behnke 2006.)

packages, the need for transition to appropriate adult generic services will become more apparent. In the UK at least, there would appear to be little prospect of this occurring at present if the patient does not have an intellectual disability. For adults with intellectual disability, mental health services are becoming aware of the psychiatric needs of this group, and if the patient requires ongoing supervision of psychotropic medication, handover to a specialist adult intellectual disability psychiatrist is usually possible. Unfortunately as this still applies to the minority, many adults find themselves not receiving an adequate level of help and support. As more FTS-affected people with ongoing mental health needs progress into adulthood, and as the awareness of FASD in particular grows, it is likely that more resources will need to be dedicated to meet their needs.

Behavioural approaches

Murphy (1991) has described a scheme for managing children with FAS, which she summarizes as the '4Ss and C' approach, that recognizes the combination of psychological difficulties such children present:

1. *Structure:* providing a clear routine and realistic choices
2. *Supervision:* depending upon the developmental needs and particular difficulties the child presents
3. *Simplicity:* use uncomplicated, clear directions and orders
4. *Steps:* use developmental rewards and repeat regularly
5. *Context:* teach skills in all life contexts and do not assume generalization or appropriateness (especially where ASD complicates the picture).

Behavioural difficulties that prove refractory to such basic advice and structure might benefit from a formal clinical psychological assessment using standard approaches such as the 'ABCs' (antecedents, behaviour and consequences) of applied behavioural analysis and treatment with appropriate contingency rewards and altered reinforcement measures, a general approach that specialist mental health teams are now commonly employing.

The role of psychotropic medication

There are no specific restrictions to the proposition of using any of the currently available and approved psychopharmacological agents in the context of addressing the mental health disorders that present within the fetal teratogen-exposed population. Different medications have, however, been shown to have differing response rates (O'Malley et al. 2000). In the past there has tended to be an over-reliance on the use of major tranquillizers (such as chlorpromazine and haloperidol) and sedative hypnotics (e.g. antihistamines) with behaviourally disturbed patients with intellectual disability, often in the absence of psychological therapies. However, modern approaches stress the use of symptom-targeted agents that are used either when other measures have failed or when combinations of drug and psychological treatments are regarded as best practice (Chandrasena et al. 2009). There is a growing trend among specialists (paediatricians and psychiatrists) when presented with a child with mental health problems that either prove refractory to other remedial measures or are themselves of sufficient intensity to merit psychopharmacological measures as a first-line measure, to characterize those groups of symptoms and signs that are causing the most distress, impairment and additional disability and select the 'best fit', most benign agent to address these. While it may be possible to accurately diagnose a formal disorder such as ADHD, in an individual with no intellectual disability, further down the ability scale, this may prove difficult. If the characteristic features are present and cannot be accounted for by other factors such as developmental delay or sensory impairments, for example, then a secure diagnosis may be made and standard treatment modalities applied. The best example of this is the most effective targeted form of medication for ADHD, namely the stimulant class of drug (methylphenidate and dexamphetamine in the UK).

There follows a brief overview of the broad classes of psychotropic agents and their applicability to mental health problems commonly associated with FTS. The literature on this is sparse. O'Malley et al. (2000) presented an overview for FASD but no such similar review exists for other FTSs. Ideas for management strategies are often extrapolated from other neurodevelopmental conditions and outcomes (Erickson et al. 2007, Leskovec et al. 2008). Without much greater amounts of directed research into this area, it is not possible to be conclusive about the statements made specifically regarding FTS.

PSYCHOSTIMULANTS

As has been discussed, the neurotoxic effects of alcohol, in particular, have been modelled in animal studies and the functional impairments reversed by amphetamine-like drugs. In the case of ADHD in association with FASD, standard psychostimulant medication such as methylphenidate and dexamphetamine may be used to treat the underlying functional impairments (inattention, poor impulse control and physical hyperactivity). The major caveat to this treatment is that these psychostimulants are controlled drugs, i.e medication with legal restrictions owing to the potential for abuse, and may be diverted by either patients or their families. Where there is a high risk of this happening, formulations that preclude easy access to the psychoactive drug, such as the Concerta XL methylphenidate delivery system, or alternative non-controlled medications, such as the noradrenergic reuptake inhibitor atomoxetine ('Strattera'), may be used instead. The usual dosage range for methylphenidate is between 15 mg and 60 mg a day in two or three divided doses. Other controlled-release preparations include 'Equasym XL' and 'Medikinet XL' capsules that contain different ratios of both immediately and long-acting smaller methylphenidate beads. These different formulations allow for the elaboration of individually tailored regimens that provide tight control of ADHD symptoms throughout the day.

ANTIPSYCHOTIC MEDICATION

Apart from their principal application in the treatment of psychotic symptoms in the context of schizophrenia or bipolar disorder, this class of agent is most commonly used in the neuro-disability field to reduce the high arousal, irritability and aggressive behaviour associated particularly with peripubertal patients with autism and intellectual disability. Currently in the UK and elsewhere, the most popular agent is risperidone and the dosage range commonly employed is between 0.5 mg and 2.5 mg a day (far lower than that used to treat psychosis), either as a once- or twice-a-day regimen. Risperidone and other antipsychotics may also be used to reduce sex drive. Antipsychotic medication should not be regarded as a first-line or sole therapeutic measure unless it is used in a crisis context. Furthermore, owing to rising levels of concern about the long-term side-effects of antipsychotic drugs – including excessive weight gain, raised levels of the hormone prolactin, cardiac arrhythmias and extrapyramidal neurological problems (parkinsonism, dystonias and tardive dyskinesia) – every attempt must be made to avoid long-term use and to consider other techniques or alternative medications to achieve the desired outcome.

ANTIDEPRESSANTS

While FASD may render older individuals more prone to develop formal clinical depression, it is the generalized anxiety, phobic anxiety and obsessive–compulsive behaviour associated with older children, adolescents and adults with autism that may respond to a selective serotonin re-uptake inhibitor such as fluoxetine hydrochloride ('Prozac') when other measures prove partially or totally ineffective. It is best to commence therapy with a low dose of the liquid formulation (5 mL/20 mg strength) such as 2.5 mL in the morning. The usual effective dose is 5–10 mL/day, but with severely anxious and obsessional individuals doses of up to 20 mL (80 mg) a day may be required. A common practice in North America is to combine a selective serotonin reuptake inhibitor and a stimulant in this context, although the efficacy of this practice has not yet received systemic evaluation.

ANXIOLYTICS

While the selective serotonin reuptake inhibitors and other antidepressant compounds may prove effective in 'trait' generalized anxiety states, the benzodiadepine anxiolytics (commonly diazepam and lorazepam) may be employed to good effect with individuals with 'state' or situationally triggered anxiety. In these circumstances, small doses of diazepam (2–5 mg) or lorazepam (1–2 mg) may be given in anticipation of predictably distressing events such as plane journeys, social gatherings, fireworks celebrations, etc. Caution needs to be applied in the context of FASD because there is a theoretical risk of social disinhibition, which may worsen established problems in this area such as inappropriate sexual approaches to vulnerable peers. Treatment should be short-term or intermittent in order to prevent problems of physiological dependence.

HYPNOTICS

No specific sleep disorders have been associated with any FTS so it is likely that any sleep-related problems encountered in this group are primarily attributable to common comorbidity factors such as intellectual disability, ADHD and autism. While there is emerging evidence for a deficiency in melatonin production in some people with ASD (Gianotti et al. 2006) and general intellectual disabilities (Braam et al. 2008), it is not clear whether this is also the case for those prenatally exposed to teratogens as a possible cause of the ASD. The most common sleep problems involve the person not settling at the desired time, repeatedly waking during the night and/or waking too early. Often this sleep disruption results in daytime sleepiness that can adversely affect demeanour, cognitive ability and daytime behaviour, thus compounding the net disability as well as contributing significantly to the overall burden of care.

Behavioural modification interventions involving the implementation of a range of techniques including strict sleep hygiene, cueing, either rapid or graded extinction methods and developmentally appropriate rewards are usually effective for the more straightforward cases. Hypnotic medication is best reserved for use in patients whose sleep problems prove refractory to these methods or in crisis situations. Melatonin is now widely used in UK paediatric and CAMHS settings for this purpose at a dose of 2–15 mg to be taken 30 minutes before settling. For best results, it is used in combination with behavioural techniques. When successful, some patients may require long-term treatment, but regular attempts to withdraw the agent ought to be built into any programme. Alternatives to melatonin in older patients are the so-called 'z' drugs (zopiclone, zolpidem and zaleplon), but these agents should not be used for longer than a few weeks because of the potential for dependence. Furthermore, they can occasionally produce states of paradoxical excitement and disinhibition, and they should not be given to patients with the night-time breathing difficulties associated with obstructive sleep apnoea.

ANTICONVULSANTS
Many drugs used in the context of epilepsy – e.g. carbamazepine, sodium valproate and lamotrigine – also have potent mood-stabilizing and explosive-anger-reduction properties and may be used where patients with FTS present difficulties of this type that prove refractory to psychological measures. The dosages used are the same as those used in the treatment of epilepsy. A trial of such therapy takes several weeks to allow a slow build-up of the dose and a period when therapeutic serum levels are operating; three or four months is advised. It should also be stated that some anticonvulsants – e.g. phenytoin, phenobarbitone and vigabatrin – may produce disinhibition, confusion and aggression in vulnerable patients and are best avoided.

Specialist clinics
Around the world different models of service delivery for people with FTS exist. Often these are in specialist centres and as yet do not have a regular place in routine neurodevelopmental clinics. For example, in the UK there are relatively few centres specializing in FASD diagnosis and management. One such example involving a psychiatric speciality clinic dedicated to a particular disorder is run by the second author in Surrey, UK. This has also served as a focus for research and training as well as a tertiary diagnostic and treatment centre. A model of service delivery was proposed in various documents, for example a review conducted into FASD by the Centers for Disease Control in the USA (National Center on Birth Defects and Developmental Disabilities 2004) and the British Medical Association in the UK (BMA Board of Science 2007). These are yet to be fully established. Given that the other FTSs with high mental-health comorbidity are an order of magnitude less prevalent than FASD, it is unlikely that similar clinics will be established for them.

Support groups for parents
The impact of having a child with FTS is almost invariably considerable. Over recent years, with growing recognition of the more common syndromes, various groups have been

established by affected families to provide a range of advice, support and educational resources. Many go further by holding regular support-group meetings and providing telephone helplines, newsletters, family activity events, conferences and training courses. Internationally there are similar organizations, each working in a complementary way, bringing together the different facets of the complex support that is needed for families and affected individuals.

The work of these groups, however, can go beyond just a support role, and increasingly they have taken on the role of lobbyist, working through political persuasion to change legislation and prevent primary and secondary harm from the effects of fetal teratogens.

Other sources of support

Alongside specific support groups, help for families whose children are suffering from the more common neuropsychological disorders associated with fetal teratogen exposure can be found in the relevant 'generic' support groups, e.g. for ADHD, autism and intellectual disabilities. Further, governments in some parts of the world are beginning to provide support for families. For example, in Britain, statutory local authority services all now have dedicated multidisciplinary teams whose brief is to support families experiencing difficulties with their children who have an intellectual disability. However, the thresholds for eligibility vary significantly between local authorities, and often children with significant disabilities who are causing major difficulties but have only a mild or moderate intellectual disability may not fulfil the specialist team's eligibility criteria.

Case example: fetal alcohol syndrome

John is a 16-year-old male, diagnosed with full FAS six years previously, who has severe intellectual disability and attends a special school. His diagnosis was delayed owing to the fact that he was previously in the sole care of his mother who was, and remains, a chronic alcoholic with a chaotic lifestyle involving frequent changes of partners and geographical location. There had been many previous involvements with social services resulting from concerns about her capacity to meet his basic needs. His birth father, with whom he had previously had little contact, agreed to take over his care when John was 9. From the outset, it was apparent that John had several areas of difficulty in addition to his intellectual disabilities: he was conspicuously socially disinhibited, he displayed impulsive sexually inappropriate behaviour towards peers of both sexes at his new special school, and his capacity to sit still and listen was conssiderably worse than that of his peers. At his first paediatric review, the characteristic facial features of FAS were detected, and a referral to a local CAMHS intellectual disability team for a psychiatric assessment revealed pronounced features of ADHD as well as a significant degree of social disinhibition and marked difficulties in terms of his ability to empathize with others, although he did not show any other features of autism. He was prescribed methylphenidate along with a recommendation that he should be supervised by adults at all times when at school and away from home. Home- and school-based observations, as well as symptom-score inventories, indicated a good response. His academic performance at school and his behaviour at home both improved, but his propensity to molest peers when even briefly out of the supervision of adults continued intermittently. This behaviour became markedly more compulsive in nature as he negotiated puberty and he was excluded from school following a serious assault on a younger boy. Developmentally sensitive counselling and tightening up the supervision arrangements as well as encouraging the normal expression of his sexual tension resulted in good control of this problem. He continues to derive benefit from immediate-release methylphenidate, although a trial of a controlled-release formulation was not successful. Plans for his transition to adult mental health services are currently underway, and the need for ongoing close supervision in situations when he is with potentially vulnerable peers is being strongly emphasized in the individualized care package.

Conclusions

Whilst certain FTSs strongly predict that affected individuals will develop disabling mental health problems, they are by no means invariable. Rather it is the complex and reciprocal interplay between an affected individual's developing damaged brain, the environment he or she experiences, and the capacity of the individual to adapt to this, that determines whether and, if so, what broad types of psychiatric problems emerge. Furthermore, those individuals with an FTS who are also comorbid for neurodevelopmental problems such as ADHD and ASD are more likely to develop mental health problems because both can adversely influence the 'brain–environment' interaction.

Early detection of the underlying condition and then prompt provision of the appropriate support and treatment should reduce the chance of problems emerging, allowing affected children to optimize their developmental potential and also reduce the burden of care their families are likely to face. Access to high-quality mental health services with 'FTS-aware' staff should help greatly in this process. Unfortunately, such services are very underdeveloped at present, meaning that children and their families effectively face a care and therapy 'lottery' in this respect, although growing interest in the field should help to improve this situation.

In parallel with improvements in health-service delivery to these patients and with growing awareness of the huge individual, family and societal costs of these essentially preventable conditions, wider and more comprehensive measures need to be taken. Prenatal exposure to alcohol is emerging as probably the single most important preventable 'environmental' cause of intellectual disability and ADHD in the UK and in many other developed societies. Given this, there ought to be a strong, coordinated educational, public health and governmental effort to take specific remedial measures that should include limiting the currently virtually ubiquitous availability of alcohol, increasing its price and giving out clear health warnings to women about the desirability of not drinking during pregnancy.

REFERENCES

American Psychiatric Association (1994) *Diagnostic and Statistical Manual of Mental Disorders, 4th edn.* Washington, DC: APA.

American Psychiatric Association (2000) *Diagnostic and Statistical Manual of Mental Disorders. 4th edn, Text Revision.* Washington, DC: APA.

Appelbaum M (1995) Fetal alcohol syndrome: diagnosis, management and prevention. *Nurse Pract* **20**: 24, 27–28, 31–33.

Astley SJ, Bailey D, Talbot C, Clarren SK (2000) Fetal alcohol syndrome (FAS) primary prevention through FAS diagnosis: II. A comprehensive profile of 80 birth mothers of children with FAS. *Alcohol Alcoholism* **35**: 509–519.

Baird G, Simonoff E , Pickles A, et al. (2006) Prevalence of disorders of the autism spectrum in a population cohort of children in South Thames: the Special Needs and Autism Project (SNAP). *Lancet* **368**: 210–215.

Barr HM, Bookstein FL, O'Malley KD, et al. (2006) Binge drinking during pregnancy as a predictor of psychiatric disorders on the structured clinical interview for DSM-IV in young adult offspring. *Am J Psychiatry* **163**: 1061–1065.

Bishop S, Gahagan S, Lord C (2007) Re-examining the core features of autism: a comparison of autism spectrum disorder and fetal alcohol spectrum disorder. *J Child Adolesc Psychol Psychiatry* **48**: 1111–1121.

BMA Board of Science (2007) *FASD: a Guide for Healthcare Practitioners.* London: BMA.

BMA Board of Science (2008) *Alcohol Misuse: Tackling the UK Epidemic.* London: BMA.

Braam W, Didden R, Smits M, Curfs L (2008) Melatonin treatment in individuals with intellectual disability and chronic insomnia: a randomized placebo-controlled study. *J Intellect Disabil Res* **52**: 256–264.

Chandrasena AN, Mukherjee RAS, Turk JT (2009) Fetal alcohol spectrum disorders: an overview of interventions for affected individuals. *Child Adolesc Ment Health* **14**: 162–167.

Chiriboga C (2003) Fetal alcohol and drug effects. *Neurologist* **9**: 267–279.

Clarke AR, Tonge BJ, Einfeld SL, Mackinnon A (2003) Assessment of change with the Developmental Behaviour Checklist. *J Intellect Disabil Res* **47**: 210–212.

Conners CK (1997) *Conners' Rating Scales—Revised.* Toronto: Multi-Health Systems.

Dean JC, Hailey H, Moore SJ, et al. (2002) Long term health and neurodevelopment in children exposed to antiepileptic drugs before birth. *J Med Genet* **39**: 251–259.

D'Onofrio BM, Van Hulle CA, Waldman ID, et al. (2007) Causal inferences regarding prenatal alcohol exposure and childhood externalizing problems. *Arch Gen Psychiatry* **64**: 1296–1304.

Erickson CA, Posey DJ, Stigler KA, McDougle CJ (2007) Pharmacological treatments of autism spectrum disorders. *Pediatr Ann* **36**: 575–585.

European Commission Health and Consumer Protection Directorate-General (2006) *Pure Alcohol Consumed, Litres per Capita, Age 15+. Health for All Database.* Geneva: WHO.

Famy C, Streissguth AP, Unis AS (1998) Mental illness in adults with fetal alcohol syndrome or fetal alcohol effects. *Am J Psychiatry* **155**: 552–554.

Fombonne E (2005) The changing epidemiology of autism. *J Appl Res Learn Disabil* **18**: 281–294.

Fryer LS, McGee CL, Matt GE, et al. (2007) Evaluation of psychopathalogical condition of children exposed to heavy prenatal alcohol. *Paediatrics* **119**: 733–741.

Gahagan S, Telfair Sharpe T, Brimacombe M, et al. (2006) Pediatricians' knowledge, training, and experience in the care of children with fetal alcohol syndrome. *Pediatrics* **118**: 657–668.

Giannotti, F, Cortesi F, Cerquiglini F, Bernabei P (2006) An open-label study of controlled-release melatonin in treatment of sleep disorders in children with autism. *J Autism Dev Disord* **36**: 741–752.

Glantz M, Chambers JC (2006) Prental drug effects on subsequent vulnerability to drug use. *Dev Psychopathol* **18**: 893–922.

Goodman R (1999) The extended version of the Strengths and Difficulties Questionnaire as a guide to child psychiatric caseness and consequent burden. *J Child Psychol Psychiatry* **40**: 791–801.

Gray R, Mukherjee RAS (2007) A psychiatrist's guide to foetal alcohol spectrum disorders in mothers who drank heavily during pregnancy. *Adv Ment Health Learn Disabil* **1**: 19–26.

House of Commons Select Committee (2009) *Alcohol.* London: The Stationery Office.

Huggins JE, Grant T, O'Malley K, Streissguth AP (2008) Suicide attempts among adults with fetal alcohol spectrum disorders: clinical considerations. *Ment Health Aspect Dev Disabil* **11**: 33–41.

International Center for Alcohol Policies (2008) *Non-commercial Alcohol in Three Regions.* Washington, DC: ICAP.

Kini U (2006) Fetal valproate syndrome: a review. *Pediatr Perinat Drug Ther* **7**: 123–130.

Leskovec TJ, Rowles BM, Findling RL (2008) Pharmacological treatment options for autism spectrum disorders in children and adolescents. *Harvard Rev Psychiatry* **16**: 97–112.

Lockhart PJ (2001) Fetal alcohol spectrum disorders for mental health professionals – a brief review. *Curr Opin Psychiatry* **14**: 463–469.

Matson JL, Minshawi NF (2006) *Early Intervention for Autism Spectrum Disorders: a Critical Analysis.* Oxford: Elsevier.

Matson JL, Neal D (2009) Diagnosing high incidence autism spectrum disorders in adults. *Res Autism Spectrum Disord* **3**: 581–589.

McGough JJ, Barkley RA (2004) Diagnostic controversies in adult ADHD. *Am J Psychiatry* **161**: 1948–1956.

McGough JJ, McCracken JT (2006) Adult attention deficit hyperactivity disorder: moving beyond DSM-IV. *Am J Psychiatry* **163**: 1673–1675 (editorial).

Mukherjee R, Hollins S, Abou-Saleh M, Turk J (2005) Low level alcohol consumption and the fetus. *BMJ* **330**: 375–376.

Mukherjee R, Hollins S, Turk J (2006) Fetal alcohol spectrum disorder: an overview. *J R Soc Med* **99**: 298–302.

Murphy MF (1991) *Hope for the FAS/FAE Child: An Educational Approach for Success in the Classroom.* Bethel, AK: Lower Kuskokwim School District.

National Center on Birth Defects and Developmental Disabilities (2004) *Fetal Alcohol Syndrome; Guidelines for Diagnosis and Referral.* Washington, DC: CDC.

National Institute for Health and Clinical Excellence (2008) *NICE Clinical Guideline 72: Attention Deficit Hyperactivity Disorder: Diagnosis and Management of ADHD in Children, Young People and Adults.* London: NICE (online at: http://www.nice.org.uk/nicemedia/pdf/CG072NiceGuidelineV2.pdf).

Oesterheld JR, Wilson A (1997) ADHD and FAS. *J Am Acad Child Adolesc Psychiatry* **36**: 1163.

O'Malley KD, Storoz L (2003) Fetal alcohol spectrum disorder and ADHD: diagnostic implications and therapeutic consequences. *Expert Rev Neurother* **3**: 477–489.

O'Malley KD, Koplin B, Dohner VA (2000) Psychostimulant clinical response in fetal alcohol syndrome. *Can J Psychiatry* **45**: 90–91.

Rutgers AH, van Ijzendoorn MH, Bakermans-Kranenburg MJ, et al. (2007) Autism, attachment and parenting: a comparison of children with autism spectrum disorder, mental retardation, language disorder, and non-clinical children. *J Abnorm Child Psychol* **35**: 859–870.

Shapiro T (2009) Psychotherapy for autism. *J Infant Child Adolesc Psychother* **8**: 22–31.

Sparrow SS, Balla DA, Cicchetti DV (1984) *Vineland Adaptive Behaviour Scales (VABS).* Circle Pines, MN: American Guidance Service.

Spohr HL, Willms J, Steinhaussen HC (2007). Fetal alcohol spectrum disorders in young adults. *J Paediatr* **150**: 175–179.

Streissguth A (2007) Offspring effects of prenatal alcohol exposure from birth to 25 years: the Seattle prospective longitudinal study. *J Clin Psychol Med Settings* **14**: 81–101.

Streissguth AP, O'Malley K (2000) Neuropsychiatric implications and long-term consequences of fetal alcohol spectrum disorders. *Semin Clin Neuropsychiatry* **5**: 177–190.

Streissguth AP, Barr HM, Kogan J, Bookstein FL (1996) *Understanding the Occurrence of Secondary Disabilities in Clients with Fetal Alcohol Syndrome (FAS) and Fetal Alcohol Effects (FAE). Final Report to the Centers for Disease Control and Prevention (CDC), August 1996. Technical Report No. 96–06.* Seattle: University of Washington, Fetal Alcohol and Drug Unit.

Streissguth, A, Barr H, Kogan J, Bookstein F (1997) Primary and secondary disabilities in fetal alcohol syndrome. In: Streissguth A, Kanter J, eds. *The Challenge of Fetal Alcohol Syndrome: Overcoming Secondary Disabilities.* Seattle: University of Washington Press, pp. 25–39.

Streissguth AP, Barr HM, Bookstein FL, et al. (1999) The long-term neurocognitive consequences of prenatal alcohol exposure: a 14-year study. *Psychol Sci* **10**: 186–190.

Tantam D, Prestwood S (1999) *A Mind of One's Own: a Guide to the Special Difficulties and Needs of the More Able Person with Autism or Asperger Syndrome. 3rd edn.* London: National Autistic Society.

Turk J (2007) Behavioural phenotypes: their applicability to children and young people who have intellectual disability. *Adv Ment Health Learn Disabil* **1**: 4–13.

Wing L (1997) The autistic spectrum. *Lancet* **350**: 1761–1766.

World Health Organization (1994) *The ICD-10 Classification of Mental and Behavioural Disorders: Diagnostic Criteria for Research.* Geneva: WHO.

Xu C, Shen RY (2001) Amphetamine normalizes the electrical activity of the dopamine neurons in the ventral tegmental area following prenatal ethanol exposure. *J Pharmacol Exper Therap* **297**: 746–752.

16

RECOMMENDED MANAGEMENT OF COMMON MEDICAL PROBLEMS IN PREGNANCY: ADVICE FROM SPECIALIST AGENCIES

Evelyne Jacqz-Aigrain and Philip M Preece

All prospective studies evaluating drug prescriptions, conducted in Europe, reported that most women receive a prescription for at least one drug during pregnancy, with a mean of 13.6 medications per woman in the study by Lacroix et al. (2000), based on French health insurance records. As more than half of all pregnancies are unplanned, millions of unborn babies are exposed to xenobiotics early during embryogenesis. The Motherisk programme in Toronto, Canada, reported that the most common drugs taken during pregnancy were analgesics, antihistamines and decongestants (Koren 2001), in most cases not prescribed by a physician but bought 'over the counter'. In addition, non-medical substances were taken, most commonly alcohol, consumed by over 50% of women in developing countries, followed by cigarettes and cannabis (Gray et al. 2009, Huizink 2009). Drugs are also prescribed by physicians later in pregnancy for acute conditions that occur similarly in non-pregnant adults, for a complication of pregnancy such as toxaemia or for chronic maternal diseases (Meadows 2001). Weighting the risk/benefit ratio of a prescription is essential to avoid potential fetal and maternal toxicity.

The potential consequences of drug exposure depend upon the drug itself, its placental transfer to the fetus and stage of pregnancy at exposure. The human teratogenic effects of thalidomide and retinoids have led the medical profession to realize how dangerous medications can be even without adverse maternal effects (Jacqz-Aigrain and Koren 2005, Rane 2006). In addition to these drastic situations, clinicians are frequently faced with a compromise situation between either a mandatory maternal treatment and its potential fetal effects or, in fewer situations, the maternal and fetal side-effects when fetal treatment is mandatory. A critically important group of women are those who need to continue drug therapy during pregnancy to ensure their health against a range of disorders. These include a large number of chronic diseases and conditions such as depression, asthma, diabetes and organ transplantation, and in these situations, the evaluation of drugs taken in pregnant women remains limited in terms of pharmacokinetics, efficacy, and maternal and fetal toxicity. Clinical trials of drugs under development rarely if ever include women of childbearing age, and

271

effective contraception is usually mandatory. Randomized control trials, which require the deliberate administration of a medicinal product to pregnant women, are often not feasible. Because little is known before marketing about the potential teratogenic and/or toxic risks of a drug during pregnancy, post-marketing surveillance is critical to the detection of drug-induced fetal effects, to provide the most up-to-date available data and to modify product labelling on the risks or absence of risks during pregnancy.

Therefore, clinicians have to deal with a large variety of situations where the mother and fetus are exposed to drugs, and the evaluation of the risk/benefit ratio of drug administration during pregnancy in individual cases often remains a challenge. Women may even be discouraged from getting pregnant, or discouraged from continuing needed therapy, although uncontrolled or suboptimal controlled conditions such as depression may affect pregnancy outcome or fetal well-being as discussed in Chapter 5.

Various sources of data are used by experts to evaluate the potential risk of exposure to a specific medicinal product, in the absence of adequate human studies. Animal studies look for possible adverse reproductive effects in humans by giving animals higher doses of a drug. Experts also consider how a drug works and its likely effects, reported experiences with similar drugs, spontaneous reports and case series of adverse events. Additionally, registries of birth defects or prospective pregnancy registries following women taking a certain drug until their pregnancy ends allow researchers to use the results to assess risks to mothers and their babies. The stage of pregnancy also influences clinical decisions. For example, after 24 weeks of pregnancy, the antibiotic tetracycline can cause permanent staining of a baby's teeth, and angiotensin-converting enzyme inhibitors or anti-inflammatory drugs can damage a baby's kidneys in the second and third trimesters of pregnancy.

Based on available data, guidances are issued by experts and made available through national health services, scientific societies and medical agencies, with detailed recommendations on how to analyse individual risks of a given drug for an individual pregnant woman and her baby and how to optimize treatment and follow-up.

In Britain the National Institute for Health and Clinical Excellence (NICE) issues clinical guidelines and recommendations about the treatment and care of people with specific diseases and conditions, including pregnancy. The number of clinical situations in pregnancy already analysed remains limited but will certainly increase in the near future. As an example, a recent reference guide, *Diabetes in Pregnancy* (NICE 2008) reviews recommendations on treatment and care of pregnant diabetic women. The guidance identifies key priorities in pre-conception, antenatal, neonatal and postnatal care that will help physicians and pregnant women. Additional documents were made available by the Food and Drug Administration (FDA) (FDA 2002, 2004, 2005, 2008) and European Medicines Evaluation Authority (EMEA) (CHMP–EMEA 2005) in order to help evaluate the risk of drugs taken during pregnancy and to provide updated information on the use of prescription drugs and biological products during pregnancy and breastfeeding. In addition, as short-comings in the labelling of prescription medicines with respect to their potential effects during pregnancy and breastfeeding are well recognized, medical agencies and the pharmaceutical industry have the common goal of improving the information available to women and their physicians in this regard (FDA 2008). The pregnancy section of the labelling will soon include

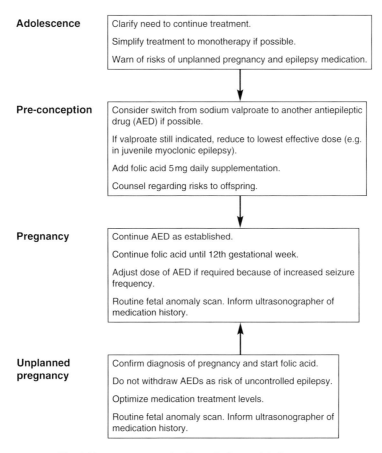

| Adolescence | Clarify need to continue treatment.

Simplify treatment to monotherapy if possible.

Warn of risks of unplanned pregnancy and epilepsy medication. |

| Pre-conception | Consider switch from sodium valproate to another antiepileptic drug (AED) if possible.

If valproate still indicated, reduce to lowest effective dose (e.g. in juvenile myoclonic epilepsy).

Add folic acid 5 mg daily supplementation.

Counsel regarding risks to offspring. |

| Pregnancy | Continue AED as established.

Continue folic acid until 12th gestational week.

Adjust dose of AED if required because of increased seizure frequency.

Routine fetal anomaly scan. Inform ultrasonographer of medication history. |

| Unplanned pregnancy | Confirm diagnosis of pregnancy and start folic acid.

Do not withdraw AEDs as risk of uncontrolled epilepsy.

Optimize medication treatment levels.

Routine fetal anomaly scan. Inform ultrasonographer of medication history. |

Fig. 16.1. Management of epilepsy before and during pregnancy.

three subsections: (1) a fetal risk summary, (2) clinical considerations with information on the use of the drug during pregnancy, and the risks of the disease itself to the mother and her baby, and (3) a description of available data; additional information will also be provided on breastfeeding.

Using the evidence reviewed in the previous chapters together with national guidance from professional bodies and specialist reports, we have attempted to produce some broad advisory algorithms. The advice may have to be modified to take account of national differences in procedure, particularly in respect of social legislation and social care practice.

The management of epilepsy reflects the clear evidence that sodium valproate, one of the most commonly used antiepileptic drugs, is associated with much higher rates of long-term problems and major malformations than other antiepileptic medications (Chapter 4). Valproate should therefore be avoided in pregnancy if possible, and, if used, the dose should be limited to <1.0 g/day (Fig. 16.1).

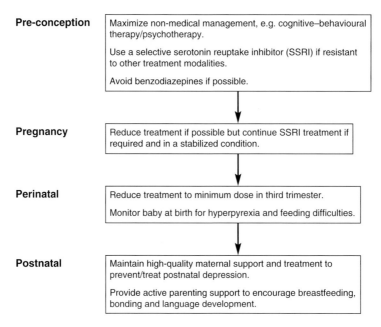

Pre-conception — Maximize non-medical management, e.g. cognitive–behavioural therapy/psychotherapy.

Use a selective serotonin reuptake inhibitor (SSRI) if resistant to other treatment modalities.

Avoid benzodiazepines if possible.

Pregnancy — Reduce treatment if possible but continue SSRI treatment if required and in a stabilized condition.

Perinatal — Reduce treatment to minimum dose in third trimester.

Monitor baby at birth for hyperpyrexia and feeding difficulties.

Postnatal — Maintain high-quality maternal support and treatment to prevent/treat postnatal depression.

Provide active parenting support to encourage breastfeeding, bonding and language development.

Fig. 16.2. Management of depression before, during and after pregnancy.

The management of depression and major psychiatric disorders is more clear. The evidence cited in Chapter 5 shows the effect of untreated depression on infant bonding and subsequent development, so treatment should be continued if required throughout pregnancy despite the short-term effects of selective serotonin reuptake inhibitors (SSRIs) in the neonatal period. Dosage may be reduced in the third trimester to minimize perinatal problems but there is little evidence to support the practice of switching to a tricyclic antidepressant and risking poor symptom control. Clearly, postnatal support to encourage bonding is important to build a strong mother–child relationship and aid long-term development (Fig. 16.2).

As discussed in Chapters 2 and 6, alcohol-related problems in women are often under-recognized and so efforts should be made to accurately assess alcohol intake in early pregnancy to allow early intervention and so minimize damage (Fig. 16.3). Clearly, in heavy alcohol users, this will not prevent fetal alcohol syndrome, as much of the damage is already established in the first few weeks of pregnancy (see Chapter 3), but early intervention may ameliorate the effects and make the long-term viability of the family more secure (see Chapter 13). Risk assessment is necessary in late pregnancy so that welfare agencies can plan for the management of the perinatal period, establish criteria for success and formulate a child protection plan. If the risks to the infant are high owing to maternal non-compliance and other risks such as domestic violence, then a robust child protection plan will be required (Fig. 16.4). Identification of problems will also allow future cases of fetal alcohol syndrome to be prevented if remedial maternal treatment proves possible.

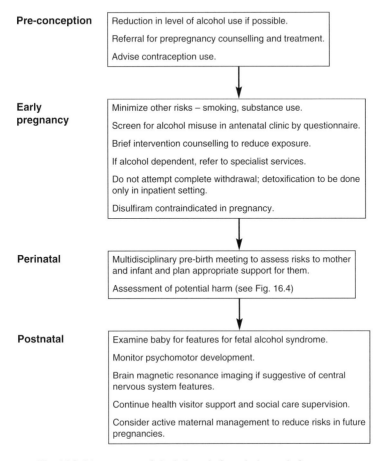

Pre-conception	Reduction in level of alcohol use if possible.
	Referral for prepregnancy counselling and treatment.
	Advise contraception use.

Early pregnancy	Minimize other risks – smoking, substance use.
	Screen for alcohol misuse in antenatal clinic by questionnaire.
	Brief intervention counselling to reduce exposure.
	If alcohol dependent, refer to specialist services.
	Do not attempt complete withdrawal; detoxification to be done only in inpatient setting.
	Disulfiram contraindicated in pregnancy.

Perinatal	Multidisciplinary pre-birth meeting to assess risks to mother and infant and plan appropriate support for them.
	Assessment of potential harm (see Fig. 16.4)

Postnatal	Examine baby for features for fetal alcohol syndrome.
	Monitor psychomotor development.
	Brain magnetic resonance imaging if suggestive of central nervous system features.
	Continue health visitor support and social care supervision.
	Consider active maternal management to reduce risks in future pregnancies.

Fig. 16.3. Management of alcohol use before, during and after pregnancy.

Similar issues arise in the management of drugs of abuse in pregnancy (Figs. 16.5, 16.6). Every opportunity should be taken to work with the mother to minimize harm to the infant and preserve the family unit if possible. Efforts should be taken to stabilize drug taking and reduce chaotic lifestyles, although in the case of opiate addiction complete withdrawal should not be attempted unless this can be achieved by the 24th week of gestation. As emphasized in Chapter 12, working with families in a respectful and positive manner is more likely to produce a positive outcome than a punitive approach is. However, these women are exposed to a complex mix of social and environmental pressures from partners and peers, which may be hard to resist without high levels of support as outlined in Chapters 12 and 14. It is clear from the evidence reviewed in Chapter 8 that opiates and cocaine are relatively weak teratogens, and the main determinant to outcome is the limitation of other lifestyle problems such as alcohol and other drug use and the building of a firm supportive family to raise the children. If these factors are not present then practitioners must take a robust

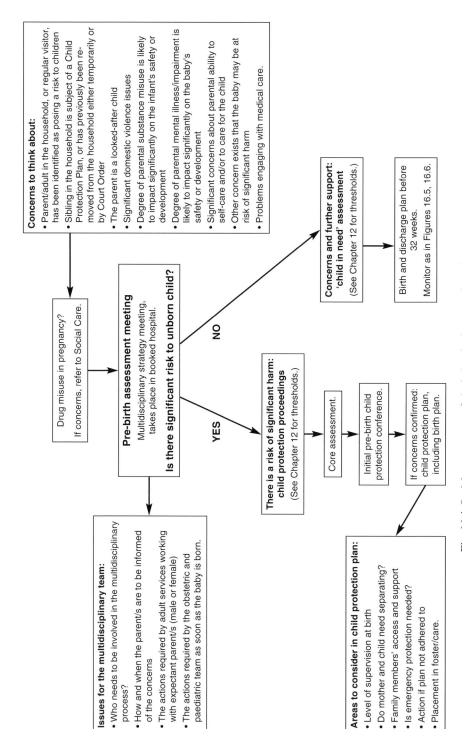

Concerns to think about:

• Parent/adult in the household, or regular visitor, has been identified as posing a risk to children
• Sibling in the household is subject of a Child Protection Plan, or has previously been re-moved from the household either temporarily or by Court Order
• The parent is a looked-after child
• Significant domestic violence issues
• Degree of parental substance misuse is likely to impact significantly on the infant's safety or development
• Degree of parental mental illness/impairment is likely to impact significantly on the baby's safety or development
• Significant concerns about parental ability to self-care and/or to care for the child
• Other concern exists that the baby may be at risk of significant harm
• Problems engaging with medical care.

Drug misuse in pregnancy?
If concerns, refer to Social Care.

Pre-birth assessment meeting
Multidisciplinary strategy meeting, takes place in booked hospital.

Is there significant risk to unborn child?

NO

YES

Concerns and further support: 'child in need' assessment
(See Chapter 12 for thresholds.)

Birth and discharge plan before 32 weeks.
Monitor as in Figures 16.5, 16.6.

There is a risk of significant harm: child protection proceedings
(See Chapter 12 for thresholds.)

Core assessment.

Initial pre-birth child protection conference.

If concerns confirmed: child protection plan, including birth plan.

Issues for the multidisciplinary team:

• Who needs to be involved in the multidisciplinary process?
• How and when the parent/s are to be informed of the concerns
• The actions required by adult services working with expectant parent/s (male or female)
• The actions required by the obstetric and paediatric team as soon as the baby is born.

Areas to consider in child protection plan:

• Level of supervision at birth
• Do mother and child need separating?
• Family members' access and support
• Is emergency protection needed?
• Action if plan not adhered to
• Placement in foster/care.

Fig. 16.4. Social management of alcohol and substance misuse in pregnancy.

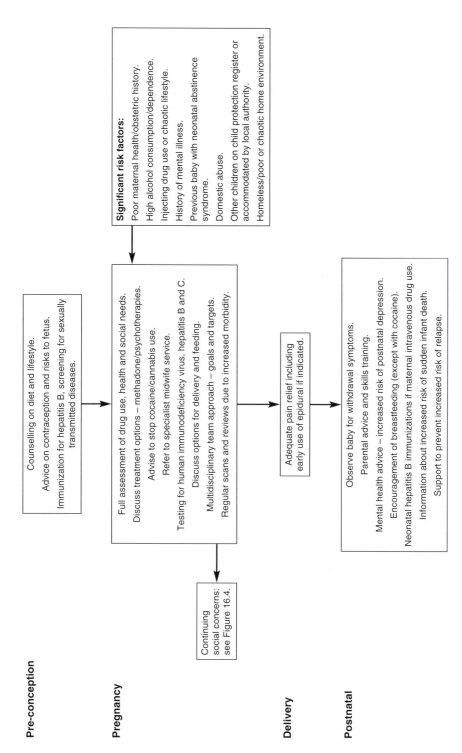

Pre-conception

Counselling on diet and lifestyle.
Advice on contraception and risks to fetus.
Immunization for hepatitis B, screening for sexually transmitted diseases.

Pregnancy

Significant risk factors:

Poor maternal health/obstetric history.
High alcohol consumption/dependence.
Injecting drug use or chaotic lifestyle.
History of mental illness.
Previous baby with neonatal abstinence syndrome.
Domestic abuse.
Other children on child protection register or accommodated by local authority.
Homeless/poor or chaotic home environment.

Full assessment of drug use, health and social needs.
Discuss treatment options – methadone/psychotherapies.
Advise to stop cocaine/cannabis use.
Refer to specialist midwife service.
Testing for human immunodeficiency virus, hepatitis B and C.
Discuss options for delivery and feeding.
Multidisciplinary team approach – goals and targets.
Regular scans and reviews due to increased morbidity.

Continuing social concerns: see Figure 16.4.

Delivery

Adequate pain relief including early use of epidural if indicated.

Postnatal

Observe baby for withdrawal symptoms.
Parental advice and skills training.
Mental health advice – increased risk of postnatal depression.
Encouragement of breastfeeding (except with cocaine).
Neonatal hepatitis B immunizations if maternal intravenous drug use.
Information about increased risk of sudden infant death.
Support to prevent increased risk of relapse.

Fig. 16.5. General management of substance misuse in pregnancy.

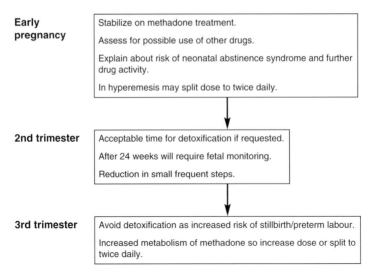

Early pregnancy	Stabilize on methadone treatment.
	Assess for possible use of other drugs.
	Explain about risk of neonatal abstinence syndrome and further drug activity.
	In hyperemesis may split dose to twice daily.

2nd trimester	Acceptable time for detoxification if requested.
	After 24 weeks will require fetal monitoring.
	Reduction in small frequent steps.

| 3rd trimester | Avoid detoxification as increased risk of stillbirth/preterm labour. |
| | Increased metabolism of methadone so increase dose or split to twice daily. |

Fig. 16.6. Treatment of opioid dependence.

approach when there is a failure to take advantage of supportive management, and take early steps to support and protect the children and not to allow institutional drift with constant attempts to 'fix the unfixable', as seen in the case history in Chapter 1 (Fig. 16.4).

We have attempted to review the subject of both therapeutic and non-therapeutic drugs and alcohol in pregnancy and the long-term outcome for the children of these pregnancies. We hope that the evidence has been thoroughly reviewed and provides a basis for advising parents and practitioners on the risks of drug administration and drug taking in pregnancy. We have concentrated on those drugs most likely to produce neurobehavioural teratogenesis but of necessity cannot review all potentially harmful agents. Not only would that require an enormous effort, but in many cases the data are not there to allow an informed judgement. The problem is illustrated well in the field of epilepsy where the production of new agents outstrips our ability to assess each one individually, and the history of teratogenesis makes it impossible to do anything other than observational research using pregnancy registers and high levels of surveillance.

REFERENCES

CHMP–EMEA (2005) *Guideline on the Exposure to Medicinal Products During Pregnancy: Need for Post-Authorisation Data.* London: Committee for Medicinal Products for Human Use, European Medicines Agency.
FDA (2002) *Guidance for Industry. Establishing Pregnancy Exposure Registries. Guideline 3626.* Rockville, MD: FDA.
FDA (2004) *Guidance for Industry. Pharmacokinetics in Pregnancy – Study Design, Data Analysis, and Impact on Dosing and Labeling. Guideline 5917.* Rockville, MD: FDA.
FDA (2005) *Reviewer Guidance. Evaluating the Risks of Drug Exposure in Human Pregnancies.* Rockville, MD: FDA.

FDA (2008) FDA proposes new rule to provide updated information on the use of prescription drugs and biological products during pregnancy and breast-feeding. FDA news release, May 28, 2008.

Gray R, Mukherjee RA, Rutter M (2009) Alcohol consumption during pregnancy and its effects on neuro-development: what is known and what remains uncertain. *Addiction* **104**: 1270–1273.

Huizink AC (2009) Moderate use of alcohol, tobacco and cannabis during pregnancy: new approaches and update on research findings. *Reprod Toxicol* **28**: 143–151.

Koren G (2001) *Maternal–Fetal Toxicology, 3rd edn.* New York: Marcel Dekker.

Jacqz-Aigrain E, Koren G (2005) Effects of drugs on the fetus. *Semin Fetal Neonatal Med* **10**: 139–147.

Lacroix I, Damase-Michel C, Lapeyre-Mestre M, Montastruc JL (2000) Prescription of drugs during pregnancy in France. *Lancet* **356**: 1735–1736.

Meadows M (2001) Pregnancy and the drug dilemma. *FDA Consumer* 35, May 2001.

NICE (2008) *Diabetes in Pregnancy. Management of Diabetes and its Complications from Pre-conception to the Postnatal Period. NICE Clinical Guideline 63.* London: National Institute for Health and Clinical Excellence.

Rane A (2006) Evaluation of fetal toxicity: human data. In: Jacqz-Aigrain E, Choonara I, eds. *Paediatric Clinical Pharmacology.* New York: Taylor & Francis/Fontis Media, pp. 299–307.

INDEX

(Page numbers in *italics* refer to figures/tables.)

changes with prenatal alcohol exposure, *111*, 114
hypoplasia, in fetal alcohol syndrome, 95, 103
reduced volume in prenatally cocaine-exposed infant, *132*, 137
Cortex, *110*
Counsellors
    alcohol, 218
    drugs, 202
Crack cocaine, *see under* Cocaine
Crack babies, 17, 130–131
Criminal activity
    and dependent drug use, 16
    of children of mothers who smoked during pregnancy, *189*
    of substance-dependent adults, 203
Crystal meth, *see* Methamphetamine

D

DAISY study, *see* Drugs and Infancy Study
Dance club culture, 14
Decongestants, 271
de Lange syndrome, *see* Cornelia de Lange syndrome
delinquency, in children of mothers who smoked during pregnancy, *189*
Depression, 2, 7, 56
    in cocaine-using women, 133–134
    management during pregnancy, *274*
    and MDMA use, 173
    in methamphetamine-using mothers, 178
    pharmacotherapy
        during pregnancy, 58–70, 271
            adverse neurocognitive outcome, *68*
            pre-conception, *274*
    untreated, 57–58
Dexamphetamine, in ADHD, 264
Desipramine, 62
Developmental delay
    antiepileptic drugs, 48
Diabetes
    drug treatment, during pregnancy, 271
        recommendations for, 272
    type II, in children of mothers who smoked during pregnancy, 186
Diazepam, 265
Diencephalon, *see under* Brain
Domestic violence/abuse, 2, 5, 16, 274
    and fetal alcohol syndrome, 224–225
    and substance misuse, 203
Dopamine, 72
    and MDMA methamphetamine, 170, 176
Doxepine, 62
Drinking, *see* Alcohol, Alcohol abuse, Binge drinking
Drug czar, 130
Drugs
    dependent use, 16

experimental use, 14
illicit, use of
    counselling, 202
    national strategy, legal vs harm reduction, 201–202
    outcomes, 17–18
    prevalence in pregnant women, 15
labelling, 272–273
misuse, parental
    and child abuse, neglect, 203–207
    external family support, 212
    family breakdown, 212–213
    interventions/treatment, 209, 211
    risk management, 204–208
    risk/resilience factors, *206*
recreational use, 14–16
soft, 14
use in pregnancy, 271
    child-care proceedings, 200
    management, 199–201, *277*
        social, *276*
    mortality, 199
    over-the-counter medicines, 271
    rate, 271
    treatment, 199
    see also individual drugs
Drugs and Infancy Study (DAISY), 172, 175–176, 177, 178–179
DSM-IV, *258*
    criteria for attention-deficit–hyperactivity disorder, *254*
Dubowitz syndrome, differential diagnosis with fetal alcohol syndrome, *91*
Dyslexia/dyspraxia, 252

E

Echocardiography, in alcohol-exposed neonate, 96, 97
Ecstasy, *see* MDMA
Embryonic development, *see* Human development, *and under* Brain
Epilepsy, 1, 44–54
    management before and during pregnancy, *273*
    preconceptional advice, 45
    see also Antiepileptic drugs
Equasym XL, 264
Examination
    of alcohol-exposed neonate, 96–97
Executive function
    influence of polydrug use, 177
    and prenatal alcohol exposure, 110, *117*, 120
    and prenatal cannabis exposure, 158–159, 161, 163–164
    and self-regulation, 242
Exencephaly, 37
Experimental use of drugs, *see under* Drugs

and specific syndromes, *see under those syndromes*
see also Psychiatric disorder, *and specific disorders*
Mental retardation, *see* Learning disability
Mesoridazine, *75*
Methadone, 8, 16, 140, 144–146, 201
    prenatal exposure
        and aggressive behaviour, 177
        and attention-deficit–hyperactivity disorder,
            146
        developmental outcome, 145
        and neonatal abstinence syndrome, 145, 202
    see also Maintenance therapy
Methamphetamine (ice, crystal meth), 169–179
    prenatal exposure
        low birthweight, 178
        neurochemical effects, 169–170
        neurocognitive effects
            in animals, 175–176
            in infants, 176–178
        neuroimaging of children, 177
        neuropsychiatric effects, 173
    sold as ecstasy, 171
    use prevalence
        in pregnant women, 171–172
        in young adults, 171
Methylphenidate, 262
    in ADHD, 264
Mice
    prenatal development, *30, 31, 32, 34, 35*
        correlation with humans, *24*
    following alcohol exposure, *35, 36, 37*
        magnetic resonance imaging, *33, 39*
    see also Animal studies
Microcephaly
    in Cornelia de Lange syndrome, *91*
    in Dubowitz syndrome, *91*
    in fetal alcohol syndrome, 94–95, 103
    in maternal phenylketonuria, fetal affects, *91*
    in Williams syndrome, 90, *91*
Midwife, specialist, 200, 201
Mirtazapine, 59
Moderate drinking, definition, 13
Morphine, 140
    neonatal abstinence syndrome, 202
    prenatal exposure in rats, 142
Mortality
    infant, and maternal smoking, 184, 185
    maternal, in fetal alcohol syndrome, 98
    see also Sudden infant death
Motherisk, 60, 271
Motor skills, and prenatal alcohol exposure, 119,
    238

N
National Institute for Health and Clinical Ex-
    cellence (NICE), 272

National Organization on Fetal Alcohol Syndrome,
    see NOFAS
Neglect, *see* Child abuse/neglect
Neocortex, *see under* Brain
Neonatal abstinence syndrome, 4, *142*, 147, 202
    breastfeeding, 202
    buprenorphine, attenuating effects, 146
    combined prenatal tobacco–opiate exposure, 146
    methadone, attenuating effects, 145
Neonate
    alcohol-exposed, examination, 96–97
Norepinephrine, and methamphetamine use, 170
Neural tube
    closure, 26, *27*
        failure, alcohol-induced, 37
    defects
        and in utero antiepileptic drug exposure, *46*
            carbamazepine, 52
        and in utero opiate exposure, 142
        and in utero valproic acid exposure, 37, 50
Neuroimaging, *see* Magnetic resonance imaging
Neuroleptics, 73–74
Nicotine, *see* Smoking (tobacco)
NOFAS/NOFAS-UK, 230
Noonan syndrome, differential diagnosis with fetal
    alcohol syndrome, *91*
Nortriptyline, 62

O
Obesity, following prenatal nicotine exposure, 185
Ocular defects
    and antiepileptic drugs, *46*, 49
    in fetal alcohol syndrome, 96
        ophthalmological evaluation, 97
    in fetal valproate syndrome, 51
Olanzapine, 72, 76
Opiates, 17
    classification, 140–141
    dependence
        maintenance therapy, 144–147
            in pregnancy, *278*
    prenatal exposure, *142*
        animal studies, 142
        attention-deficit–hyperactivity disorder, 143
        cocaine–opiate combination, 143
        developmental outcome, 142–144
        fetal abstinence syndrome, 142
        intrauterine growth retardation, 142
        low birthweight, 142
        and maternal HIV infection, 142
        neonatal abstinence syndrome, 142, 202
        neurodevelopmental outcome, 142–144
        preterm birth, 142
        stillbirth, 142
        sudden infant death syndrome, 142
    use in pregnant women, 141–142

Venlafaxine, 59, 67–69
Vermilion border, *see* Upper lip
Vigabatrin, 266
Violence
    alcohol-related, 223, 260
        risk of poor outcomes in children, 211
    in cocaine-using women, 139
    domestic, 2, 5, 131
    and substance misuse, 209
Visual impairments, *see* Ocular defects
Visuospatial skills, and prenatal alcohol exposure, 118
Vitamin K deficiency, 47

in fetal hydantoin syndrome, 49

W
Warning labels, on alcoholic beverages, 19, *220*, 220–221, 229
White matter, *see under* Brain
Williams syndrome, in differential diagnosis of fetal alcohol syndrome, 90, *91*

Z
'Z' drugs (zopiclone/zolpidem/zaleplon), 266
Ziprasidone, 72
Zuclopenthixol, *75*

Recent titles from Mac Keith Press www.mackeith.co.uk

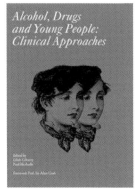

Alcohol, Drugs and Young People: Clinical Approaches
Eilish Gilvarry and Paul McArdle (Eds) Foreword by Prof. Sir Alan Craft
Clinics in Developmental Medicine no. 172
2007 248pp hardback 978-1-898683-47-6 £60.00 / €72.00 / US$110.00

In this comprehensive account of the misuse of drugs by young people, an international group of authors from the fields of addiction and adolescence review the short-term effects and long-term harms of drugs of abuse on the child or adolescent (including on the fetus when used in pregnancy). The authors also discuss evidence-based approaches to treatment and prevention. The book will be of interest to professionals in education, general practice, paediatrics, adolescent psychiatry and addiction.

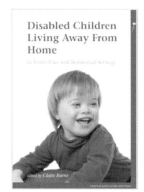

Disabled Children Living Away From Home in Foster Care and Residential Settings
Claire Burns (Ed)
A practical guide from Mac Keith Press
2009 148pp softback 978-1-898683-58-2 £20.00 / €24.00 / US$34.95

This book uniquely addresses the double needs of disabled children living away from home, providing practical guidance for the whole team responsible for the care of the child. The contributors consider the key issues that must be addressed when these children move from the family home to new accommodation. They provide insights into the difficulties that these children face and look at how the standards of care that they receive might be improved.

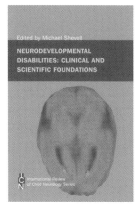

Neurodevelopmental Disabilities: Clinical and Scientific Foundations
Michael Shevell (Ed)
International Reviews in Child Neurology
2009 504pp softback 978-1-898683-67-4 £75.00 / €90.00 / US$119.95

This book takes a comprehensive approach to the challenges of neurodevelopmental disabilities. The contributors not only set out our understanding of the scientific basis of these disorders and their underlying causes but also address medical management, rehabilitation, public policy, and ethics.

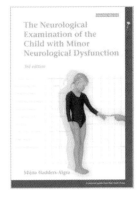

The Neurological Examination of the Child with Minor Neurological Dysfunction 3rd edition

Mijna Hadders-Algra Foreword by Prof. Bert Touwen
A practical guide from Mac Keith Press
2010 168pp softback 978-1-898683-98-8 £49.95 / €60.00 / US$72.00

Bert Touwen's classic handbook has been updated to reflect contemporary clinical practice. This refined, sensitive and age-appropriate technique is designed to take into account the developmental aspects of the child's rapidly changing nervous system. The accompanying CD-ROM contains videos illustrating typical and atypical performance and also provides an electronic assessment form.

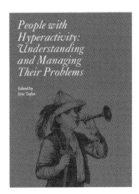

People with Hyperactivity: Understanding and Managing Their Problems

Eric A. Taylor (Ed)
Clinics in Developmental Medicine no. 171
2007 260pp hardback 978-1-898683-46-9 £65.00 / €78.00 / US$119.95

This book provides a practical, comprehensive and evidence-based approach to managing ADHD and hyperkinetic disorder. It explains the scientific basis for understanding these conditions and gives practical guidance on how to treat them. The book includes fact sheets and questionnaires to be photocopied for parents and teachers.

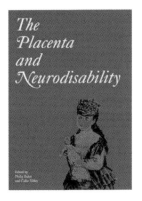

The Placenta and Neurodisability 2nd edition

Philip Baker and Colin Sibley (Eds)
Clinics in Developmental Medicine no. 169
2006 172pp hardback 978-1-898683-44-5 £45.00 / €54.00 / US$82.95

This detailed account of placental lesions that affect normal structure and function demonstrates how impaired placental function may contribute to deviant fetal growth and altered brain development. It outlines the processes that lead to brain injury, and shows how such early effects on brain development lead to disability in later childhood.

Other recent titles from Mac Keith Press

An Atlas of Neonatal Brain Sonography Paul Govaert and Linda S de Vries 2010 400 pages hardback 978-1-898683-56-8 £149.50 €179.40 US$240.00

Comorbidities in Developmental Disorders Martin Bax and Christopher Gillberg (Eds) 2010 176pp softback 978-1-907655-00-5 £59.95 / €72.00 / US$95.95

Inflammatory and Autoimmune Disorders of the Nervous System in Children Russell C. Dale and Angela Vincent (Eds) 2010 448pp hardback 978-1-898683-66-7 £110.00 / €132.00 / US$199.95

Physiotherapy and Occupational Therapy for People with Cerebral Palsy Karen Dodd, Christine Imms and Nicholas F. Taylor (Eds) 2010 256 pages softback 978-1-898683-68-1 £29.95 / €36.00 / US$39.99

Visual Impairment in Children due to Damage to the Brain Gordon Dutton and Martin Bax (Eds) 2010 224pp hardback 978-1-898683-86-5 £80.00 / €96.00 / US$135.00